OXFORD MEDICAL PUBLICATIONS

Obstetric Medicine

T0177519

Oxford Specialist Handbooks in Obstetrics and Gynaecology

Series editor | Sally Collins
Obstetric Medicine *Charlotte Frise and Sally Collins*
Urogynaecology *Helen Jefferis and Natalia Price*

Oxford Specialist Handbooks in Obstetrics and Gynaecology

Obstetric Medicine

Charlotte Frise

Consultant Obstetric Physician
Oxford University Hospitals NHS Foundation Trust,
Oxford, UK and
Imperial College Healthcare NHS Trust, London, UK
Honorary Senior Clinical Lecturer
Nuffield Department of Women's and
Reproductive Health
University of Oxford, Oxford, UK

Sally Collins

Consultant Obstetrician and Subspecialist in
Maternal and Fetal Medicine
Oxford University Hospitals NHS Foundation Trust,
Oxford, UK
Associate Professor of Obstetrics
Nuffield Department of Women's and
Reproductive Health
University of Oxford, Oxford, UK

OXFORD
UNIVERSITY PRESS

OXFORD
UNIVERSITY PRESS

Great Clarendon Street, Oxford, OX2 6DP,
United Kingdom

Oxford University Press is a department of the University of Oxford.
It furthers the University's objective of excellence in research, scholarship,
and education by publishing worldwide. Oxford is a registered trade mark of
Oxford University Press in the UK and in certain other countries

© Oxford University Press 2020

The moral rights of the authors have been asserted

First Edition published in 2020

Impression: 1

Published in the United States of America by Oxford University Press
198 Madison Avenue, New York, NY 10016, United States of America

British Library Cataloguing in Publication Data
Data available

Library of Congress Control Number: 2019913738

ISBN 978–0–19–882154–0

Printed and bound in China by
C&C Offset Printing Co., Ltd.

CF: to Matthew, Emilia, Alexander, and Oliver who fill my life with joy.
SC: to David, Lexi, and Bea for letting me do this again when I promised not to.

Preface

Obstetric medicine is a small specialty with a big remit, covering all medical conditions that can affect women of childbearing age. This book therefore hopes to rise to the challenge of including a large amount of information in a small package, to be of use to both trainees in medicine and obstetrics, as well as specialists in the field. Included here are both practical approaches to common questions that arise in pregnancy such as palpitations, isolated proteinuria, and headache, but also details of important conditions less commonly encountered and potentially unfamiliar.

Charlotte Frise
Sally Collins
2019

Preface

Acknowledgements

CF: a big thank you to Bruno and Susanna Brunskill who provided time, space, childcare, and sustenance in what was a crazily busy time of life. Thank you also to Catherine Nelson-Piercy, Catherine Williamson, Lucy Mackillop, and Mandish Dhanjal, for their support from the very start of my career in obstetric medicine. I would not be writing this book if it were not for their mentoring, education, and encouragement.

CF and SC: we are very grateful to all those who reviewed our chapters. They were Rebecca Black, Victoria Blackwell, Jane Collier, Anjali Crawshaw, Jeremy Dwight, Deborah Hay, Karin Hellner, Victoria Hogarth, Tim Littlewood, Philippa Matthews, Carolyn Millar, Elizabeth Orchard, Ketan Shah, Srilakshmi Sharma, May Ching Soh, Gaya Thanabalasingham, Tom Vale, Kate Wiles, and Michael Yousif. We can't thank you enough!

We also would like to thank the staff at Oxford University Press for their patience and kindness throughout all the personal difficulties we experienced during the writing of this book, especially Helen Liepman and Elizabeth Reeve. A special mention has to go to Sylvia Warren who was tirelessly supportive, encouraging, and whose excellent editing skills kept us on track.

Contents

Contents

Contributor

Katherine Talbot
Specialty Registrar in Obstetrics and Gynaecology Health Education
England, Thames Valley, UK

Symbols and abbreviations

💣	controversial topic
⮎	cross-reference
⚠	warning
▶	important
▶▶	don't dawdle
🐾	website
↓	decreased
↑	increased
→	leads/leading to
↔	normal
♀	female
♂	male
1°	primary
2°	secondary
∴	therefore
ACE	angiotensin-converting enzyme
ACE-I	angiotensin-converting enzyme inhibitor
AChR	acetylcholine receptor
ACS	acute coronary syndrome
ACTH	adrenocorticotropic hormone
ADH	antidiuretic hormone
ADHD	attention deficit hyperactivity disorder
AED	antiepileptic drug
AFLP	acute fatty liver of pregnancy
AIHA	autoimmune haemolytic anaemia
AKI	acute kidney injury
ALT	alanine aminotransferase
AML	acute myeloid leukaemia
ANCA	antineutrophil cytoplasmic antibody
APC	activated protein C
APS	antiphospholipid syndrome
APTT	activated partial thromboplastin time
ARB	angiotensin receptor blocker

AS	aortic stenosis
ASD	atrial septal defect
AST	aspartate transaminase
AVM	arteriovenous malformation
AV	atrioventricular
AVSD	atrioventricular septal defect
BCG	bacillus Calmette–Guérin
BD	bis in die (twice a day)
BHIVA	British HIV Association
BII	blood, injury, and injection
BMI	body mass index
BP	blood pressure
BSS	Bernard–Soulier syndrome
BTS	British Thoracic Society
CAP	community-acquired pneumonia
cART	combination antiretroviral therapy
CCP	cyclic citrullinated peptide
CF	cystic fibrosis
CFU	colony-forming unit
CKD	chronic kidney disease
CMV	cytomegalovirus
COPD	chronic obstructive pulmonary disease
CPR	cardiopulmonary resuscitation
CSF	cerebrospinal fluid
CTG	cardiotocography
CTPA	computed tomography pulmonary angiogram
CVS	chorionic villus sampling
CVST	cerebral venous sinus thrombosis
CXR	chest X-ray
DBP	diastolic blood pressure
DIC	disseminated intravascular coagulation
DKA	diabetic ketoacidosis

DM	diabetes mellitus
DMARD	disease-modifying antirheumatic drug
dsDNA	double-stranded deoxyribonucleic acid
DVT	deep venous thrombosis
DXA	dual-energy X-ray absorptiometry
EBV	Epstein–Barr virus
ECG	electrocardiogram
ECT	electroconvulsive therapy
EDS	Ehlers–Danlos syndrome
EF	ejection fraction
eGFR	estimated glomerular filtration rate
EGPA	eosinophilic granulomatosis with polyangiitis
ERCP	endoscopic retrograde cholangiopancreatography
ESC	European Society of Cardiology
EUPD	emotionally unstable personality disorder
FBC	full blood count
FBS	fetal blood sampling
FEV_1	forced expiratory volume in 1 second
FMF	familial Mediterranean fever
FNAIT	fetal/neonatal alloimmune thrombocytopenia
FSE	fetal scalp electrode
FSH	follicle-stimulating hormone
FVC	forced vital capacity
GAD	generalized anxiety disorder
GAS	group A Streptococcus
GBS	group B Streptococcus
G-CSF	granulocyte colony-stimulating factor
GDM	gestational diabetes mellitus
GFR	glomerular filtration rate
GGT	gamma-glutamyl transferase
GH	growth hormone or gestational hypertension
GHRH	growth hormone-releasing hormone

GI	gastrointestinal
GPA	granulomatosis with polyangiitis
GT	Glanzmann thrombasthenia
GTT	glucose tolerance test
Hb	haemoglobin
HbA1c	glycated haemoglobin
HBc	hepatitis B core antigen
HBeAg	hepatitis B e antigen
HBs	hepatitis B surface antibody
HBsAg	hepatitis B surface antigen
HBV	hepatitis B virus
HCG	human chorionic gonadotropin
HCV	hepatitis C virus
HD	haemodialysis
HDU	high dependency unit
HELLP	haemolysis, elevated liver enzymes, and low platelet count
HLA	human leucocyte antigen
HLH	haemophagocytic lymphohistiocytosis
HNIG	human normal immunoglobulin
HR	heart rate
HSV	herpes simplex virus
HUS	haemolytic uraemic syndrome
IBD	inflammatory bowel disease
ICD	implantable cardiac defibrillator
ICP	intrahepatic cholestasis of pregnancy
IE	infective endocarditis
IIH	idiopathic intracranial hypertension
IM	intramuscular
INR	international normalized ratio
IOP	intraocular pressure
ITP	immune thrombocytopenia
ITU	intensive therapy unit
IU	international unit
IUGR	intrauterine growth restriction

IV	intravenous
IVC	inferior vena cava
IVF	*in vitro* fertilization
IVIg	intravenous immunoglobulin
JVP	jugular venous pressure
kPa	kilopascal
LCH	Langerhans cell histiocytosis
LDH	lactate dehydrogenase
LFT	liver function test
LH	luteinizing hormone
LMWH	low-molecular-weight heparin
LV	left ventricle/ventricular
LVS	low vaginal swab
MAHA	microangiopathic haemolytic anaemia
MCV	mean cell volume
MDT	multidisciplinary team
MHA	Mental Health Act
MI	myocardial infarction
MMF	mycophenolate mofetil
MMR	measles, mumps, and rubella
MOH	major obstetric haemorrhage
MPA	microscopic polyangiitis
MR	modified release *or* magnetic resonance
MRCP	magnetic resonance cholangiopancreatography
MRI	magnetic resonance imaging
MTCT	mother-to-child transmission
NAFLD	non-alcoholic fatty liver disease
NMO	neuromyelitis optica
NO	nitric oxide
NSTEMI	non-ST elevation myocardial infarction
NYHA	New York Heart Association
OCD	obsessive–compulsive disorder
OD	omne in die (once a day)
PA	posteroanterior
$PaCO_2$	arterial partial pressure of carbon dioxide
PAI	Plasminogen activator inhibitor
PaO_2	arterial partial pressure of oxygen

PAPP-A	pregnancy-associated plasma protein A
PBC	primary biliary cholangitis
PCI	percutaneous coronary intervention
PCOS	polycystic ovarian syndrome
PCR	protein / creatinine ratio *or* polymerase chain reaction
PD	peritoneal dialysis
PDA	persistent ductus arteriosus
PEP	polymorphic eruption of pregnancy
PET	positron emission tomography
PFO	patent foramen ovale
PG	pemphigoid gestationis
PH	pulmonary hypertension
PHE	Public Health England
PLGF	placental growth factor
PNH	paroxysmal nocturnal haemoglobinuria
PO	per os (by mouth)
PPH	postpartum haemorrhage
PRES	posterior reversible encephalopathy syndrome
PsA	psoriatic arthritis
PSC	primary sclerosing cholangitis
PT	prothrombin time
PTU	propylthiouracil
QDS	quater die sumendum (four times a day)
RA	rheumatoid arthritis
RCo	ristocetin co-factor
RCOG	Royal College of Obstetricians and Gynaecologists
RCVS	reversible cerebral vasoconstriction syndrome
RR	respiratory rate
RTA	renal tubular acidosis
RUQ	right upper quadrant
RV	right ventricle/ventricular
S1	first heart sound
S2	second heart sound
SAH	subarachnoid haemorrhage
SBP	systolic blood pressure

SC	subcutaneous		TPMT	thiopurine S-methyltransferase
SCH	subclinical hypothyroidism		TPO	thyroid peroxidase
sFlt-1	soluble fms-like tyrosine kinase 1		TSH	thyroid-stimulating hormone
SGA	small for gestational age		TTP	thrombotic thrombocytopenic purpura
SIGN	Scottish Intercollegiate Guidelines Network		TWI	T-wave inversion
SLE	systemic lupus erythematosus		U&E	urea and electrolytes
SPECT	single-photon emission computed tomography		UC	ulcerative colitis
			UDCA	ursodeoxycholic acid
SSRI	selective serotonin reuptake inhibitor		UK	United Kingdom
			USA	United States of America
SpO$_2$	oxygen saturation measured by a pulse oximeter		USS	ultrasound scan
			UTI	urinary tract infection
STEMI	ST elevation myocardial infarction		V/Q	ventilation/perfusion
			VC	vital capacity
STI	sexually transmitted infection		VEGF	vascular endothelial growth factor
SVC	superior vena cava		VL	viral load
SVT	supraventricular tachycardia		VP	ventriculoperitoneal
T1DM	type 1 diabetes mellitus		VSD	ventricular septal defect
T2DM	type 2 diabetes mellitus		VTE	venous thromboembolism
T$_3$	triiodothyronine		VT	ventricular tachycardia
T$_4$	thyroxine		VWD	von Willebrand disease
TB	tuberculosis		VWF	von Willebrand factor
TDS	ter die sumendum (three times a day)		VZIG	varicella zoster immune globulin
			VZV	varicella zoster virus
TFT	thyroid function test		WBC	white blood cell
TGA	transposition of the great arteries		WHO	World Health Organization
ToF	tetralogy of Fallot		WPW	Wolff–Parkinson–White

Hypertensive disorders of pregnancy

Physiology and blood pressure measurement

Basic physiology
BP follows a distinct course during pregnancy:
- ↓ in early pregnancy until 24 wks (↓ in vascular resistance)
- ↑ after 24 wks until delivery (↑ in stroke volume)
- ↓ after delivery, but may peak again 3–4 days postpartum

> ⚠ Be aware of the pregnant ♀ with a 'normal' booking BP (≥120/80 mmHg), she may have previously undetected essential hypertension.
>
> Especially important in older pregnant ♀.

Blood pressure measurement
- BP must be measured correctly to avoid falsely ↑ or ↓ readings that may influence clinical management
- BP should be measured sitting or in the supine position with a left-sided tilt (to avoid compression of the inferior vena cava by the pregnant uterus, which ↓ blood flow to the heart and consequently stroke volume and → falsely ↓ BP) with the upper arm at the level of the heart
- Use the correct cuff size (a normal adult cuff is usually for an upper arm of ≤34 cm); if too small, may → a falsely ↑ BP reading
- The diastolic BP should be taken as Korotkoff V (the absence of sound), rather than Korotkoff IV (muffling of sound), which was previously used, unless the sound is heard all the way down to 0

> ⚠ Be aware of automated BP monitors:
> - They may under-record BP especially in pre-eclampsia
> - If unsure, check with manual sphygmomanometer

Hypertensive disorders in pregnancy

Hypertension
- ↑ arterial BP > normal range
- Normal BP in pregnancy is <120/80 mmHg
- Hypertension is graded as mild, moderate, or severe (Table 1.1)

Table 1.1 Grades of hypertension in pregnancy

	Systolic BP (mmHg)	Diastolic BP (mmHg)
Hypertension	140–159	90–109
Severe hypertension	≥160	≥110

Hypertensive disorders of pregnancy
- One of the most common medical problems in pregnancy
- High rate of recurrence in subsequent pregnancies

Definitions of hypertensive disorders of pregnancy	
Gestational hypertension (⊋ see p. 6)	• New-onset hypertension after 20 wks with no other features of pre-eclampsia

Pre-eclampsia (⊋ see p. 8)	• Hypertension after 20 wks *And*
	 • One or more of the following:
	  • Proteinuria
	  • Other maternal organ dysfunction, e.g. renal insufficiency (biochemical markers > the normal range in the absence of an alternative cause)
	  • Utero-placental dysfunction (fetal growth restriction)

HELLP (⊋ see p. 14)	• Evidence of:
	  • Haemolysis (elevated LDH, fragments on blood film, ↓ Hb)
	  • Elevated liver enzymes
	  • Low platelets

Pre-existing hypertension

Background
- Diagnosis suggested by:
  - Evidence of hypertension before pregnancy
  - If the BP at the 1st trimester booking visit is inappropriately 'normal' (physiological changes should result in a BP that is lower in the 1st trimester than in the non-pregnant ♀, i.e. <120/80 mmHg)
  - ↑ BP at <20 wks
- If 'gestational' hypertension persists for >3 mths postpartum, it is likely to be underlying hypertension rather than pregnancy related
- A careful assessment for 2° causes is required (Table 1.2)

Preconception
- Look for 2° causes and treat before conception
- Optimize BP control (target <135/85 mmHg)
- Review medications:
  - Stop ACE-I, ARB, or chlorothiazide
  - Start pregnancy-appropriate alternatives (➲ see table 1.7)
- Discuss risks in pregnancy:
  - Pre-eclampsia
  - IUGR
- Discuss aspirin prophylaxis (start at 12 wks)
- Discuss dietary modification and weight loss if obese
- Discuss exercise

In pregnancy
- Increase or initiate treatment if BP>140/90mmHg
- Target BP ≤135/85mmHg
- Consider PLGF-based testing if pre-eclampsia suspected

Table 1.2 Secondary causes of hypertension

		Clinical features	Diagnostic test
Cardiovascular	Aortic coarctation	• Radioradial and/or radiofemoral delay • Chest radiograph may show rib notching	• MR angiogram
Endocrine	Cushing's syndrome	• Examination may show buffalo hump, striae, centripetal obesity • Blood tests may show hyperglycaemia, hypokalaemia	➔ See p. 425
	Conn's syndrome	• No specific findings on examination • Blood tests show hypokalaemia in 40%	➔ See p. 427
	Phaeochromocytoma	• Examination may show a sinus tachycardia/tachyarrhythmia, postural hypotension may be present	➔ See p. 432
	Hyperparathyroidism	• No specific findings on examination • Bloods will show hypercalcaemia	• Serum calcium • Serum phosphate • Parathyroid hormone level
Renal	Renovascular e.g. renal artery stenosis	• Examination may reveal a renal bruit	• USS (asymmetric kidney size) • MR angiogram
	Glomerular disease	• Examination may show features of conditions associated with glomerular disease • Proteinuria and/or haematuria may be present on urine dipstick	• Renal biopsy
	Polycystic kidney disease		• Imaging, e.g. USS

Gestational hypertension

Background
- Seen in ≤20% of otherwise uncomplicated pregnancies
- Often appears late in 3rd trimester or in the early postpartum period
- May take 6–12 wks to return to normal
- Often recurs in subsequent pregnancies

Diagnosis
- ↑ BP at >20 wks
- Without coexistent proteinuria or evidence of other maternal organ dysfunction

Risk factors
- Obesity
- T2DM
- Previous diagnosis of PCOS

⚠ 10–50% of ♀ diagnosed with GH go on to develop pre-eclampsia.

▶ Close monitoring is therefore advised.

▶ Consider PLGF-based testing after 20 wks if pre-eclampsia suspected

---

Risk factors for GH developing into pre-eclampsia
- Gestational age of <34 wks at diagnosis
- Mean SBP >135 mmHg on 24 hr BP monitoring
- Abnormal uterine artery Doppler indices
- ↑ serum urate level

Management
- Management based on severity (Table 1.3)

> **Isolated new-onset proteinuria**
> ➔ See 'Proteinuria', p. 188.

Table 1.3 Suggested management of GH by severity

	Hypertension	Severe hypertension
BP	140/90 to 159/109 mmHg	≥160/110 mmHg
Mandatory admission	No	Yes (until BP below 160/110 mmHg, when can be managed as hypertension)
Treatment Target BP ≤135/85 mmHg	Yes if BP remains above 140/90 mmHg	Yes
BP measurement	Once or twice a week until BP 135/85 mmHg or less	Every 15–30 minutes until BP under 160/110 mmHg
Dipstick test for proteinuria (automated strip reading device)	Each visit	Daily
Blood tests	At presentation: FBC, U+E, LFTs Weekly thereafter Consider PLGF-based testing if possible pre-eclampsia	At presentation FBC, U+E, LFTs Repeat weekly

Source: data from NICE Hypertension in pregnancy guidelines. ⌖ https://www.nice.org.uk/guidance/ng133

Pre-eclampsia

Background
- Affects 2–4% of all pregnancies
- Probably related to abnormally shallow placentation
- Can have both fetal and maternal consequences
- The speed of deterioration varies greatly:
  - Prediction of rapid or slower deterioration is not possible
- The only treatment is delivery of the placenta

International Society for the Study of Hypertension in Pregnancy (ISSHP) diagnostic criteria for pre-eclampsia

- >20 wks' gestation
  And
- Hypertension
  And
- One or more of the following:
  - Proteinuria (≥300 mg/day or PCR >30 mg/mmol)
  - Evidence of maternal organ dysfunction, e.g. renal or hepatic
  - Utero-placental dysfunction (fetal growth restriction)

Clinical features

Symptoms
- Headache, esp. frontal (but very common without pre-eclampsia)
- Visual disturbance (esp. flashing lights)
- Abdominal pain in epigastrium or RUQ
- Nausea and vomiting
- Rapid development of oedema (esp. face)
- ⚠ Symptoms usually occur only with severe disease

Signs
- Hypertension (>140/90 mmHg; severe if ≥160/110 mmHg)
- Proteinuria
- Facial oedema
- Epigastric/RUQ tenderness
- Confusion
- Hyperreflexia and/or clonus
- Uterine tenderness or vaginal bleeding (sign of placental abruption)
- Fetal growth restriction on USS, particularly if <36 wks and abnormal uterine artery Doppler indices

Risk factors for the development of pre-eclampsia

Moderate risk
- 1st pregnancy
- Age ≥40 yrs
- Pregnancy interval >10 yrs
- Family history of pre-eclampsia
- BMI ≥35 kg/m^2 at 1st visit
- Multiple pregnancy

High risk
- Hypertensive disease during previous pregnancy
- Chronic kidney disease
- Autoimmune disease, e.g. SLE, APS
- T1DM or T2DM
- Chronic hypertension
- History of severe/early-onset pre-eclampsia

Differential diagnoses for pre-eclampsia
- AFLP
- HUS/TTP
- SLE
- Catastrophic APS
- Severe viral infection, e.g. HSV
- Sepsis

Measures to prevent pre-eclampsia

Pre-pregnancy
- Ensure appropriate levels of exercise
- Encourage weight loss if obese

In pregnancy
- 75–150 mg aspirin:
  - From 12 wks if one high risk factor or ≥2 moderate-risk factors
  - 150 mg OD may be preferable but only one study so far
- Calcium:
  - High dietary intake → low frequency of hypertensive disorders of pregnancy (epidemiological evidence)
  - >1 g/day ↓ incidence of pre-eclampsia by >50%
  - Ca^{2+} supplements include varying amounts of elemental Ca^{2+}
  - ◌ See p. 441 for calcium/vitamin D combinations

  ◌ No evidence for benefit of vitamin C or E

Management of pre-eclampsia

Pre-eclampsia at term
- Deliver the baby (and the placenta—this is the definitive treatment):
  - Fetal assessment and maternal condition determine the urgency
  - Mode of delivery can be vaginal or caesarean depending on severity of maternal illness and fetal well-being
- Antihypertensives aiming to ↓ BP to ≤135/85 mmHg
- Fluid restriction may be appropriate if renal dysfunction until spontaneous onset of diuresis
⚠ Anticipate ↑ BP if endotracheal intubation performed
⚠ Do not routinely give ergometrine (can cause significant ↑ BP)

Pre-eclampsia pre-term
- Management will depend on the severity, gestation, and estimated fetal weight (Table 1.4):
  - Fetuses are usually not considered viable at <500 g irrespective of gestation
- Hospital admission is advisable, usually until delivery
- Outpatient management/day leave may be considered if:
  - BP stable and ≤135/85 mmHg
  - No concerns for maternal or fetal wellbeing
  - Not at high risk of adverse events (e.g. using a risk prediction model such as fullPIERS)
- Regular review of symptoms
- Regular BP measurement:
  - Exact frequency depends on severity
- Antihypertensives to ↓ BP to ≤135/85 mmHg (➔ see table 1.7)
- VTE risk assessment ± prophylaxis
- Regular assessment of fetal well-being:
  - CTG at diagnosis and as clinical situation dictates
  - USS (frequency will depend on severity)

Investigations
- Blood tests should include:
  - FBC
  - Coagulation
  - U&Es
  - LFTs
  - ± Urate (not included in all guidelines)
- Arterial blood gas analysis if severe pre-eclampsia is suspected
- Capillary glucose if AFLP or HELLP is suspected

Table 1.4 Suggested management of pre-eclampsia by severity

	Hypertension	Severe hypertension
BP	140/90 to 159/109 mmHg	≥160/110 mmHg
Mandatory admission	Yes if: • Clinical concerns re mother • Clinical concerns re baby • High risk of adverse events (e.g. using fullPIERS model)	Yes
Treatment Target BP ≤135/85 mmHg	Yes if BP remains above 140/90 mmHg	Yes
BP measurement	At least every 48 hours (more often if an inpatient)	Every 15–30 minutes until BP under 160/110 mmHg then x4/day whilst inpatient
Dipstick test for proteinuria (automated strip reading device)	Only if clinically indicated (e.g. diagnostic uncertainty)	Only if clinically indicated (e.g. diagnostic uncertainty)
Blood tests	Twice weekly FBC, U+E, LFTs	Three times a week FBC, U+E, LFTs

Source: data from NICE Hypertension in pregnancy guidelines. ℅ https://www.nice.org.uk/guidance/ng133

Table 1.5 Women who need additional fetal monitoring

History	Imaging recommendation	Frequency
• Previous severe eclampsia • Pre-eclampsia needing birth before 34/40 • Pre-eclampsia with baby's birth weight <10th centile • Intrauterine death • Placental abruption	• USS fetal growth and amniotic fluid volume assessment • Umbilical artery Doppler assessment	• 28–30/40 • Or at least 2 wks before previous gestational age of onset if <28/40 • Repeat 4/52 later

Source: data from NICE Hypertension in pregnancy guidelines. ℅ https://www.nice.org.uk/guidance/ng133

Severe pre-eclampsia

⚠ Defined as the occurrence of systolic BP ≥160 mmHg or diastolic BP ≥110 mmHg in the presence of significant proteinuria and/or evidence of maternal organ dysfunction.

Features

- Severe headache
- Visual disturbance, e.g. blurring, flashing lights
- Severe epigastric or RUQ pain ± vomiting
- Papilloedema
- Signs of clonus (≥3 beats)
- Liver tenderness
- Platelets <100 × 10⁹/L
- Abnormal liver enzymes (ALT or AST >70 IU/L)

Severe pre-eclampsia at term

- Deliver the baby (and the placenta—this is the definitive treatment):
  - Likely but not always by caesarean
- Aggressive antihypertensives aiming to ↓ BP to ≤135/85 mmHg
- Fluid restriction to avoid pulmonary oedema
- ⚠ Anticipate ↑ BP if endotracheal intubation performed
- ⚠ Do not routinely give ergometrine (causes significant ↑ BP) and avoid carboprost if possible

Severe pre-eclampsia pre-term

- Delivery may be delayed with intensive monitoring if <34 wks

---

Indications for immediate delivery

- Worsening thrombocytopenia or coagulopathy
- Severe and/or significantly worsening hepatic or renal function
- Severe maternal symptoms especially epigastric pain with abnormal LFTs
- Developing eclampsia or HELLP
- Fetal reasons in a viable fetus (abnormal CTG or USS findings)

Indications for magnesium sulfate administration

- Prevention of seizures in ♀ with severe pre-eclampsia
- Treatment of seizures in ♀ with eclampsia
- Fetal neuroprotection before preterm delivery:
  - 26–33⁺⁶ wks
  - Can be considered prior to this and up to 36 wks

↪ NICE (2015). Preterm labour and birth (NG25): ♪ https://www.nice.org.uk/guidance/ng25

Complications of pre-eclampsia

Central nervous system
- Seizures (eclampsia)
- Intracranial haemorrhage
- Cerebral oedema
- Posterior reversible encephalopathy syndrome
- Cortical blindness
- Retinal oedema
- Retinal detachment

Renal
- Renal cortical necrosis
- Renal tubular necrosis

Respiratory
- Pulmonary oedema
- Laryngeal oedema

Liver
- HELLP syndrome
- Hepatic infarction
- Hepatic haematoma and capsular rupture

Coagulation
- DIC
- Microangiopathic haemolysis

Placenta
- Infarction
- Placental abruption

HELLP syndrome

Background
- A serious complication manifesting as
  - Haemolysis (H)
  - Elevated liver enzymes (EL)
  - Low platelets (LP)
- Regarded as a variant of severe pre-eclampsia
- Incidence estimated to be 5–20% of pre-eclamptic pregnancies
- Variants may only have two of the three components, e.g. ELLP (elevated liver enzymes and low platelets)
- In its severest form, maternal mortality has been reported to be 1% and perinatal mortality 10–60%
- Eclampsia may coexist
- Hypertension and/or proteinuria may be absent
- Immediate delivery is indicated

Investigations
- FBC
- Blood film
- LDH
- LFTs
- U&Es
- Urate
- For treatment, see Table 1.6

Postnatal management
- ➔ See p. 19.

Table 1.6 Treatment of severe pre-eclampsia or HELLP syndrome

Type of treatment	Specific drug	Doses	Indications	Cautions	Side effects
Antihypertensives	Labetalol IV	**Bolus:** 20 mg IV then double after 10 mins, to a max. single dose of 80 mg or total dose of 300 mg **Infusion:** 20 mg/hr, doubling rate every 30 mins if target BP not achieved, max. 160 mg/hr	• Severe hypertension despite oral therapy • Unable to take oral antihypertensives	• Contraindicated in asthma	• Bradycardia
	Hydralazine IV	**Bolus:** 5–10 mg IV/IM, then further 5–10 mg every 20–30mins (max. effect of bolus after 15–20 mins) **Infusion:** 0.5–10 mg/hr IV	• Labetalol contraindicated • Labetalol not adequately controlling BP	• Consider up to 500 mL crystalloid fluid preload if concerns about hypovolaemia	• Facial flushing • Headache • Tachycardia • Dizziness • Nausea and vomiting
	Magnesium sulfate	**Bolus:** 4 g IV over 5–15 mins then **Infusion:** 1 g/hr for 24 hrs **Further boluses:** 2–4 g over 5–15 mins if recurrent seizures	• Hypertensive disorders • Severe pre-eclampsia • HELLP syndrome • Eclampsia • Established preterm labour or planned preterm delivery within 24 hrs	• Need close monitoring for toxicity (observations and reflexes at least every 4 hrs) • May cause a deterioration in neurological conditions such as myasthenia gravis, use with extreme caution and specialist input	• Warm/flushed feeling • Nausea or vomiting • Muscle weakness • Hypotension • Dizziness, drowsiness, or confusion • Headache

(Continued)

Table 1.6 (Contd.)

Type of treatment	Specific drug	Doses	Indications	Cautions	Side effects
Steroids	Betamethasone	12 mg IM (two doses, 24 hrs apart)	• If birth likely within 7 days, offer 24/7 days, offer 24/40 • Consider 34–36/40 40–33⁺⁶/40 • Up to 39/40 if elective caesarean section	Women on therapeutic anticoagulation	• Hyperglycaemia • Hypertension • Euphoria • Difficulty sleeping
	Dexamethasone	6 mg IM (four doses, 12 hrs apart)	As for betamethasone. IV can be given if IM contraindicated	The preparation used must not include the sulphite preservative NNF60211 as this may be neurotoxic to the fetus	
Fluids	Depends on local policy	Limit maintenance fluids to 80 mL/hr unless ongoing loss (e.g. bleeding)	Do not give volume expansion to women with severe pre-eclampsia	Do not preload prior to spinal or epidural	• Volume expansion

Eclampsia

Background
Defined as the occurrence of a tonic–clonic seizure in association with a diagnosis of pre-eclampsia.
- Complicates 1% of cases of pre-eclampsia
- Tonic–clonic seizures are followed by a post-ictal phase
- May be the 1st presentation of pre-eclampsia
- Seizures:
  - Can occur antepartum, intrapartum, or postpartum
  - Arise following hypoxia and localized vasoconstriction
  - Often preceded by headache and hyperreflexia
  - Complications include haemorrhagic or ischaemic stroke

⚠ Eclampsia is a sign of severe disease: most ♀ who die do so from associated complications of severe pre-eclampsia such as blood loss, intracranial haemorrhage, or HELLP.

Principles of management
- Manage the seizure (usually self-limiting)
- Reduce the risk of further seizures ($MgSO_4$)
- Control the BP (antihypertensives)
- Deliver the baby

Management of eclampsia

⚠ This is an obstetric emergency.

Seizure

- Call for help and apply basic principles of airway, breathing, and circulation plus IV access
- Most eclamptic fits are short-lasting and terminate spontaneously
- $MgSO_4$ is the drug of choice for both control of fits and preventing (further) seizures:
  - A loading dose of 4 g should be given over 5–10 min followed by an infusion of 1 g/hr for 24 hrs
  - If more fits occur, another 2 g can be given as a bolus (therapeutic range for Mg^{2+} is 2–4 mmol/L)
  - In repeated seizures, use diazepam (if still fitting, the patient may need intubation, ventilation, and imaging of head to rule out a cerebral haemorrhage)

⚠ Mg^{2+} toxicity is characterized by confusion, loss of reflexes, respiratory depression, and hypotension

- Assessment of reflexes every hour for Mg^{2+} toxicity
- ⚠ Use biceps if epidural *in situ*
- Halve/stop infusion if oliguric (<20 mL/hr) or raised creatinine and seek senior/renal advice
- ⚠ If toxic give 1 g calcium gluconate over 10 min

Maternal observations

- Strict monitoring of the ♀ is mandatory
- Pulse, BP, RR, and oxygen saturations every 15 min
- Measure hourly urine output

Blood pressure

- If hypertensive, give BP-lowering drugs:
  - Oral nifedipine MR
  - IV labetalol

Renal

- Fluid restrict the patient to 80 mL/hr or 1 mL/kg/hr due to the risk of pulmonary oedema (even if oliguric the risk of renal failure is small); monitor the renal function with the creatinine
- A CVP line may be needed if there has been associated maternal haemorrhage and fluid balance is difficult or if the creatinine rises

Fetus and delivery

- The fetus should be continuously monitored with CTG
- Deliver fetus once the mother is stable
- Vaginal delivery is not contraindicated if cervix is favourable
- 3rd stage should be managed with 5–10 U oxytocin, rather than Syntometrine® or ergometrine which causes ↑ BP

➲ NICE (2010). Hypertension in pregnancy: diagnosis and management (CG107): ℅ http://www.nice.org.uk/guidance/cg107

Postnatal management of pre-eclampsia and HELLP

- Review medications:
  - Replace methyldopa with alternative agent
  - Gradual ↓ in antihypertensive dose
  - Ensure consistent advice with respect to breastfeeding
- DVT prophylaxis with LMWH can be given as long as platelets >75 × 10^9/L (and no other contraindications are present)
- Regular BP review

⚠ Further assessment for underlying essential hypertension is required if BP does not return to normal in <3 mths

Management of acute kidney injury in severe PET
- ⚠ Transient oliguria is common in 1st 24 hrs postpartum
- Usually gets worse after delivery before improving
- In healthy ♀ renal recovery occurs in most cases
- Classical changes on renal biopsy include glomerular endotheliosis
- Often multifactorial, e.g. a PPH in a ♀ with pre-eclampsia

Advice for future pregnancies
Gestational hypertension in previous/current pregnancy
- 1 in 5 women will develop some form of hypertension in a future pregnancy
- 1 in 7 women will develop GH again
- 1 in 14 women will develop pre-eclampsia
Pre-eclampsia in previous/current pregnancy
- 1 in 5 women will develop some form of hypertension in a future pregnancy
- 1 in 8 women will develop GH
- 1 in 6 women will develop pre-eclampsia (1 in 3 if delivery was between 28–34 wks; 1 in 4 if delivery was between 34–37 wks)

Pre-eclampsia and cardiovascular disease in later life
- ♀ with a history of pre-eclampsia have an ↑ risk of cardiovascular disease including:
  - Hypertension (4× ↑ risk)
  - Ischaemic heart disease (2× ↑ risk)
  - Stroke (2× ↑ risk)
- Counselling should focus on appropriate risk-reduction strategies:
  - Exercise
  - Weight management
  - Not smoking
- Encourage engagement with healthcare for appropriate screening

Antihypertensives in pregnancy

See Table 1.7.

Table 1.7 Antihypertensives and their use in pregnancy

Type of treatment	Specific drug	Doses	Contraindications	Possible side effects
β blockers	Methyldopa	250 mg–1 g TDS	Avoid if liver dysfunction Avoid if postpartum	Hepatic dysfunction, depressant
	Atenolol	12.5–100 mg OD	Asthma	Possible association with IUGR with 1st trimester use
	Labetalol	100–800 mg TDS		Neonatal bradycardia is not usually a problem
Calcium channel blockers	Nifedipine modified release	Up to 90 mg in 2–3 divided doses		Loading dose of MgSO₄ with calcium channel blocker can cause profound hypotension, → watershed infarcts and fetal loss
	Sublingual nifedipine	Not recommended in pregnancy.		Risk of hypotensive stroke at watershed areas in brain, and lack of placental perfusion
	Amlodipine	5–10 mg once daily	Longer time of onset compared to nifedipine so not as useful in acute setting	Can be continued during pregnancy and lactation
α blockers	Doxazosin	2–16 mg total daily dose	Avoid in heart failure from obstructive lesions such as aortic stenosis	Postural hypotension
	Prazosin	1–20 mg total daily dose		
Diuretics	Furosemide	10–80 mg daily, can be divided (higher doses required in renal impairment)	Avoid in pre-eclampsia	Association with growth restriction
ACE-I	Enalapril Captopril	If breastfeeding: Enalapril 2.5–20 mg BD Captopril 12.5–50 mg BD	Do not use in pregnancy (fetotoxic if used in second/third trimester; no increase (↑) in congenital malformations with first trimester use if data corrected for underlying ↑ BP)	1st trimester teratogenesis Later—oligohydramnios, fetal and neonatal renal failure Renal function monitoring required when used postnatally

PLGF-based testing

- Soluble fms-like tyrosine kinase 1 (sFlt-1) is a tyrosine kinase protein
- Acts as an antagonist of placental growth factor (PLGF) and vascular endothelial growth factor (VEGF) binding and sequestering them from circulation
- It is upregulated in pregnancy but especially so in pre-eclamptic pregnancies
- Often used to rule out pre-eclampsia in ♀ with borderline ↑ BP
- Helpful where the diagnosis is uncertain, or with medical conditions where the features overlap those of pre-eclampsia (e.g. lupus flare)

sFlt-1/PLGF ratio

- An ↑ sFlt-1/PLGF ratio may be seen before pre-eclampsia presents clinically
- A ratio of ≤38 is widely accepted as ruling out the condition
- Less than 34 wks:
  - Ratio of 38–85   Excludes pre-eclampsia, but high likelihood of developing this in next 4 weeks
  - Ratio of ≥ 85   Pre-eclampsia likely
- 34 weeks or more:
  - Ratio of 38–110   Excludes pre-eclampsia, but high likelihood of developing this in next 4 weeks
  - Ratio of ≥ 110   Pre-eclampsia likely

PLGF testing

PLGF <12 pg/ml	Highly abnormal: pre-eclampsia likely
PLGF 12–100 pg/ml	Abnormal: suggestive of pre-eclampsia
PLGF >100 pg/ml	Normal: pre-eclampsia unlikely

Cardiology

Physiological changes

- Pregnancy is associated with global haemodynamic changes
- These occur early and gradually return to normal after delivery
- Peripheral vasodilatation → ↓ systemic vascular resistance
- Cardiac output ↑ by:
  - 40% during pregnancy (↑ heart rate and ↑ stroke volume)
  - 15% in the 1st stage of labour
  - 50% in the 2nd stage of labour
- After the 3rd stage there is further ↑ cardiac output due to ↑ venous return from:
  - Relief of vena caval obstruction
  - Tonic uterine contraction (expels blood into systemic circulation)
- ↓ BP in pregnancy, lowest towards the middle of the 2nd trimester
- Colloid osmotic pressure ↓ causing ↑ susceptibility to pulmonary oedema
- ↑ LV wall thickness and mass
- Plasma volume expansion
- ↑ cholesterol (50%)
- ↑ triglycerides (300%)

Changes on clinical examination

- Hyperdynamic circulation
- Ejection systolic (flow) murmur
- Elevated JVP
- A 3rd heart sound (S3; occurs after the 2nd heart sound, S2)
- Apex beat is forceful, displaced
- Premature atrial and ventricular ectopics
- Resting heart rate may ↑ by 10–20 beats per minute

Investigations

- CXR:
  - ↑ cardiothoracic ratio and vascular markings (hila can look bigger)
- ECG (➔ see Fig. 2.1):
  - Tachycardia, small Q waves, and TWI in lead 3 and aVR
  - Can see left axis deviation and ST sagging
- Echocardiogram:
  - Mild mitral, tricuspid, and pulmonary regurgitation can be a normal finding but aortic regurgitation is usually abnormal
  - LV is hyperdynamic

General management principles

Preconception

- Imaging
- Assessment of functional status (NYHA functional classification)
- Consider surgical intervention
- Adjust medications if needed
- Assess level of maternal risk for each specific condition (WHO classification, see Table 2.1)
- Contraceptive discussion where avoidance of pregnancy is advisable

---

NYHA functional classification for cardiac disease

I   No symptoms and no limitation in ordinary physical activity
II Mild symptoms (mild breathlessness and/or angina) and slight limitation during ordinary activity
III Marked limitation in activity due to symptoms even during less than ordinary activity. Comfortable at rest
IV Severe limitations. Symptoms even at rest. Mostly bedbound

Criteria Committee, New York Heart Association Inc. (1964) *Diseases of the Heart and Blood Vessels: Nomenclature and Criteria for Diagnosis*, 6th edition. Little, Brown and Co.

Antenatal

- Management as part of a MDT
- Echocardiography regularly if at risk of deterioration
- Fetal echocardiography if congenital heart disease present
- Monitoring for factors that may worsen maternal condition (e.g. anaemia, arrhythmias)
- Fetal growth scans

At delivery

- Aim for a vaginal delivery unless clear indications for caesarean section are present, e.g.:
  - Aortic size (thresholds are condition dependent)
  - Aortic dissection
  - Very poor LV function
- Careful positioning to avoid aortocaval compression
- Consider limiting the 2nd stage
- Consider invasive monitoring
- Active management of 3rd stage of labour
- Strict fluid balance
- Medication plan:
  - Avoid ergometrine if BP changes or coronary spasm could worsen the maternal condition
  - Avoid PGF2α
- Cautious use of oxytocin which can cause ↓ BP:
▶ One alternative to the normal bolus is a bolus of 2–5 units followed by an infusion of 40 IU/hr

Table 2.1 Modified WHO classification of maternal risk (examples included here, please see ESC guidelines for full list)

WHO I: no ↑ in maternal mortality, no/mild ↑ in morbidity

- Uncomplicated, small, or mild pulmonary stenosis, PDA, or mitral valve prolapse
- Atrial or ventricular ectopics
- Successfully repaired ASD, VSD, PDA, anomalous pulmonary venous drainage

---

WHO II: small ↑ risk of maternal mortality or moderate ↑ in morbidity

- Unoperated ASD or VSD
- Repaired ToF
- Most arrhythmias
- Turner's syndrome without aortic dilatation

WHO II or III (depending on individual)

- Mild LV impairment (EF >45%)
- Hypertrophic cardiomyopathy
- Native or tissue valvular heart disease that is not class I or IV
- Marfan or other aortic syndrome without aortic dilatation
- Aorta <45 mm associated with bicuspid aortic valve
- AVSD

WHO III: significantly ↑ risk of maternal mortality or severe morbidity

- Moderate LV impairment (EF 30–45%)
- Previous peripartum cardiomyopathy with no residual LV dysfunction
- Mechanical valve
- Systemic RV
- Fontan circulation
- Cyanotic heart disease (uncorrected)
- Moderate mitral stenosis
- Severe asymptomatic AS
- Moderate aortic dilatation
- VT

WHO IV: extremely high risk of maternal mortality or severe morbidity, pregnancy contraindicated

- Pulmonary arterial hypertension
- Severe systemic ventricular dysfunction (LVEF <30%)
- Previous peripartum cardiomyopathy with residual impairment of LV function
- Severe mitral stenosis
- Severe symptomatic AS
- Marfan syndrome with aorta >45 mm
- Native severe coarctation

Source: ESC 2018 pregnancy guidelines
https://academic.oup.com/eurheartj/article/39/34/3165/5078465

Ischaemic heart disease

Background

- Ischaemic heart disease is a broad term encompassing both chronic angina and acute ischaemic events ('acute coronary syndrome')
- Traditional risk factors include:
  - ↑ BP
  - Family history of vascular disease
  - DM
  - Smoking
  - Hypercholesterolaemia
- ⚠ Absence of risk factors does not exclude ischaemic heart disease
- Ischaemic heart disease in pregnancy is associated with:
  - ↑ age
  - ↑ parity
  - Obesity
  - Ethnicity
  - Physical inactivity
- Both atherosclerotic lesions and vessel dissection can cause myocardial ischaemia in pregnancy:
  - Atherosclerotic lesions are a more common cause of myocardial ischaemia than vessel dissection during pregnancy
  - Incidence of dissection ↑ in the 3rd trimester (left anterior descending > right coronary artery > circumflex)
  - Dissection more common than atherosclerotic lesions postpartum
- Ischaemic events, irrespective of aetiology, are associated with significant maternal mortality, particularly postpartum

---

Differential diagnosis for an ↑ troponin level in pregnancy

Associated with chest pain

- Myocardial infarction:
  - Atherosclerosis
  - Coronary artery dissection
  - Coronary artery embolism (e.g. from a PFO)
- Vasoconstriction from drugs (e.g. ergometrine, cocaine)
- Hypercoagulation
- Coronary artery spasm
- Myopericarditis
- Pulmonary embolism
- Takotsubo cardiomyopathy
- SVT with very fast rate

Not associated with chest pain

- Any condition causing myocardial dysfunction (e.g. severe sepsis)
- Pregnancy-related conditions such as pre-eclampsia

⚠ Troponin is NOT ↑ in normal pregnancy, at vaginal delivery, or caesarean section.

Management of an acute coronary syndrome

Background
- Combination of acute chest pain, with ECG changes and cardiac enzyme elevation consistent with acute damage to the myocardium
- The term 'acute coronary syndrome' (ACS) includes:
  - ST elevation myocardial infarction (STEMI)
  - Non-ST elevation myocardial infarction (NSTEMI)
  - Unstable angina

Clinical assessment
- Careful history and examination with consideration of other causes

Investigations
- ECG: repeat if any suspected abnormalities
- Bloods: FBC, troponin, renal function, LFTs

Treatment
- Oxygen
- Analgesia: morphine if necessary
- GTN: sublingual spray or tablet
- Aspirin: 75 mg daily can be used at any time in pregnancy, one-off dose of 300 mg is not contraindicated (➲ see 'Ischaemic stroke', p. 227)

Intervention
- ST elevation on ECG:
  - Immediate ('primary') percutaneous coronary intervention (PCI), i.e. angiography ± stent insertion
  - Thrombolysis can be performed if PCI not available
- Dynamic ischaemic changes on ECG, e.g. ST ↓ or TWI:
  - Discuss with cardiology about PCI and timing
- Dual antiplatelet therapy indicated for atherosclerotic events:
  - 75 mg clopidogrel preferred to ticagrelor (➲ see p. 29)
- Consider β blocker (e.g. bisoprolol)
- Avoid ACE-I until after delivery
- Do not check lipids during pregnancy
- Avoid statins:
  - Generally contraindicated in pregnancy
  - If deemed advisable, then pravastatin may be used
- The type of stent should be discussed with Cardiology:
  - In contrast to drug-eluting stents, a bare metal stent does not require dual antiplatelet therapy for a year (2nd agent can be stopped near delivery, with ↓ risk of haemorrhage)
  - New guidelines for ACS outside pregnancy advocate new-generation drug-eluting stents (which require a shorter duration of dual antiplatelet therapy); this may be useful in pregnancy

Myocardial infarction

Management of a patient with previous MI

- Pre-pregnancy assessment including:
  - Cardiology review
  - Echocardiography
  - Exercise testing
- Review medications:
  - Ensure cessation of agents including ACE-I, statin, and spironolactone (and start alternatives if indicated)
  - Modification of agents such as clopidogrel instead of ticagrelor
- Aspirin 75 mg OD throughout pregnancy
- 2nd antiplatelet agent (i.e. clopidogrel) to continue in pregnancy if indicated by previous event or intervention

Ticagrelor in pregnancy

- Ticagrelor is an antiplatelet agent similar to clopidogrel
- Recent guidelines recommend ticagrelor in preference to clopidogrel for high-risk lesions in non-pregnant individuals
- Animal models show no adverse fetal effects with equivalent doses
- At doses 2–3× higher, fetal growth and development was affected
- There has been one case report of ticagrelor use throughout pregnancy with a good pregnancy outcome.

Delivery in a ♀ with recent myocardial infarction

- Review medication before delivery, i.e. antiplatelet agents
- Consider limiting length of 2nd stage
- Avoid ergometrine

Troponin rise and normal coronary arteries on angiography

- Pre-eclampsia
- Pulmonary embolism
- Severe decompensated AS
- Coronary arteritis esp. polyarteritis nodosa
- Coronary embolus 2° to paradoxical embolus, intramural thrombus or vegetation
- Severe anaemia
- Thyrotoxicosis
- Phaeochromocytoma
- Cocaine
- Amphetamines

⊖ ESC guidelines on acute MI in patients presenting with ST-segment elevation: ℳ https://www.escardio.org/Guidelines/Clinical-Practice-Guidelines/Acute-Myocardial-Infarction-in-patients-presenting-with-ST-segment-elevation-Ma

ECG changes in pregnancy and STEMI

See Figs. 2.1–2.3.

Normal pregnancy changes

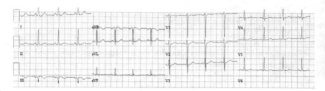

Fig. 2.1 Normal pregnancy changes. Reproduced from Adamson D. et al. (2011) *Heart Disease in Pregnancy* Oxford University Press: Oxford with permission from Oxford University Press.

Example of an inferolateral STEMI

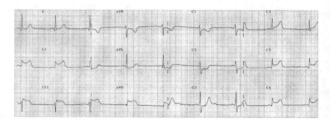

Fig. 2.2 Example of an inferolateral STEMI. Reproduced from Olson K. (2014) *Oxford Handbook of Cardiac Nursing* Oxford University Press: Oxford with permission from Oxford University Press.

Example of an anterior STEMI

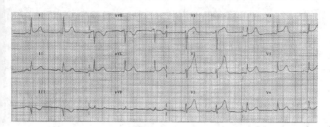

Fig. 2.3 Example of an anterior STEMI. Reproduced from Olson K. (2014) *Oxford Handbook of Cardiac Nursing* Oxford University Press: Oxford with permission from Oxford University Press.

Persistent ductus arteriosus

The ductus arteriosus connects the descending aorta to the pulmonary artery and normally closes at birth. Failure to close results in a left-to-right shunt which can cause heart failure in childhood and pulmonary hypertension. Small ducts can be incidental findings. See Fig. 2.4.

- Usually the diagnosis is made and treated in childhood (most common in preterm infants)
- Most multifactorial and probably a combination of a genetic tendency and environmental factors, e.g. *in utero* (maternal rubella infection) or at time of delivery (preterm delivery)
- Can be associated with:
  - VSD
  - Pulmonary stenosis
  - Coarctation of the aorta
- Examination may reveal:
  - Machinery murmur at the 2nd left intercostal space (or outer border of clavicle)
  - Heaving apex beat
  - A systolic or diastolic thrill at the 2nd intercostal space
  - Collapsing pulse

Management of PDA in pregnancy

- Haemodynamically insignificant with no pulmonary hypertension:
  - No impact on pregnancy
- Haemodynamically significant, i.e. associated with LV dilation and/or dysfunction:
  - Can develop heart failure in pregnancy
- PDA and presence of pulmonary hypertension:
  - Should be viewed as very high risk and counselled against pregnancy

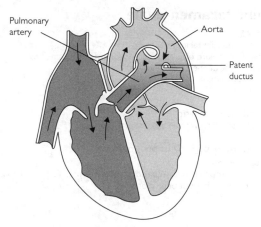

Fig. 2.4 Persistent ductus arteriosus. Reproduced from Myerson S. G. et al. (2009) *Emergencies in Cardiology* 2nd Ed. Oxford University Press: Oxford with permission from Oxford University Press.

Patent foramen ovale

See Fig. 2.5.
- Very common septal lesion
- Results from failure of embryonic closure of the foramen ovale
- Found in 20% of the healthy population
- Associated with:
  - Migraine
  - Stroke
  - Paradoxical embolism
- May be associated with an atrial septal aneurysm

Management of PFO in pregnancy
- Closure is rarely indicated
- Thromboprophylaxis is required if history of paradoxical embolus and the lesion has not been closed

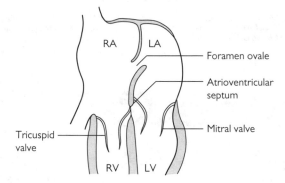

Fig. 2.5 Patent foramen ovale. Reproduced from Archer and Manning (2018) *Fetal Cardiology* 2nd Ed. Oxford University Press: Oxford with permission from Oxford University Press.

Atrial septal defect

• Types of ASD are classified by septal location (Table 2.2 and Fig. 2.6)

Table 2.2 Types of ASD

Ostium primum	• Defect in the atrial primum septum, with formation at the level of the mitral and tricuspid valves
	• Cleft in mitral valve, which often → mitral regurgitation
	• Usually requires surgical closure
Ostium secundum	• Most common type
	• Hole in the secundum septum
	• Transcatheter closure possible
Sinus venosus	• Inferior (IVC) or superior (SVC) defect
	• Superior defect associated with anomalous pulmonary venous drainage

• All involve blood flow from left to right resulting in ↑ size of the right atrium and ventricle
• Signs on examination may include:
    • A fixed split 2nd heart sound with pulmonary flow murmur
    • Atrial flutter/fibrillation and a left parasternal heave
• ASD closure recommended if a significant shunt is present, or right heart dilatation
• An uncorrected ASD can be associated with:
    • Right heart failure
    • Paradoxical embolism
    • Arrhythmias such as AF
    • Pulmonary hypertension

At delivery

• Shunt may reverse and therefore saturations drop
• Risk of air embolism, preventative filters should be used on IV lines
• If complications are present:
    • Consider limiting 2nd stage of labour
    • Lower threshold for instrumental assistance

Management of ASD in pregnancy

- If small and uncomplicated:
  - No excess maternal risk
  - Paradoxical embolism and arrhythmias very uncommon
- If closed with no complications (including pulmonary hypertension), can be treated as normal
- Consider aspirin 75 mg OD if recently closed
- Thromboprophylaxis if:
  - ♀ at high risk of VTE
  - If the ASD has resulted in enlarged atria
  - Atrial arrhythmias

⚠ If pulmonary hypertension present, ♀ should be counselled against pregnancy.

Atrial septal defects

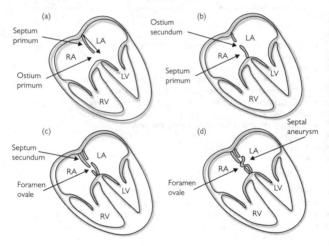

Fig. 2.6 Atrial septal defects. Reproduced from Khavandi A. (2014) *Essential Revision Notes for the Cardiology KBA* Oxford University Press: Oxford with permission from Oxford University Press.

Ventricular septal defect

- Can be part of complex congenital heart disease including:
  - ToF
  - Truncus arteriosus
  - Double-outlet RV
- Can also be associated with:
  - PDA
  - Pulmonary stenosis
  - ASD
  - Coarctation of the aorta
  - Tricuspid atresia
  - Transposition of the great arteries
  - Pulmonary atresia

Types of VSD

Type 1 (infundibular)
- Septal defect above and anterior to the crista supraventricularis

Type 2 (membranous)
- Septal defect of the membranous septum; the commonest defect

Type 3 (inlet)
- Septal defect beneath the mitral and tricuspid valve

Type 4 (muscular)
- Septal defects away from the valves, which can be small or large

Atrioventricular VSD (Gerbode defect)
- Caused by a membranous septal defect between the LV and right atrium

VSDs can also be classified by size, i.e. restrictive/small, or non-restrictive/large defects. The latter are closed in childhood to prevent the development of pulmonary hypertension.

Complications

- Aortic regurgitation
- Endocarditis
- Pulmonary hypertension
- Thromboembolism
- Arrhythmia
- LV or RV dysfunction

Management of VSD in pregnancy

- Fetal echocardiography
- If surgically closed with no residual complications, or restrictive and no sequelae, ♀ can be treated as normal in pregnancy
- Otherwise can be monitored in each trimester, with echocardiography for assessment of pulmonary pressures

⚠ If pulmonary hypertension is present, ♀ should be counselled against pregnancy.

Ventricular septal defect
See Fig. 2.7.

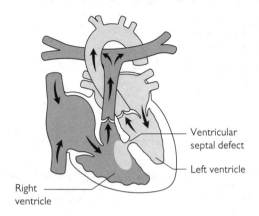

Ventricular
septal defect

Left ventricle

Right
ventricle

Fig. 2.7 Diagram of a ventricular septal defect. Reproduced from Myerson
S. G. et al. (2009) *Emergencies in Cardiology* 2nd Ed. Oxford University Press: Oxford
with permission from Oxford University Press.

Atrioventricular septal defect

Background

- Most commonly found in association with trisomy 21
- Term encompasses a variety of atrial septal lesions, that can be associated with VSDs, and/or lesions of the mitral/tricuspid valves
- They are often identified and corrected surgically in childhood

Management of AVSD in pregnancy

- Arrhythmias and atrioventricular valve regurgitation have been described
- Follow-up every trimester is advised in ESC guidelines unless significant valve issues are present, which require more frequent review (e.g. every 2–4 wks)

→ ESC 2018 pregnancy guidelines: ℜ https://academic.oup.com/eurheartj/article/39/34/3165/5078465

Eisenmenger's syndrome

See Fig. 2.8.
- When shunt reversal occurs, e.g. in uncorrected VSD
- Associated with significant maternal mortality:
  - Inability to ↑ cardiac output
  - Prone to sudden death from ischaemia
  - Paradoxical embolism
- ↓ BP can result in shunt reversal:
  - ↓ in cardiac output and therefore ↑ cyanosis
  - Close attention should be paid to bleeding and cardiovascular stability at delivery
- IV prostacyclins, sildenafil, or inhaled NO can be of benefit (but watch for the development of methaemoglobinaemia)

Effects in pregnancy

- Miscarriage is common, which correlates with the degree of maternal hypoxia
- Higher risk of bleeding
- Fetal outcomes are poor when maternal saturation <85%

⚠ Caution is required when administering IV medications due to the risk of a paradoxical air embolism, preventative filters should be used.

Unrestrictive VSD

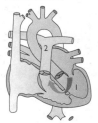
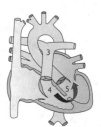

1. Large shunt from LV to RV
2. Excessive pulmonary blood flow

3. Progressive "damage" to pulmonary vasculature
4. Elevation of pulmonary artery & RV pressures
5. Pressure equalisation & reversal of shunt leading to desaturation

Fig. 2.8 Diagram illustrating the progressive reversal of a left-to-right shunt and Eisenmenger syndrome. Reproduced from Hezelgrave N. et al. (2015) *Challenging Concepts in Obstetrics and Gynaecology: Cases with Expert Commentary* Oxford University Press: Oxford with permission from Oxford University Press.

Transposition of the great arteries

The RV pumps blood into the aorta and the LV connects to the pulmonary trunk (Fig. 2.9).

Atrial switch

- Creates baffles (artificially created vascular tunnels)
- Mustard procedure uses either synthetic or pericardial tissue baffles, to allow systemic venous return into the LV (Fig. 2.10)
- Senning procedure baffle is endogenous tissue which connects the systemic venous return into the LV
- The result is a systemic RV and tricuspid valve
- Complications include baffle stenosis, tricuspid regurgitation, heart failure, and arrhythmias

Arterial switch

- Replaced Mustard and Senning procedures in the late 1980s
- Usually performed in early infancy
- Involves surgically resecting the aorta and pulmonary artery and anastomosing to the anatomically correct ventricle (Table 2.3)
- The coronary arteries are reattached to the newly formed aorta
- Can be complicated by stenoses at any of the anastomosis sites, but low rate of arrhythmias and ventricular dysfunction

Table 2.3 Surgically corrected TGA in pregnancy

	Assessment	Risks
Atrial switch		
Pre-pregnancy	• Ensure up-to-date assessment of baffle patency • Check ventricular function and tricuspid regurgitation • Cardiac MRI • Cardiopulmonary exercise test	
During pregnancy	• Check for arrhythmias • Check ventricular function	• Arrhythmias • Heart failure • ↓ in functional status
Fetus		• Premature delivery • Growth restriction • ↑ mortality rate
Arterial switch		
During pregnancy	• Check for regurgitant neoadjuvant valve • Check abnormalities of coronary artery reimplantation	• ↑ risk of stenosis • ↑ risk of occlusion • Ventricular outflow tract obstruction • Pulmonary artery stenosis

Transposition of the great arteries

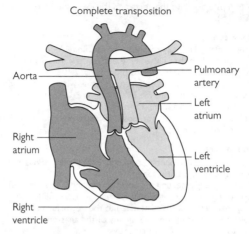

Complete transposition

Fig. 2.9 Diagram illustrating transposition of the great arteries. Reproduced from Myerson S. G. et al. (2009) *Emergencies in Cardiology* 2nd Ed. Oxford University Press: Oxford with permission from Oxford University Press.

Mustard/Senning (interatrial repair)

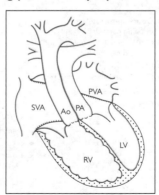

Fig. 2.10 Surgical approaches to complete transposition of the great arteries. Ao, aorta; LV, left ventricle; PA, pulmonary artery; RV, right ventricle; PVA, pulmonary venous atrium; SVA, systemic venous atrium. Reproduced from Adamson D. et al. (2011) *Heart Disease in Pregnancy* Oxford University Press: Oxford with permission from Oxford University Press.

Congenitally corrected transposition of the great arteries

- The left and right ventricles are reversed:
  - **Left** ventricle receives blood from the **right** atrium and connects to the pulmonary trunk
  - **Right** ventricle receives blood from the **left** atrium and connects to the aorta
- Patients have a systemic RV
- Can occasionally present in pregnancy

Complications of congenitally corrected TGA in pregnancy

- Generally fewer than those in ♀ with TGA:
  - RV failure and tricuspid regurgitation
  - Pulmonary oedema from RV volume overload
  - Arrhythmias especially heart block
  - Impaired functional status
- Fetal effects:
  - Association with small-for-gestational-age babies
  - Congenital heart disease

Congenitally corrected TGA
See Fig. 2.11.

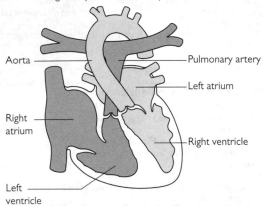

Fig. 2.11 Features of congenitally corrected transposition of the great arteries.
Reproduced from Myerson S. G. et al. (2009) *Emergencies in Cardiology* 2nd Ed.
Oxford University Press: Oxford with permission from Oxford University Press.

Cyanotic heart disease

⚠ ♀ with high pulmonary pressures should be counselled against pregnancy.

Pregnancy in ♀ with cyanotic heart disease without pulmonary vascular disease

- Systemic vascular resistance ↓ in pregnancy can cause an ↑ right-to-left shunt with resulting ↑ cyanosis
- ↓ oxygen saturation and ↑ haemoglobin concentration (as a result of hypoxia) is associated with a ↓ chance of a live birth

---

Risks of cyanotic heart disease in pregnancy

Fetal risks
- Intrauterine death
- Prematurity
- Low birthweight (correlates to oxygen saturation)

Maternal risks
- Haemorrhage
- Paradoxical embolism
- Impaired renal function
- Heart failure
- Arrhythmias
- Endocarditis

Tetralogy of Fallot

- Four main features (Fig. 2.12):
  - VSD with a right-to-left shunt
  - RV outflow tract obstruction
  - Over-riding of aorta
  - 2° RV hypertrophy
- It may also be associated with:
  - An ASD
  - A right-sided aortic arch
  - Left-sided SVC
  - Hypoplastic pulmonary arteries

Surgical correction

- Usually involves:
  - Temporary measure in infancy: shunt to increase pulmonary blood flow e.g. Blalock–Taussig shunt
  - Later complete repair with closure of the VSD and relief of the outflow tract obstruction with a transannular patch

⚠ A transannular patch can cause significant pulmonary regurgitation and RV failure ∴ pulmonary valve replacement before pregnancy may be indicated.

Pregnancy

Uncorrected

- A few are identified in adulthood and present in pregnancy with:
  - ↑ cyanosis
  - Arrhythmias
  - Heart failure
- Associated with significant maternal and fetal mortality

Surgically corrected

- Pregnancy usually occurs without complication

Management of ToF in pregnancy

- Pre-pregnancy counselling
- Genetic assessment (15% have DiGeorge syndrome)
- Regular echocardiography
- Fetal echocardiography
- Regular assessment of fetal growth
- Monitor for arrhythmias (risk of atrial and ventricular tachyarrhythmias and bradycardia, particularly complete heart block with surgically corrected ToF)
- Anticoagulation with prophylactic LMWH if residual shunt (risk of paradoxical embolus)
- Oxygen if cyanosis present

Tetralogy of Fallot
See Fig. 2.12.

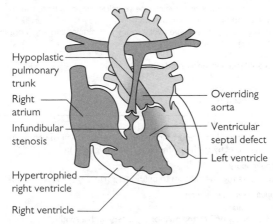

Fig. 2.12 Tetralogy of Fallot. Reproduced from Myerson S. G. et al. (2009) *Emergencies in Cardiology* 2nd Ed. Oxford University Press: Oxford with permission from Oxford University Press.

Univentricular heart

See Fig. 2.13.
- A variety of conditions in which one ventricle supports both the systemic and pulmonary circulation
- Lesions usually present when very young and require surgery (Fontan procedure)
- Causes include:
  - Hypoplastic left heart syndrome
  - Double-inlet LV
  - Tricuspid atresia
  - Unbalanced AVSD

Fontan procedure

There are several procedures included in this label, where venous blood is diverted directly to the pulmonary artery (Fig. 2.14):

Atriopulmonary
- Connects the right atrium to pulmonary artery

Cavopulmonary circulation
- Extracardiac:
  - Connects IVC to the pulmonary artery with a synthetic conduit
- Intracardiac:
  - Uses an intra-atrial conduit to divert blood from the IVC to the pulmonary artery

---

Complications of a Fontan procedure

- Ventricular dysfunction and AV valve regurgitation
- Atrial arrhythmias
- Thrombosis
- Cyanosis from right-to-left shunting
- Infection
- Systemic complications, e.g. cirrhosis and protein-losing enteropathy

Management of pregnancy post Fontan procedure

- Pre-pregnancy assessment involves:
  - Ensuring up-to-date assessment of ventricular function
  - Cardiac MRI
  - Cardiopulmonary exercise testing
- Anticoagulation:
  - Therapeutic or prophylactic LMWH
- 4-weekly assessment of maternal condition and fetal growth
- ↑ risk of miscarriage and preterm delivery
- No contraindication to vaginal delivery, early epidural advisable
- Lateral position in labour recommended

⚠ There is a risk of impairment of functional capacity that may not recover entirely after pregnancy.

Univentricular heart

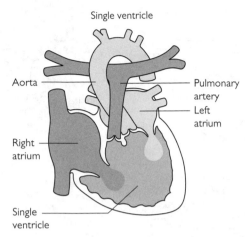

Fig. 2.13 Univentricular heart. Reproduced from Myerson S. G. et al. (2009) *Emergencies in Cardiology* Oxford University Press: Oxford with permission from Oxford University Press.

Fontan procedure

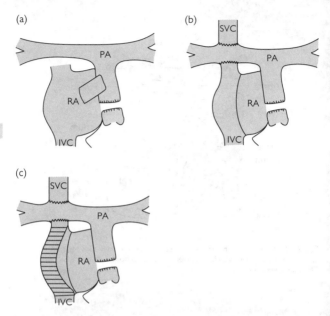

Fig. 2.14 Diagrams illustrating various types of Fontan operation.
(A) Atriopulmonary Fontan. (B) Total cavopulmonary connection (TCPC, lateral tunnel). (C) TCPC (extracardiac conduit). Reproduced from Myerson S. G. et al. (2009) *Emergencies in Cardiology* Oxford University Press: Oxford with permission from Oxford University Press.

Pulmonary stenosis

- Common cause of congenital heart disease
- Can be seen in Noonan's syndrome

Management of pulmonary stenosis in pregnancy

- If RV function normal, pregnancy is usually well tolerated
- If a significant gradient across the valve is present (>50 mmHg):
  - Ideally surgery should be performed before conception
  - If surgery has not been performed, clinic review every 4 wks is advised
- Balloon valvuloplasty has been performed in pregnancy in ♀ with severely symptomatic pulmonary stenosis which is unresponsive to medical therapy

Noonan's syndrome

- Autosomal dominant condition
- Features include:
  - Short stature
  - Pectus excavatum
  - Developmental delay
  - Bleeding disorders
  - Characteristic facial appearance
- Congenital heart defects in 50–80%, including:
  - Pulmonary stenosis
  - Hypertrophic cardiomyopathy
  - AVSD

Ebstein's anomaly

The tricuspid valve is displaced towards the apex of the RV, → right atrial enlargement and tricuspid regurgitation.

Causes

- Can be associated with:
  - Maternal lithium use in pregnancy
  - Other abnormalities such as an ASD or WPW syndrome

Surgical correction

- Surgical prior to correction should be considered if:
  - Cyanosis is present
  - Exercise capacity is ↓
  - Severe tricuspid regurgitation

Risks of pregnancy with Ebstein's anomaly

Maternal risks

- ⚠ Symptomatic ♀ should be advised against pregnancy
- In the absence of cyanosis or right heart failure, ♀ do well
- Potential complications:
  - Heart failure
  - ↑ cyanosis
  - Arrhythmias
  - Paradoxical embolus
  - Infective endocarditis

Fetal risks

- If maternal cyanosis is present, ↑ risk of
  - Low birthweight babies
  - Preterm birth
  - Fetal loss

Investigations

- CXR can show cardiomegaly
- ECG changes may include tall and broad P waves, ↑ PR interval, right bundle branch pattern, and 'fragmented' QRS complex

---

Management of Ebstein's anomaly in pregnancy

- Review at least every 4 weeks and monitor for complications
- Thromboprophylaxis should be considered if ASD also present
- Regular fetal growth scans

Mitral stenosis

- Commonly caused by rheumatic fever
- Less commonly mitral annular calcification or congenital stenosis
- Normal valve area is 4–6 cm^2:
  - Pregnancy usually tolerated well if the valve area >1.5 cm^2
  - ESC guidelines advise valve replacement prior to pregnancy in ♀ with severe mitral stenosis, i.e. <1.0 cm^2
- Diastolic filling time is prolonged in mitral stenosis:
  - ↑ reliance on left 'atrial kick' for adequate LV filling
  - If tachycardia develops, the diastolic filling time is ↓, or if the atrial kick is lost, e.g. if AF develops, rapid decompensation can occur
- Signs of severity include:
  - Signs of pulmonary hypertension (loud P2, RV heave)
  - Signs of right heart failure with no other cause (hepatomegaly, ↑ JVP/ features of tricuspid regurgitation, oedema, ascites)
  - Longer duration of murmur
  - Reduced time between S2 and opening snap
- CXR shows upper lobe congestion and LA enlargement causing a double silhouette; 2° pulmonary haemosiderosis

Management of mitral stenosis in pregnancy

- Echocardiography and clinical assessment every 2–4 wks (Tables 2.4 and 2.5)
- Medical therapy for symptoms or clinically significant pulmonary hypertension (systolic pulmonary artery pressure ≥50 mmHg):
  - Diuretics
  - β blockade to control heart rate and ↑ diastolic filling time
- Anticoagulation:
  - Therapeutic LMWH if history of embolic events, a left atrial appendage thrombus is present, or AF present
  - Consider in ♀ in sinus rhythm with significant MS and spontaneous echocardiographic contrast in left atrium, left atrium ≥60 mL/m^2, or heart failure
- Treatment of AF with β blockade and/or digoxin:
  - Consider cardioversion
- If symptomatic despite maximal medical treatment, percutaneous mitral commissurotomy can be performed in pregnancy

Management at time of delivery

- Risk of pulmonary oedema is greatest at the time of labour
- Positioning in labour to avoid being supine or in the lithotomy position
- Vaginal delivery with epidural analgesia is advised, with a limited 2nd stage
- Careful fluid balance and cautious fluid supplementation

Table 2.4 Echocardiographic assessment of mitral stenosis

	Valve area (cm²)	Gradient (mmHg)
Mild	1.6–2.0	<5
Moderate	1.0–1.5	5–10
Severe	<1.0	>10

Table 2.5 Clinical assessment of mitral stenosis

Symptoms	• Breathlessness
	• Orthopnoea
	• Paroxysmal nocturnal dyspnoea
	• Palpitations
	• Systemic embolism
	• Hoarse voice (recurrent laryngeal nerve compression)
	• Dysphagia (left atrial compression of oesophagus)
	• Cough (can be haemoptysis; white/pink frothy sputum suggests pulmonary oedema)
Signs	• Malar flush
	• AF
	• Mid to late rumbling diastolic murmur at apex (can be exaggerated by exercise)
	• Palpable S1 (tapping apex beat)
	• Pulmonary oedema
	• Loud S1
	• Opening snap (opening of stenosed valve; heard after a loud S2 at apex in lateral decubitus position)
	↑ severity suggested by:
	• Signs of pulmonary hypertension (loud P2, RV heave)
	• Right heart failure (tricuspid regurgitation, peripheral oedema, hepatomegaly)

Complications of mitral stenosis in pregnancy

Maternal
- Left atrial enlargement
- AF
- Systemic embolization
- Pulmonary hypertension
- Right heart failure

Fetal
- Preterm delivery
- IUGR
- Stillbirth

Aortic stenosis

- Common causes include:
  - Accelerated calcification of a bicuspid aortic valve
  - Rheumatic heart disease
  - Degeneration of calcified valve
- Symptoms develop when gradient is severe and include exertional:
  - Chest pain
  - Breathlessness
  - Syncope
- The chest pain may sound ischaemic in nature:
  - Can be associated with ischaemic ECG changes resulting from ↑ myocardial oxygen demand
- LV failure can occur in decompensated severe AS
- Signs of severe AS include:
  - A slow rising pulse
  - Narrow pulse pressure
  - Quiet S2
  - A 'heaving' apex beat

Supravalvular AS

- Much less common
- More likely to be above the coronary arteries and not have the same ischaemic sequelae to the myocardium
- May → ischaemic symptoms in limbs

Echocardiographic changes

- Severe stenosis is a valve area of <1 cm^2, or if the mean gradient is >50 mmHg (measured when not pregnant)
- Gradient across the aortic valve is affected by ↑ cardiac output as pregnancy progresses, so an ↑ in the gradient is to be expected, and the absence of an ↑ is concerning
- Aortic valve gradient is an unreliable marker of the severity of AS in the context of impaired LV function and the valve area should be assessed

---

Pre-conceptual considerations in AS

- Pregnancy is not contraindicated even in severe AS if:
  - Asymptomatic
  - No LV impairment
  - Normal exercise test
- Aortic valve replacement should be considered with:
  - Critical AS (valve area of <0.7 cm^2, or if the mean gradient is >50 mmHg) even in the absence of symptoms
  - Symptomatic severe AS
  - LV dysfunction
  - Onset of features of LV failure

Management of AS in pregnancy

- In severe AS, monthly or bimonthly clinical evaluation with echocardiography is indicated (Table 2.6)
- In individuals with severe symptoms despite medical therapy, percutaneous valvuloplasty can be considered
- Potential fetal complications include IUGR and preterm birth, more commonly in ♀ with severe AS
- Fetal echocardiography advised due to potential inheritance, e.g. bicuspid aortic valve
- Anaesthetic considerations: aim to avoid BP fluctuations (epidural preferred to spinal)
- Vaginal delivery not contraindicated, but adequate analgesia and maintenance of normal BP is important
- In symptomatic severe AS, caesarean delivery is preferred

Table 2.6 Echocardiographic assessment of severity in AS

	Valve area (cm²)	Gradient (mmHg)
Mild	>1.5	<25
Moderate	1.0–1.5	25–50
Severe	<1.0	>50
Critical	<0.7	>80

Differential diagnosis of ejection systolic murmur

Physiological
- Flow murmur

Subvalvular outflow obstruction
- Hypertrophic cardiomyopathy

Valvular
- AS
- Pulmonary stenosis

Supravalvular
- Williams syndrome (in >95% of affected individuals, mutation in *ELN* gene which codes for the protein elastin):
  - Typical facies
  - Loud A2
  - Thrill

Mitral regurgitation

- Asymptomatic, mild mitral regurgitation is not an uncommon finding on echocardiography
- Mild/moderate regurgitation is usually well tolerated in pregnancy because of the ↓ in systemic vascular resistance
- Moderate/severe MR can result in heart failure

Overview

- Most common cause in pregnancy is mitral valve prolapse
- Other causes include:
  - Ischaemic heart disease
  - Infective endocarditis
  - 2° to LV dilatation
  - Associated with Ehlers–Danlos syndrome, Marfan syndrome, and pectus excavatum
- Prolapse of the mitral valve is a common finding (about 2% of normal population) and results from displacement of an abnormal mitral valve leaflet into the left atrium during systole
- If severe, LV enlargement and systolic dysfunction can occur and may therefore warrant valve replacement

Examination

- Pansystolic murmur at the apex
- In mitral valve prolapse the murmur may be late systolic and associated with a mid-systolic click; in such cases the mitral regurgitation is not usually haemodynamically severe

Management of mitral regurgitation in pregnancy

- In ♀ with acute severe regurgitation refractory to medical therapy for heart failure, surgery may be unavoidable
- Monitor with echocardiography every trimester in mild/moderate regurgitation, more often if severe
- Concerning features include:
  - Any decline in LV function from normal
  - ↑ systolic LV dimensions
- Vaginal delivery with early epidural with low threshold for assisted 2nd stage is usually appropriate

Tricuspid regurgitation

- An element of mild tricuspid regurgitation is present in many normal people on echocardiography
- 1° tricuspid regurgitation may be due to Ebstein's anomaly or endocarditis
- 2° tricuspid regurgitation due to left-sided valve disease or pulmonary hypertension is more common and is managed according to the 1° condition

Aortic regurgitation

- Mild or moderate regurgitation is well tolerated in pregnancy as a result of the ↓ systemic vascular resistance
- Severe regurgitation can result in heart failure

Causes of aortic regurgitation

Abnormal valve
- Infective endocarditis
- Congenital bicuspid valve
- Rheumatic fever

Normal valve, but abnormal aorta
- Aortic root dilatation
- Acute aortic dissection
- Aortitis, e.g. in giant cell arteritis, Takayasu arteritis, syphilis
- Ankylosing spondylitis

Symptoms
- May be asymptomatic
- Symptoms of consequences such as heart failure

Signs
- Collapsing pulse
- Wide pulse pressure
- Hyperdynamic ± displaced apex
- Early diastolic murmur most easily heard in expiration at when sitting forward, at lower left sternal edge
- An additional diastolic murmur can sometimes be heard at the apex, and results from the blood hitting the mitral valve from the aorta and the left atrium simultaneously ('Austin Flint' murmur)
- Sometimes an ejection systolic murmur can also be heart at the base (which can be loud)

Investigations
- Echocardiography
- CXR:
  - May show a large heart ('cor bovinum')

Management of aortic regurgitation in pregnancy
- Mild/moderate: likely to tolerate pregnancy well
- Severe (symptoms or LV dysfunction): diuretics, treatment of arrhythmias, vasodilators (hydralazine and nitrates)
- Surgery is only needed in the acute setting, e.g. acute valve dysfunction in endocarditis or dissection

Prosthetic heart valves

△ ♀ with prosthetic heart valves usually have normal cardiac function, so can adapt well to the physiological demands of pregnancy.

△ The problems that these ♀ encounter in pregnancy are from the thrombotic risks of pregnancy and the use of anticoagulation.

Decisions about which valve to use in ♀ of childbearing age should include alternatives such as the Ross procedure for aortic disease (pulmonary autograft to replace the aortic valve, and a pulmonary graft inserted) or transcatheter valve implantation (pulmonary valves).

Bioprosthetic valves

- Do not require therapeutic anticoagulation unless there is a history of associated arrhythmias
- Aspirin 75 mg OD recommended for all ♀
- ↑ chance of valve degeneration in pregnancy

Metal valves

- Need therapeutic anticoagulation throughout pregnancy, in addition to aspirin 75 mg OD

Warfarin

- Warfarin is preferable to LMWH to prevent thrombosis of a **metal heart valve** and is the main treatment in the non-pregnant population
△ Warfarin crosses the placenta and is known to be teratogenic
- Associated with miscarriage
- Fetal exposure in 1st trimester can result in:
  - Nasal bone hypoplasia
  - Shortened fingers
  - Microcephaly
  - Ventriculomegaly
  - Congenital cardiac abnormalities
- Thought to be dose dependent, with ↓ rates of embryopathy occurring with a daily dose of <5 mg of warfarin
△ Later in pregnancy, warfarin use can also cause complications:
  - Fetal haemorrhage (including intracranial haemorrhage)
  - Occurs due to the relative deficiency of vitamin K in the fetus the fetal INR is greater than maternal INR

Low-molecular-weight heparin

- Does not cross the placenta
- Is appropriate for many conditions in pregnancy (treatment of VTE)
- Is not associated with fetal complications

△ In ♀ with metal heart valves, LMWH is inferior to warfarin for prevention of thrombosis thus ↑ maternal morbidity and mortality
- See Table 2.7

Antenatal anticoagulation for metal heart valves

Options include:
- LMWH throughout pregnancy (deemed highest risk to the mother)
- If a ♀ is particularly high risk, or is on a low daily dose, i.e. <5 mg warfarin per day:
  - Warfarin throughout pregnancy
- If a ♀ is on high daily dose, i.e. >5 mg warfarin per day, changing between the two drugs can be considered:
  - LMWH from positive pregnancy test to 12 wks
  - Warfarin in wks 12–36
  - LMWH 36 wks until delivery

➔ ESC 2018 pregnancy guidelines: https://academic.oup.com/eurheartj/article/39/34/3165/5078465

Table 2.7 Suggested target anti-Xa levels if on LMWH

	Peak (4–6 hrs post dose)	Trough
Aortic valve replacement	0.8–1.2 IU/mL	≥0.6 IU/mL
Mitral valve or right-sided valve replacement	1.0–1.2 IU/mL	≥0.6 IU/mL

Source: data from ESC 2018 pregnancy guidelines https://academic.oup.com/eurheartj/article/39/34/3165/5078465

Management of peripartum anticoagulation

Delivery

- Induction of labour at 37–38 wks suggested:
  - Enables planning of timing of LMWH doses
  - ↓ the risk of delivery occurring when fully anticoagulated
- Regional anaesthesia contraindicated <24 hrs after therapeutic dose of LMWH

�• No pregnancy-specific guidelines are available regarding intrapartum LMWH if labour is long.

⚠ If ♀ spontaneously labour within 2 wks of warfarin cessation, a caesarean delivery is advisable to ↓ risk of fetal intracranial haemorrhage due to the likelihood of the fetus still having a high INR.

Anticoagulation after delivery

▶ In a non-pregnant setting, treatment-dose LMWH is withheld for 48 hrs after surgery, with prophylactic LMWH doses being given instead **but** there is no evidence that this is appropriate in pregnancy especially as the prothrombotic changes are maximal around the time of delivery.

Possible options for anticoagulation after delivery

These include:

Day of delivery
- No LMWH, or prophylactic dose 4–8 hrs after delivery for most ♀
- Therapeutic-dose LMWH in highest risk ♀ (ESC 2018 guidelines)

Day 1 post delivery
- Higher doses (i.e. therapeutic doses) can be considered provided there are no concerns regarding ongoing bleeding
- Dose may be divided depending on individual circumstances

Day 2 post delivery
- Usually appropriate to restart therapeutic dose

⚠ There is a significant risk of bleeding, irrespective of anticoagulant regimen so care should be in an appropriately monitored setting
- Both LMWH and warfarin can be used in breastfeeding
- It is advisable to wait for 7–10 days post-delivery before restarting warfarin because of the risk of late PPH

⊖ ESC 2018 pregnancy guidelines: ℛ https://academic.oup.com/eurheartj/article/39/34/3165/5078465

If bleeding, or delivery imminent, and fully anticoagulated

Warfarin

- Prothrombin complex concentrate:
  - Dose determined by weight
  - Do not need to wait for INR result before administering, it will return to normal within 15–20 mins
- Vitamin K 5–10 mg IV
- Cross-match blood

LMWH

- Discuss with haematologist about giving protamine sulfate
- Cross-match blood

Pulmonary hypertension

Symptoms
- Breathlessness without other cause of cardiac or respiratory disease
- Symptoms of right heart failure including:
  - Abdominal distension (↑ girth > than gestational age)
  - Oedema
- Syncope, pre-syncope, or chest pain can also occur

Signs
- Mild PH will not cause any abnormalities on clinical examination
- Advanced PH can be associated with:
  - RV heave
  - Loud 2nd (pulmonary) heart sound
  - ↑ JVP
  - Signs of right heart failure including hepatomegaly, which may be pulsatile, peripheral oedema, and ascites

Diagnosis
- ECG is often abnormal showing features including:
  - P pulmonale
  - Right axis deviation
  - RV hypertrophy
  - RV strain
  - Right bundle branch block
  - QTc prolongation (indicator of severe disease)

⚠ A normal ECG does not exclude the diagnosis
- Right heart catheterization:
  - Mean pulmonary artery pressure >25 mmHg at rest, **or** >30 mmHg on exercise
  - With pulmonary wedge pressure <15 mmHg
- Echocardiography:
  - Systolic pulmonary artery pressure can be estimated from tricuspid regurgitant velocity if tricuspid regurgitation is present
  - Enlarged RA and RV (suggestive not diagnostic features)
- CXR:
  - Features of PH can be present in up to 90%
  - Other respiratory conditions that contribute to development of PH may also be identified on a plain CXR
- Lung function tests can be performed to look for underlying causes
- Imaging (V/Q scan or CTPA) to assess for underlying thromboembolism

Classification
See Box 2.1.

Box 2.1 Classification of pulmonary hypertension

Pulmonary arterial hypertension
- Idiopathic
- Heritable, e.g. *BMPR2* mutation
- Drugs, e.g. fenfluramine, dexfenfluramine
- Other conditions, e.g. HIV infection, portal hypertension, schistosomiasis, congenital heart disease

Pulmonary vaso-occlusive disease and/or pulmonary capillary haemangiomatosis
- Idiopathic
- Heritable, e.g. *EIF2AK4* mutation
- Drugs, toxins, or radiation
- Associated with connective tissue disease and HIV infection

Pulmonary hypertension 2° to left heart disease
- Systolic or diastolic dysfunction
- Valvular disease

Pulmonary hypertension 2° to lung disease or hypoxia
- Chronic obstructive airways disease
- Interstitial lung disease
- Sleep-disordered breathing
- Alveolar hypoventilation disorders, e.g. chest wall deformities, neuromuscular weakness, central alveolar or obesity-related hypoventilation
- Chronic exposure to high altitude

Pulmonary hypertension 2° to chronic thromboembolic disease

Multifactorial
- Haematological, e.g. chronic haemolytic anaemia, myeloproliferative disease, splenectomy
- Systemic disorders, e.g. sarcoidosis, LCH, neurofibromatosis, lymphangioleiomyomatosis, vasculitis
- Metabolic disorders, e.g. glycogen storage disorders, Gaucher's disease
- Other, e.g. tumour obstruction, fibrosing mediastinitis, chronic renal failure

Source: data from Galiè N et al. (2015) 2015 ESC/ERS Guidelines for the diagnosis and treatment of pulmonary hypertension. *Eur Resp J* 46:903–975.

Pulmonary hypertension in pregnancy

- Physiological changes in the cardiovascular system (↑ blood volume and ↑ cardiac output) require a well-functioning RV

△ Irrespective of aetiology, PH is very high risk in pregnancy and associated with significant maternal mortality
- Highest risk time is 1st few days postpartum
- Mortality rate was thought to be up to 50% but recent data appears to show it is more like 20–30%
- Contraception and pregnancy should be discussed with any ♀ of childbearing age with PH
- In all pregnancies, termination must be discussed and offered
- PH should be looked for in any ♀ of childbearing age with a condition that can cause it
- Hormonal changes also influence the pulmonary vasculature
- In PH, there is a fixed pulmonary vascular resistance and an inability to ↑ pulmonary blood flow

Management of pulmonary hypertension in pregnancy

- Care should be coordinated in a centre with expertise in PH
- Consider prophylactic LMWH if poor RV function or factors that ↑ their thrombotic risk such as AF
- Oxygen
- Regular fetal growth scans
- Regular echocardiography
- Diuretics may be required (some use the IVC dimensions to guide this treatment)
- Routine use of a Swan–Ganz catheter for monitoring is not required and may ↑ the risk of arrhythmias

At delivery

- Spinal or epidural is viewed in many centres as mandatory
- Avoid suddenly ↑ vagal tone and venous return, e.g. ergometrine
- Avoid PGF2α which can cause pulmonary vasoconstriction
- Delivery and postnatal care needs to be in a location where tight BP control and careful fluid balance can occur
- ☙ Mode of delivery is controversial:
  - Many undergo caesarean with epidural anaesthesia as a result of preterm delivery and the ability to maintain careful control of the anaesthesia
  - Vaginal delivery is possible and can be supported in many ♀ with PH
- Timing of delivery—many advocate delivery by 36 wks' gestation
- Very careful fluid balance should be maintained
- ☙ Some advocate significant diuresis post delivery (up to 5 L in the 1st 3 days postpartum)
- Careful haemostasis as any bleeding risks decompensation
- Continue anticoagulation postnatally

Medications used in pulmonary hypertension

Prostanoids
- Iloprost (can be nebulized)

Phosphodiesterase inhibitor
- Sildenafil

Calcium channel antagonists
- Amlodipine
- Nifedipine

Endothelin antagonists
- Bosentan
- Macitentan

✒ NB There are some fetal concerns with agents such as bosentan from animal models, so this agent is often discontinued after conception. However, if this agent has helped this could be used, particularly after the 3rd trimester, as the likely benefit is > the theoretical risks based on animal studies.

➔ ESC 2015 pulmonary hypertension guidelines: ℗ https://www.escardio.org/Guidelines/ Clinical-Practice-Guidelines/Pulmonary-Hypertension-Guidelines-on-Diagnosis-and-Treatment-of

Aortopathies

⚠ Pregnancy ↑ the likelihood of aortic dissection.

Marfan syndrome

- Autosomal dominant resulting from a defect in the *FBN1* gene
- Diagnosis made by the Ghent criteria, which gives weight to a variety of clinical findings alongside the family history
- (➔ Ghent criteria can be found at: ℒ https://www.marfan.org/dx/rules)

Classical features

- ↑ arm span
- Pectus carinatum or pectus excavatum
- Ectopia lentis
- Dilation or dissection of the ascending aorta
- Mitral valve prolapse
- Spontaneous pneumothorax
- Dural ectasia

Cardiac complications

- Vessel dissection, particularly aortic
- Mitral valve prolapse/regurgitation
- Arrhythmias

Obstetric complications

- Premature rupture of membranes

Loeys–Dietz syndrome

- Relatively recently described syndrome associated with mutations in components of the TGFβ pathway
- Originally described phenotype included:
  - Generalized arterial tortuosity
  - Hypertelorism
  - Bifid or broad uvula
  - Cleft palate
- Cases are ↑ being identified which lack these features
- Syndrome is associated with vessel dissection which can occur at an earlier age (including in childhood) compared to Marfan syndrome

Management of aortopathies in pregnancy

▶ Aortic root replacement may be appropriate preconception to ↓ the risk of dissection (Table 2.8).

- Assessment of vascular tree (ideally pre-pregnancy)
- Counselling about inheritance
- MDT including cardiology, obstetrics, and neonatology
- Optimize medication, e.g. change from losartan to a β blocker (if regular periods and pregnancy testing, then continue losartan until test is positive, otherwise change in advance of conception)
- Excellent BP control
- Counselling about ↑ risk of aortic dissection (further ↑ if aortic dilatation present or if family history of dissection)
- Regular assessment of aortic diameters with echocardiography or cardiac MRI
- Delivery in a centre with access to cardiothoracic surgery and neonatal intensive care
- Individualized delivery plan:
  - Timing and mode of delivery depends on obstetric history and degree of aortic abnormality (Table 2.9); caesarean delivery is not mandatory

Table 2.8 European guidelines for consideration of aortic root replacement in Marfan and Loeys–Dietz syndromes

Non-pregnant population	
Consider surgery	• Maximum aortic diameter >50 mm
	• Maximum aortic diameter >45 mm with other risk factors
	• Family history of dissection
	• Yearly growth >2–3 mm
	• Severe aortic regurgitation
If contemplating pregnancy	
Marfan syndrome	• Consider surgery if maximum aortic diameter >45 mm
Loeys–Dietz syndrome	• No cut-off for aortic root diameter

The North American guidelines differ from the European guidelines and advocate a lower threshold for intervention in Loeys–Dietz syndrome:

◗ European guidelines: ℛ https://www.escardio.org/Guidelines/Clinical-Practice-Guidelines/Aortic-Diseases

◗ North American guidelines: ℛ https://insights.ovid.com/crossref?an=00000539-201008000-00011

Table 2.9 Mode of delivery by aortic root diameter

Aortic diameter	Recommendation
<40 mm	• Vaginal delivery
40–45 mm	• Consider either vaginal delivery with epidural and expedited 2nd stage, or caesarean section
>45 mm	• Caesarean section advised

See also ℬ https://www.escardio.org/Guidelines/Clinical-Practice-Guidelines/Cardiovascular-Diseases-during-Pregnancy-Management-of

Coarctation of the aorta

- A narrowing of the aorta
- Usually identified (and corrected) in childhood:
  - These are usually associated with aortic arch abnormalities
- Can present in adulthood, often with hypertension:
  - These tend to have stenosis in the descending aorta, distal to the left subclavian artery
- Associated with a bicuspid aortic valve in up to 85% of cases
- Also associated with:
  - Turner's syndrome
  - VSD
  - PDA
  - Mitral valve dysfunction (stenosis or regurgitation)
- ↑ risk of congenital heart disease in the offspring of mothers with coarctation

Symptoms
- Headache
- Intermittent claudication

Signs
- LV hypertrophy
- Palpable collaterals
- Systolic murmur (mid systolic) anteriorly or posteriorly in the chest
- Systolic thrill in suprasternal notch
- Bruits over scapulae, anterior axillary areas, and left sternal edge

Investigations
- CXR can show rib notching
- ECG may show LV hypertrophy

Preconception
- If corrected, cardiac MRI to establish the success of correction and presence of any complications
- If uncorrected, there is a risk of ↑ BP and heart failure (risk is related to the gradient)
- Risk of aortic dissection so careful BP control is required
- Intracranial aneurysms are 5× more common with aortic coarctation

---

Complications following surgical correction of aortic coarctation

- Re-coarctation
- ↑ BP even in the absence of re-coarctation
- Aneurysm formation at site of previous repair
- Risk ↑ if a patch repair was performed

Other aortic pathologies

See Table 2.10.

Bicuspid aortic valve

- Associated with an ↑ risk of aortic regurgitation, aneurysm formation, and aortic dissection
- Echocardiography may miss distal ascending aortic dilatation so MRI may be required
- Aortic diameter >50 mm is a contraindication to pregnancy

Turner's syndrome

- Spontaneous pregnancy is unlikely (<2%) given the associated ovarian abnormalities and premature ovarian failure
- However, pregnancies are becoming more common due to ART using egg donation

⚠ There is a significant risk of aortic root dilatation and dissection in pregnancy

⚠ Concern regarding maternal deaths following aortic root dilatation in Turner's ♀ led the French Agence de la biomédecine to issue guidelines regarding pregnancy and Turner's syndrome (⅋ http://www.cngof.asso.fr/D_TELE/RPC_Turner_et_gro_090723_en.pdf)

⚠ **Pregnancy is not advisable if:**
  - Aortic size index (ASI) >2.5 cm/m²
  - ASI 2–2.5 cm/m² with risk factors such as coarctation or hypertension, or history of a previous dissection

💣 There is not a consensus as to whether actual aortic size should be used, or ASI, i.e. corrected for weight and height.

Ehlers–Danlos syndrome type 4 (vascular EDS)

- ↑ risk of large artery rupture and dissection including aorta
- ↑ risk of uterine rupture in labour
⚠ Pregnancy usually advised against.

Familial thoracic aortic aneurysm and/or dissection (FTAAD)

- A number of mutations have been identified in this condition including *ACTA2*, *SMAD3*, and *MYH11*
- Presentation is heterogeneous and not all affected individuals have a mutation identified
- Pregnancy is high risk and associated with ↑ risk of dissection

---

Pre-pregnancy considerations after aortic surgery

- Consider the underlying disorder:
  - Assess the maternal risk of pregnancy
  - Plan appropriate management
- Assessment of aortic valve function and appearance of aorta adjacent to the graft using echocardiography and/or cardiac MRI
- If reimplantation of coronary arteries was performed, need to be aware of risk of anastomosis stenoses

Table 2.10 Summary of aortic conditions affecting pregnancy

	Location of aneurysms	Comorbidities	Advise against pregnancy if
Low risk of aortic dissection (<1%)			
Bicuspid AV	• Ascending aorta	• AS or regurgitation	• Ascending aorta >50 mm
High risk of aortic dissection (1–10%)			
Marfan syndrome	• Everywhere	• Dural abnormalities • Mitral regurgitation • Heart failure • Arrhythmias	• Ascending aorta >45 mm • Ascending aorta >40 mm and family history of dissection or sudden death
Loeys–Dietz syndrome	• Everywhere	• Dural abnormalities • Mitral regurgitation	• Ascending aorta >45 mm • Ascending aorta >40 mm and family history of dissection or sudden death
Turner's syndrome	• Ascending aorta • Aortic arch • Descending aorta	• Low height • Infertility • Hypertension • Diabetes • Bicuspid aortic valve	• ASI >25 mm^2
Vascular EDS	• Everywhere	• Dural abnormalities • Uterine rupture	• All ♀

Source: data from European Society of Cardiology guidelines
https://academic.oup.com/eurheartj/article/39/34/3165/5078465

Heart failure

The clinical syndrome of signs of fluid overload in the context of an abnormally functioning heart.

- Presence of normal LV systolic function on echocardiography does not exclude diagnosis as diastolic dysfunction can also occur
- It is important to distinguish 'heart failure' from pulmonary oedema
- Echocardiographic appearances of the LV change in normal pregnancy so it is important that echocardiography is performed by someone experienced and familiar with pregnancy-related changes
- Symptoms can ↑ in pregnancy as a result of the ↑ demand on the heart, this classically occurs in the 1st trimester or at 27–30 wks

Left ventricular systolic dysfunction

Causes in pregnancy
- Underlying cardiomyopathy:
  - Dilated cardiomyopathy
  - Previous ischaemia
- Rate related, i.e. poorly controlled tachyarrhythmias
- New cardiomyopathy:
  - Peripartum cardiomyopathy
  - New presentation of ischaemic or dilated cardiomyopathy

Management
- Maintenance of normovolaemia
- Diuresis with furosemide
- Consideration of use of a mineralocorticoid receptor antagonist, e.g. eplerenone rather than spironolactone (former theoretically preferable as it lacks the anti-androgen effects of the latter)
- β blocker
- LMWH prophylaxis if EF greatly ↓ (thresholds vary)

Pulmonary oedema

- Pregnant ♀ are more inclined to pulmonary oedema (↓ oncotic pressure)
- Should be considered even in the absence of known cardiac disease
- Pulmonary oedema can occur with a structurally normal heart, so the absence of abnormalities on echocardiography does not exclude the diagnosis

⚠ Excessive IV fluid administration in pre-eclampsia is an important iatrogenic cause of pulmonary oedema so careful fluid monitoring ± restriction is advised until diuresis occurs.

Investigations
- CXR
- Echocardiogram

Management
- Identify and treat the underlying cause
- Diuresis with furosemide
- Fluid restriction
- Supportive care

Causes of pulmonary oedema

Non-cardiogenic causes
- Excessive fluid administration
- Pre-eclampsia
- Drugs:
  - Steroids
  - NSAIDs (diclofenac)
- Tocolytics
- Infection:
  - Pyelonephritis
  - Chorioamnionitis
  - Appendicitis

Cardiogenic causes
- Cardiac ischaemia
- Peripartum cardiomyopathy
- Undiagnosed congenital heart disease
- Other causes of cardiomyopathy (e.g. rate related)

Peripartum cardiomyopathy

An idiopathic cardiomyopathy presenting with heart failure 2° to LV systolic dysfunction towards the end of pregnancy or in the months following delivery.

- No other cause of heart failure is identified
- Remains a common misdiagnosis, on review other causes of heart failure are often identified, such as:
  - A missed ischaemic event
  - Undiagnosed dilated cardiomyopathy
  - LV dysfunction from sepsis or pre-eclampsia
- ⚠ It is a diagnosis of exclusion
- Incidence 1 in 3000–15,000 pregnancies, and varies geographically (is as high as 1 in 300 in Haiti)
- The aetiology is unknown; autoimmunity, viral infection, high prolactin, and fetal microchimerism have all been suggested

Clinical features

- Presenting symptoms can include breathlessness, pleural effusions, peripheral oedema, and embolic phenomena
- LV may not be dilated but EF nearly always <45%

Risk factors for peripartum cardiomyopathy

- Tocolytics
- Multiple pregnancy
- Gestational hypertension or pre-eclampsia
- African origin
- Gravida
- Parity
- Extremes of age

Management of peripartum cardiomyopathy

- Optimize medical treatment including β blockade and diuresis
- If postpartum, also consider ACE-I
- If occurs antenatally, delivery is indicated
- Prophylactic LMWH
- Close monitoring postpartum
- ☀ Prolactin has been implicated in the aetiology:
  - In some series, breastfeeding appears to be associated with ↑ LV EF recovery, so cessation is not advocated at present
  - Bromocriptine shows some promise and consideration of its use is suggested in the ESC 2018 guidelines

Subsequent pregnancies

- Good outcomes are seen when cardiac dysfunction has resolved by 6 months postpartum
- Morbidity and mortality are associated with a persistently impaired EF or a LV end-diastolic diameter of >60 mm (which also correlates with BMI)

● ESC 2018 pregnancy guidelines: ⬥ https://academic.oup.com/eurheartj/article/39/34/3165/5078465

Hypertrophic cardiomyopathy

Definition: an asymmetrical ↑ in myocardial thickness in the absence of another cause such as ↑ BP.

- Inheritance is autosomal dominant in about 60% of cases, but penetrance is variable
- Many ♀ are asymptomatic

Clinical features

Symptoms of LV outflow tract obstruction
- Breathlessness
- Chest pain
- Syncope
- Palpitations

Signs
- Double apical impulse
- Systolic thrill over the left sternal edge
- 4th heart sound
- Ejection systolic murmur at left 3rd interspace (inspiration can → a pronounced ↓ in volume of the murmur)

ECG changes
- LV hypertrophy
- Q waves
- Conduction defects

Echocardiography
- Asymmetric septal hypertrophy (apical is more common in Japan)
- Systolic anterior motion of anterior leaflet of mitral valve

Complications
- Arrhythmias
- Endocarditis
- Sudden death

⚠ An implantable defibrillator may be indicated if sustained ventricular arrhythmias or a strong family history of sudden cardiac death.

Management of hypertrophic cardiomyopathy in pregnancy

Antenatal management
- Pregnancy usually well tolerated if asymptomatic before conception
- Maternal death is rare
- Risk of sudden death is not ↑ by pregnancy
- Asymptomatic ♀ do not require any treatment
- Careful screening for arrhythmias should be undertaken
- β blockade should be continued if taking prior to conception
- β blockade should be initiated if there is a significant LV outflow tract gradient, or if symptoms develop (diuretics may also be required in the latter setting)
- If AF develops, prompt pharmacological treatment or electrical cardioversion is advised

Intrapartum management
- Careful fluid balance:
  - Keep normovolaemic
- Regional anaesthesia/analgesia may result in vasodilation which may be poorly tolerated
- Valsalva manoeuvres may ↓ preload and worsen symptoms
- Vaginal delivery is often preferred
- β blockers can be continued

Dilated cardiomyopathy

Where there is systolic dysfunction of the LV ± RV, or unexplained ventricular dilatation in the absence of other causes (e.g. ↑ BP, coronary artery disease).
- A significant proportion are inherited
- Can be idiopathic, but can also occur in other medical conditions

---

Causes of dilated cardiomyopathy

- Idiopathic
- Familial
- Genetic
- Infective:
  - Viral (e.g. Coxsackie B)
  - TB
- Toxins:
  - Alcohol
  - Drugs (e.g. anthracyclines)
- Cardiac:
  - Tachyarrhythmias
  - Myocardial ischaemia
- Nutrition:
  - Niacin deficiency
  - Thiamine deficiency

Pre-pregnancy advice

- Risk of irreversible deterioration in LV function
- Most are advised against pregnancy
- Potentially better outcomes if condition is stable and asymptomatic over many years
- Poor prognostic indicators include:
  - Very poor EF, i.e. <20%
  - Poor performance status pre-pregnancy (NYHA class III or IV)
  - ↓ BP

Management in pregnancy

- Diuretics:
  - Furosemide
  - Eplerenone could be considered if a mineralocorticoid receptor antagonist is warranted (spironolactone has anti-androgen activity so may affect masculinization of a ♂ fetus)
- Vasodilators
- Cautious β blockade
- Anticoagulation

Restrictive cardiomyopathy

Dysfunction caused by a rigid, stiff myocardium, resulting from infiltration of abnormal material or fibrosis.
- Can present with heart failure
- Atrial arrhythmias are common

Causes of restrictive cardiomyopathy

- Idiopathic
- Familial
- Infiltrative:
  - Amyloid
  - Sarcoid
  - Gaucher's disease
- Endomyocardial conditions:
  - Hypereosinophilic syndrome
  - Endomyocardial fibrosis
- Storage disorders:
  - Haemochromatosis
  - Fabry's disease
  - Glycogen storage disorders
- Other conditions:
  - Carcinoid
  - Systemic sclerosis

Clinical features
- ECG:
  - No specific changes
- Echocardiography:
  - Typical pattern involves a LV that looks normal
  - Biatrial enlargement
- Cardiac MRI shows a similar pattern, but can give more detail about the myocardial appearance and therefore help identify a specific cause

---

Management of restrictive cardiomyopathy in pregnancy

- Very few reported cases of restrictive cardiomyopathy in pregnancy
- Supportive treatment including diuretics

⚠ Pregnancy is likely to be high risk (as it is unlikely a stiff ventricle can cope well with the ↑ cardiac output of pregnancy).

Takotsubo cardiomyopathy

The rapid development of systolic dysfunction in the absence of coronary artery disease.

- Has been reported in a wide range of individuals, some with an identifiable stressful precipitant, some without
- Thought to account for up to 10% of young ♀ with suspected ACS
- Imaging findings are characteristic with abnormal contraction of the mid and upper parts of the ventricle with apical sparing (likened to a Japanese fishing pot used to trap octopus, hence the name; see Fig. 2.15)
- Most likely explanation is that this is catecholamine mediated, hence the alternative name of 'stress cardiomyopathy'

Management of Takotsubo cardiomyopathy in pregnancy

- There have been a small number of cases of this reported in pregnancy and 1 probable case developing at the time of caesarean section
- An ↑ troponin level can occur
- Arrhythmias can also occur
- Recurrence can be seen in 5–10% of individuals and is not entirely prevented by β blockade

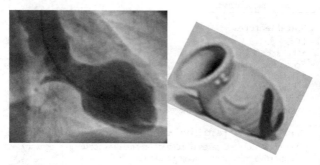

Fig. 2.15 Left ventriculography from a 65-year-old ♀ who presented as a primary angioplasty call showing a typical apical ballooning with dynamic proximal ventricular contraction. This patient had unobstructed coronaries. On the right, a picture of a Japanese fishing pot with a narrow neck and wide base that is used to trap octopus. Reproduced from Zamorano J. L. et al. (2015) *The ESC Textbook of Cardiovascular Imaging* 2nd Ed. Oxford University Press: Oxford with permission from the European Society of Cardiology.

Other cardiomyopathies

Arrhythmogenic right ventricular cardiomyopathy

A condition where the RV myocardium is progressively replaced by fibrofatty tissue.

- Leading cause of sudden cardiac death in young people and athletes
- Most common presentation is palpitations or syncope on exertion
- Often autosomal dominant
- Ventricular arrhythmias and ventricular dysfunction can occur and may require pathway ablation and/or an implantable defibrillator
- ECG changes include TWI in leads V1–V3

Management of arrhythmogenic right ventricular cardiomyopathy in pregnancy

- Anti-arrhythmic treatment may need to be ↑ during pregnancy
- Implantable defibrillators can be placed in pregnancy if required
- Emergency pathway ablation can also be performed if medical treatment is not sufficient to control arrhythmias

Left ventricular non-compaction

- A rare cardiomyopathy seen both in children and adults
- Myocardium is abnormal, with a thin epicardial layer and a non-compacted endocardial layer, with prominent trabeculations
- Thought to result from abnormal development in the fetus
- This is ↑ recognized as a result of improved imaging techniques, i.e. echocardiography and cardiac MRI
- Heart failure, thromboembolism and arrhythmias can occur

Management of left ventricular non-compaction in pregnancy

- A small number of cases in pregnancy have been reported
- Outcome is dependent on pre-pregnancy status; if asymptomatic before with minimal complications, pregnancy is usually relatively well tolerated
- Thromboprophylaxis should be considered but full anticoagulation is not advised for all cases

Assessment of palpitations

▶ Most important diagnostic feature is the history.

Features that ↑ likelihood of a pathological tachyarrhythmia

- Sudden rather than gradual onset/offset
- Occurrence at rest rather than on exertion
- Nature of heart rate (ask to tap out), e.g.:
  - Fast and regular
  - Fast and irregular
  - Big beat and then a pause (often reflects ectopy)
- Associated breathlessness, syncope, or chest pain
- No features that are more suggestive of other diagnoses, e.g. nausea/vomiting and prolonged recovery are more common in vasovagal syncope than syncope due to an arrhythmia

Other important aspects of the assessment

- Symptoms or signs of an underlying cause such as:
  - Hyperthyroidism
  - Pulmonary embolism
- Risk factors for tachyarrhythmias:
  - Caffeine
  - Alcohol
  - Drugs
- Family history of cardiac disease or sudden cardiac death
- Any abnormality on cardiac examination

Investigations

- Bloods:
  - FBC
  - TFTs
- ECG
- Ambulatory ECG monitoring:
  - Duration depends on the frequency of the episodes
- Echocardiogram:
  - If underlying structural heart disease or ventricular dysfunction is suspected

---

Sinus tachycardia

- Commonest cause of tachycardia in pregnancy
- Relevant investigations include Hb and TFTs to exclude anaemia and hyperthyroidism as contributory factors
- Sinus tachycardia in the setting of other symptoms should not be ignored and may represent other underlying pathology such as pulmonary embolism
- An isolated, asymptomatic sinus tachycardia does not cause harm to mother or fetus so pharmacological therapy is not indicated
- Sometimes the sinus tachycardia may be 'inappropriate' but even in this setting, the benefits of β blockade are not clear and so conservative management and reassurance can appropriately be the mainstay of treatment

---

Ventricular ectopy
- Normal frequency of ectopy is 200–500 beats/day
- ↑ risk of LV dysfunction if:
  - Ectopy >15% or 10,000 beats/day
  - Non-outflow tract origin
  - QRS is broad on a baseline ECG

▶ Echocardiogram is only required if ectopy burden is significant or other suspicions of underlying structural heart disease.

▶ Cardiac MRI is particularly poor in the presence of a high ectopy burden so this should be treated before an MRI is undertaken.

Atrial arrhythmias

See Table 2.11.

Atrial tachycardia

- Uncommon but occur more frequently with structural heart disease
- Difficult to diagnose, may be wrongly labelled sinus tachycardia
- Risk of a tachycardia-related cardiomyopathy:
  - Echocardiographic monitoring is recommended
- Ambulatory ECG monitoring may aid diagnosis as atrial tachycardia has a different pattern throughout the day to sinus tachycardia
- Aggressive rate control required if LV EF compromised

Atrial fibrillation/flutter

- Uncommon in pregnancy
- Previously thought to mostly occur in structural heart disease, but more cases now reported in absence of structural heart disease (so may reflect the changing health status of pregnant ♀ and ↑ maternal age)
- Needs urgent treatment in conditions such as mitral stenosis, where arrhythmia development can cause a rapid deterioration in cardiac function

Diagnosis of AF or atrial flutter

- ECG:
  - Irregular QRS complexes without a P wave before each complex (AF)
  - Organized atrial activity, reflected by regular P waves, but these are not followed each time by a QRS complex (atrial flutter)

Table 2.11 Management of atrial arrhythmias in pregnancy

Rhythm control	• DC cardioversion if haemodynamically unstable
	  • Signs of heart failure or ↓ BP
	• Pharmacological cardioversion
	  • Flecainide
	  • Amiodarone (used in acute setting if other agents fail, not for regular use in pregnancy as can be fetotoxic)

Rate control	• Digoxin[a] • β blockade[a] (not in ♀ with history of asthma) • Verapamil
Anticoagulation	• Therapeutic LMWH if high risk • Prophylactic LMWH if low risk
Radiofrequency catheter ablation	• Can be a successful curative measure for atrial flutter or those arrhythmias associated with an accessory pathway • Usually delayed until after delivery

[a] Larger doses may be required in pregnancy because of ↑ metabolism and clearance.

Pre-excitation syndromes

Wolff–Parkinson–White syndrome

WPW syndrome: an accessory pathway **and** a resulting AV re-entrant tachycardia.

WPW abnormality: a delta wave alone, without a history of tachyarrhythmia.

- Can cause pre-excited AF
- If AV nodal blocking medications are given, can degenerate into ventricular fibrillation (↑ conduction through accessory pathway)
- ECG shows a short PR interval **and**
  - A left-sided accessory pathway (type A WPW) with a delta wave positive in V1
    Or
  - A right-sided accessory pathway (type B WPW) with negative delta waves in V1 and V2 and positive in V4–V6

Management of WPW syndrome in pregnancy
- Regular review
- If symptoms ↑, ambulatory monitoring may be beneficial to establish whether symptoms represent pathological arrhythmia prior to ↑ or altering therapy

Treatment options for WPW syndrome in pregnancy
- DC cardioversion
- Pharmacological including:
  - Flecainide
  - Sotalol
  - Disopyramide
  - (Amiodarone in an emergency setting only)

Lown–Ganong–Lavine syndrome
- Another cause of pre-excitation
- ECG shows a short PR interval and normal QRS complexes
- Principles of management are the same as in WPW

Supraventricular tachycardia

- Most common tachyarrhythmia in pregnancy
- Less common than ectopy and sinus tachycardia, so empirical treat
  ment before diagnosis confirmed is not usually advised
- The description encompasses a variety of abnormal rhythms including:
  - Atrial tachycardia which involves the AV node (AV nodal re-entrant
    tachycardia; P wave is present)
  - Atrial tachycardia that does not require the AV node as are
    transmitted by an accessory pathway (AV re-entrant tachycardia;
    P wave is absent)

Treatment of an acute SVT in pregnancy

- Vagal manoeuvres
- Adenosine may stop the episode (normal doses can be used)
- β blockade, e.g. with oral bisoprolol or IV metoprolol
- Verapamil can be used (oral or IV)

Prophylaxis for SVT

- Advisable if recurrent episodes, or severe episode
- β blocker
- Verapamil (up to 240 mg in 3–4 divided doses)
- If difficult to treat, consideration of catheter ablation

Ventricular tachycardia

Causes
See Table 2.12.

Idiopathic VT
- Normal ECG between episodes
- Normal echocardiogram, cardiac MRI, and stress test

Repetitive monomorphic VT
- Can be treated with:
  - Adenosine
  - β blocker
  - Verapamil
- Ablation can be considered if medical treatment fails or the EF is ↓

Table 2.12 Causes of ventricular tachycardia

Structurally normal heart	Structurally abnormal heart
• Idiopathic	• Hypertrophic cardiomyopathy
• Long QT syndrome	• Congenital heart disease
• Brugada syndrome	• Arrhythmogenic RV cardiomyopathy

High-risk features
- Family history of sudden death
- Syncope or haemodynamic compromise
- Sustained or polymorphic VT
- Heavy ectopy burden

Treatment
- DC cardioversion
- Pharmacological:
  - Lidocaine 1st choice agent in pregnancy
  - Amiodarone in emergency
- If this fails, overdrive pace:
  - Temporary pacing wire at rate 10/20/30 beats > rate
  - Check for capture, then ↓ rate to normal after a few beats
- β blockade:
  - Essential if underlying structural heart disease
- Consider an ICD:
  - Indications same as in non-pregnant population but there is a high recovery rate after delivery for those arrhythmias that develop during pregnancy

Brugada syndrome

- Rare channelopathy, resulting from mutations in the cardiac voltage-gated Na^+ channel
- Associated with sudden cardiac death from tachyarrhythmias
- Two typical patterns of ECG changes, mainly seen in V1/2 in association with a pseudo right bundle pattern:
  - **Type 1**: ST elevation (with upward convexity) and TWI
  - **Type 2**: ST elevation with saddle ST-T wave changes, which → a positive or biphasic T wave
- Ajmaline challenge used to unmask Brugada syndrome

Management of Brugada syndrome in pregnancy
- High-risk cases may require an ICD
- Avoid medications that could be arrhythmogenic

⮱ Advice on these medications can be found at: ℬ https://www.brugadadrugs.org

Long QT syndrome

- Abnormal repolarization of the myocardium manifests as an abnormally long QT interval on ECG:
  - Normal QT interval corrected for rate is <0.45–0.46 s in ♀
- Associated with sudden death from ventricular arrhythmias
- In ♀ with high-risk features (family history, or symptoms such as syncope) then there is no specific QT cut-off and dynamic testing should be considered
- Causes include:
  - Congenital
  - Drugs, e.g. anti-arrhythmics, some antihistamines, and some antibiotics including macrolides
    ➔ For a full list see ⟲ https://www.crediblemeds.org
- Risks from ventricular arrhythmias, in particular torsades de pointes, may be ↓ in pregnancy as a result of the ↑ heart rate (which ↓ the QT interval) but the reverse is true in the postpartum period where risk of VT is ↑

Management of long QT syndrome in pregnancy

- β blockers are advised but do not entirely protect against arrhythmia development
- Guidelines recommend consideration of an ICD in addition to a β blocker, if an individual has a pathogenic mutation and the QT is >500 ms, even if asymptomatic
- A low-grade exercise test can be used to look at the QT dynamics if there is doubt about the phenotype
- If either parent is positive for a long QT-associated mutation then a neonatal ECG should be performed
- Anaesthetic considerations:
  - Avoid any medications that can prolong the QT interval
  - Avoid hypothermia
  - Do not stop β blocker
- Consider genetic testing and cord blood testing

Bradyarrhythmias

These are unusual in pregnancy, but a pacemaker can be inserted in pregnancy if required for a pathological bradycardia.

Permanent pacemakers

- Majority of ♀ with pacemakers have them implanted before conception
- Small number of ♀ may need pacemakers in pregnancy for pathological bradyarrhythmias (ideally inserted after 1st trimester due to radiation exposure of the procedure)
- Pacemaker checks should occur at normal frequency
- Adjustment of rate is not routinely required in pregnancy, however pacemaker-dependent ♀ with symptoms such as syncope or pre-syncope may benefit from an ↑ in the rate

Implantable defibrillators

- Similar advice applies for ♀ with ICDs as in ♀ with permanent pacemakers
- Pregnancy does not ↑ the risk of complications

⚠ ♀ with one of these devices should be referred to an obstetric anaesthetist and obstetrician prior to delivery to ensure magnet availability (to disable tachyarrhythmia detection if needed during a procedure where electromagnetic interference is likely, i.e. with diathermy at time of surgery).

▶ If a magnet is to be used, the response of the ICD/permanent pacemaker to the magnet should be tested before the procedure is started.

Cardiac transplantation

- May be performed for peripartum cardiomyopathy, but the majority of cases are performed for other reasons unrelated to pregnancy
- The heart is denervated, which has some important consequences:
  - ↑ resting heart rate which does not respond to exercise or hypovolaemia
  - May not experience ischaemic pain in the event of MI
  - Can contribute to ↑ BP (can be worse with calcineurin inhibitors)
- Transplant recipients have accelerated coronary artery disease (up to 40% 3 years after transplantation) so recipients have regular angiography
- In some transplant recipients, persistent sinoatrial node dysfunction can occur, requiring a permanent pacemaker
- In some countries the unintended pregnancy rate is up to 50% in ♀ with cardiac transplants, emphasizing the need for early discussion about contraception and pre-pregnancy counselling

Pre-pregnancy recommendations

- Consider the underlying reason for the transplant
- As with other solid organ transplants it is advisable to delay conception until ♀ has been in good health for a year (i.e. not necessarily 1 year post procedure)
- ↑ BP should be well controlled
- No episodes of rejection in the preceding year
- The immunosuppressive regimens for cardiac transplants use the same agents as for other solid organ transplants in pregnancy
- ► Avoid MMF and sirolimus

Management of a ♀ with cardiac transplant in pregnancy

- A high level of suspicion for ischaemia is required, in the absence of typical symptoms
- Pacemaker checked regularly
- Risks to the mother include:
  - Gestational hypertension or pre-eclampsia
  - Toxicity from immunosuppressive agents
  - Infection
- Risks to the fetus include:
  - IUGR
  - Preterm delivery
- It is not a contraindication to vaginal delivery
- There are no reports of recurrence of peripartum cardiomyopathy in a transplant patient, but the numbers of subsequent pregnancies are small

Acute pericarditis

Background

- Most common cause of pericardial disease in ♀ of childbearing age
- Inflammation of the pericardial sac around the heart
- Most commonly virally mediated (e.g. Coxsackie virus, echovirus, or adenovirus) or no cause is identified
- Poor prognostic factors include:
  - Associated fever
  - Subacute onset
  - Large effusion
  - Tamponade
  - Lack of response to therapy after 1 week

Clinical features

- Chest pain:
  - Typically central
  - May be pleuritic
  - ↑ on lying down
  - ↓ by sitting and leaning forward
- Examination may be normal
- Pericardial friction rub may be present but its absence does not exclude the diagnosis

Investigations

- ECG:
  - Concave ST elevation and PR depression are the classic changes
  - Later TWI can occur, which then normalizes after several weeks

Management of acute pericarditis in pregnancy

- NSAIDs up until 24–28 wks
- Colchicine:
  - Commonly viewed as contraindicated in pregnancy (although no adverse pregnancy outcomes have been shown in ♀ on colchicine for familial Mediterranean fever)
- Aspirin:
  - High doses advocated in non-pregnant individuals are higher than most feel appropriate to use in pregnancy
- Paracetamol
- Prednisolone:
  - Preferred treatment later in pregnancy

Diagnostic criteria for acute pericarditis

Inflammatory pericardial syndrome with at least 2 of:
- Pericardial chest pain
- Pericardial rub
- New widespread ST elevation or PR depression on ECG
- Pericardial effusion

Additional supporting findings
- Elevation of inflammatory markers (CRP, ESR, WBC count)
- Evidence of pericardial inflammation on imaging

⊃ ESC 2015 pericardial diseases guidelines: ℛ https://www.escardio.org/Guidelines/Clinical-Practice-Guidelines/Pericardial-Diseases-Guidelines-on-the-Diagnosis-and-Management-of

Constrictive pericarditis

- Results from pericardial scarring and restricts cardiac filling
- Typical echocardiographic features include:
  - Pericardial thickening
  - Moderate biatrial enlargement
  - Abnormal ventricular septal motion in diastole with inspiration

Causes

- Idiopathic
- Post-cardiac surgery
- TB
- Connective tissue disease:
  - Rheumatoid arthritis
  - Scleroderma
- Mediastinal irradiation
- Other causes:
  - Neoplasia
  - Drugs, e.g. amiodarone

Management of constrictive pericarditis in pregnancy

- Medical therapy including diuretics
- Consideration of pericardiectomy or pericardial window depending on severity and gestation

---

Pericardial effusion

Hydropericardium
- The most common pericardial abnormality in pregnancy, found in up to 40% of pregnant ♀ in the 3rd trimester
- Usually asymptomatic and occasionally is associated with non-specific ECG changes

Haemopericardium
- Following trauma or aortic dissection

Exudative
- Metastatic disease
- Acute pericarditis

Transudative
- Heart failure
- Nephrotic syndrome

⚠ Cardiac tamponade may be indicated by:
- ↑ JVP
- Pulsus paradoxus (drop in systolic BP >10 mmHg on inspiration)
- Kussmaul's sign (↑ JVP with inspiration)

Infective endocarditis

An infection of the cardiac endocardium, which commonly affects the native valves but can also affect mechanical valves and other intracardiac devices.

Causative organisms

- *Staphylococcus aureus*
- *Viridans streptococci*
- *Streptococcus bovis*
- Community-acquired enterococcus without a 1° focus
- HACEK organisms:
  - *Haemophilus aphrophilus*
  - *Aggregatibacter actinomycetemcomitans*
  - *Cardiobacterium hominis*
  - *Eikenella corrodens*
  - *Kingella kingae*

Treatment

- Medical
- Antibiotic treatment depending on the microorganism
- Long duration of parenteral antibiotic therapy
- Surgical management is undertaken for:
  - Infection not controlled with medical treatment
  - Valvular dysfunction causing cardiac failure
  - Prevention of embolic events if the vegetation is of large size

Complications

- Uncontrolled infection
- Heart failure from valvular dysfunction
- Embolic events such as ischaemic stroke or transient ischaemic attack, intracranial haemorrhage, and abscess formation
- Splenic complications such as infarcts or abscesses
- Myocarditis
- Conduction abnormalities
- Acute kidney injury
- Musculoskeletal symptoms such as arthralgia and myalgia

Management of infective endocarditis in pregnancy

- No role for antibiotic prophylaxis at delivery
- Rare but associated with maternal and fetal morbidity and mortality
- Pregnancy does not alter the diagnosis or management
- Imaging can be performed as required, with the exception of PET/ CT which would usually be avoided
- Any delivery decision is individualized, depending on the gestation, severity of infection, and the timing of any potential surgical intervention

Diagnosis of infective endocarditis

See Table 2.13 and Box 2.2.

Table 2.13 Diagnosis of infective endocarditis

Definite IE	
Clinical criteria	• 2 major criteria OR • 1 major and 3 minor criteria OR • 5 minor criteria
Pathological criteria	• Microorganisms on culture or histological examination of vegetation, embolized vegetation, or intracardiac abscess specimen • Pathological lesions; vegetation or intracardiac abscess confirmed on histology to show active endocarditis
Possible IE	
Clinical criteria	• 1 major and 1 minor criterion OR • 3 minor criteria
Not IE	
Clinical criteria	• Firm alternate diagnosis OR • Resolution of symptoms suggesting IE with antibiotic therapy for ≤4 days
Pathological criteria	• No pathological evidence of IE at surgery or postmortem, with antibiotic therapy for ≤4 days

Box 2.2 Criteria for diagnosing infective endocarditis

Major criteria
- Blood cultures positive for IE
- Microorganisms consistent with IE from 2 separate blood cultures
- Microorganisms consistent with IE from persistently positive blood cultures
- 2 or more positive blood cultures taken over 12 hrs apart
  OR
- All of 3 or majority of 4 blood cultures over at least an hour
- Single positive culture for *Coxiella burnetii* or phase 1 antibody titre >1:800

Imaging criteria
- Echocardiogram positive for IE
- Vegetation
- Abscess, pseudoaneurysm, intracardiac fistula
- Valvular perforation or aneurysm
- New partial dehiscence of prosthetic valve
- Abnormal activity around site of prosthetic valve as detected by PET/CT or radiolabelled leucocytes SPECT/CT
- Definite paravalvular lesions on cardiac CT

Minor criteria
- Predisposition such as underlying cardiac condition or IV drug use
- Fever >38°C
- Vascular phenomena including those on imaging only (major arterial emboli, septic pulmonary infarcts, infectious aneurysms, intracranial haemorrhage, conjunctival haemorrhage, Janeway lesions)
- Immunological phenomena including glomerulonephritis, Osler's nodes, Roth's spots, rheumatoid factor
- Microbiological evidence including positive cultures that do not meet the specifics of a major criterion, or serological evidence of infection with organism consistent with IE

➔ See ESC 2015 guidelines on infective endocarditis: https://www.escardio.org/Guidelines/Clinical-Practice-Guidelines/Infective-Endocarditis-Guidelines-on-Prevention-Diagnosis-and-Treatment-of

Cardiac arrest in pregnancy

⚠ Immediate maternal resuscitation is vital

Airway
Open airway with head tilt and chin lift; jaw thrust may be required.

Breathing and signs of life
Look listen and feel (with or without a pulse check) for 10 secs.

⚠ If no signs of life, not breathing or very abnormal breathing (agonal breaths), or no pulse—call for help/put out cardiac arrest call and start CPR.

> ### Resuscitation of the pregnant ♀
>
> ⚠ If >20 wks the uterus must be manually displaced or it will cause aortocaval compression:
> * This can be performed by cupping the abdomen in 1 or 2 hands and drawing the uterus towards the left of the mother (Fig. 2.16)
>
> ⚠ If CPR is required at >20 wks, resuscitative caesarean must be performed if there has been >4 mins of continuous CPR (i.e. 5 mins after the arrest):
> * This is for maternal resuscitation purposes, not for fetal reasons
> * It does not require transfer to theatre or GA
> * In a cardiac arrest the blood loss is minimal
> * If resuscitation is successful, the ♀ can be transferred to theatre for anaesthesia and closure afterwards
>
> ⚠ Additional causes to consider in pregnancy:
> * Underlying/undiagnosed cardiac disease
> * Amniotic fluid embolism
> * Toxins including high spinal block, local anaesthetic toxicity (consider treatment with Intralipid®)
>
> ▶▶ CPR and resuscitation is otherwise as per the Resuscitation Council (UK) adult life support guidelines (Fig. 2.17).

(a)

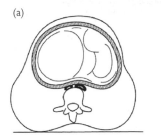

(b)

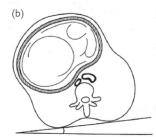

Fig. 2.16 Diagrams demonstrating how uterine displacement relieves aortocaval compression. Reproduced from Clyburn P. et al. (2008) *Obstetric Anaesthesia* Oxford University Press: Oxford with permission from Oxford University Press.

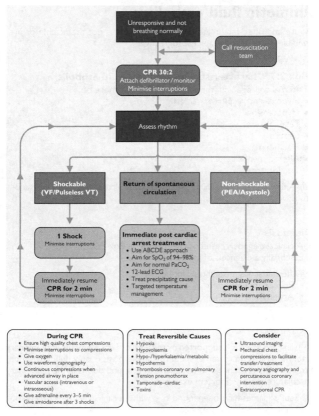

Fig. 2.17 Adult Advanced Life Support algorithm. Reproduced with the kind permission of the Resuscitation Council (UK).

Amniotic fluid embolism

A rare and often fatal maternal complication. It is not predictable or preventable, and is usually rapidly progressive.

> **Box 2.3 Characteristics of amniotic fluid embolism**
> Maternal collapse with the acute onset of 1 of more of:
> - Hypoxia and respiratory arrest
> - Hypotension
> - Fetal distress
> - Seizure
> - Haemorrhage
> - Altered mental status
> - Cardiac arrest
>
> ⚠ Although only 12% will present with DIC, virtually all cases will go on to develop it within 4 hrs.

Diagnosis
- A clinical diagnosis based on the features in Box 2.3.
- Essentially a diagnosis of exclusion

▶ Differential diagnosis should include:
  - Pulmonary embolism
  - Anaphylaxis
  - Sepsis
  - Eclampsia
  - MI

⚠ Clinical diagnosis is supported by retrieval of fetal elements in pulmonary artery aspirate and maternal sputum. The diagnosis is only definitively confirmed by the presence of fetal squamous cells and debris in the pulmonary vasculature at a postmortem examination.

☛ Fetal squames have been found in ♀ without clinical features of amniotic fluid embolism so their presence alone is not diagnostic.

Investigations
- Arterial blood gas
- Electrolytes including calcium and magnesium levels
- FBC (↑ WBC count)
- Coagulation profile
- CXR (pulmonary oedema)
- ECG (ischaemia and infarction)

Management of amniotic fluid embolus

- Rapid maternal resuscitation/CPR
- Admission to intensive care unit with senior input from obstetrics, anaesthetics, and haematology
- Treatment of complications:

Respiratory compromise

- O_2 to maintain saturation close to 100% (helps to prevent neurological impairment from hypoxia)
- Pulmonary artery wedge pressure monitoring may assist in the haemodynamic management (now infrequently required):
  - Blood aspirated via the catheter can be examined to aid with the diagnosis

Circulatory compromise

- Fluid resuscitation is imperative to counteract hypotension and haemodynamic instability
- For refractory hypotension, direct-acting vasopressors, such as phenylephrine, are required to optimize perfusion pressure
- Inotropic support may be needed

Coagulopathy

- DIC should be managed with the help of a haematologist
- Plasma exchange techniques may be helpful in clearing fibrin degradation products from the circulation.

Fetal distress

- If not yet delivered, continuous fetal monitoring is indicated

Respiratory

Respiratory changes in pregnancy

Oxygen consumption
- Progressive ↑ of O_2 consumption by 30–40%:
  - ↑ metabolic needs of fetus, placenta, and uterus
  - ↑ cardiac and respiratory work
- ↑ in CO_2 production mirrors O_2 consumption

Thoracic anatomy
- The rib cage circumference ↑ by 5–7 cm
- Capillary engorgement of the nasal and oropharyngeal mucosae and larynx starts in the 1st trimester and continues throughout pregnancy:
  - Nasal breathing may become more difficult
  - ↑ epistaxis
- Large airways dilate possibly enhanced by β-adrenergic activity induced by progesterone

Lung volume
- ↑ tidal volume (500–700 mL)
- Functional residual capacity ↓ from 20 wks onwards:
  - ↓ to 80% of the non-pregnant volume by term

Ventilation
- No change in respiratory rate
- Minute ventilation ↑ by 45% during pregnancy as a result of ↑ tidal volume
- Mild, chronic respiratory alkalosis
- Progesterone stimulates respiratory drive and sensitivity to CO_2
- Brainstem is sensitive to progesterone (protects fetus against acidosis):
  - ↑ PaO_2
  - Drives left shift of fetal Hb

Shortness of breath
- Also known as 'physiological breathlessness of pregnancy'
- Reported by 70% of healthy pregnant ♀ during activities of daily living
- Can start as early as the 1st trimester

👉 May be due to an ↑ awareness of the physiological hyperventilation of pregnancy or ↑ perception of discomfort due to an ↑ in minute ventilation.

Respiratory infections

Bacterial pneumonia

- Pregnancy does not alter the incidence of pneumonia
- Independent risk factors include asthma and antenatal steroids
- Pathogens are the same as in the non-pregnant population:
  - *Streptococcus pneumoniae*
  - *Haemophilus influenza*
  - *Moraxella catarrhalis*
  - *Staphylococcus aureus*
  - *Klebsiella pneumoniae*
  - 'Atypical organisms' can include *Mycoplasma pneumoniae* and *Legionella pneumoniae*

Viral pneumonia

- Most common causes are influenza and varicella infection
- Can be more severe than in the non-pregnant population

Influenza

➡ See also p. 459 and Table 3.1.
- Influenza in pregnancy can be more severe than in non-pregnant individuals and has an associated ↑ mortality
- Advise all pregnant ♀ to receive the influenza vaccination
- Antiviral treatment may be indicated, see local guidelines for up-to-date advice
- Oseltamivir and zanamivir can be used in pregnancy if required

Table 3.1 H1N1 influenza and pregnancy

Seasonal	Swine flu
More severe in elderly	More severe in young
Rarely cause diarrhoea and vomiting	Often causes diarrhoea and vomiting
Infectious	Very infectious
↑ severity in pregnancy	

Varicella

- ➡ See also p. 464.
- Pneumonitis occurs in 10% of ♀ who develop 1° varicella infection in pregnancy:
  - Associated with significant mortality, especially in the 3rd trimester
  - Admission is indicated if ♀ develop respiratory symptoms in the presence of varicella infection
- Vaccination in pregnancy is not advised

➡ RCOG (2015). Chickenpox in pregnancy (green-top guideline no. 13): ⌘ https://www.rcog.org.uk/en/guidelines-research-services/guidelines/gtg13/

Management of respiratory infections in pregnancy
- Tools to assess severity, e.g. CURB65 should not be used
- Titrate O_2 to obtain oxygen saturation of 94–98%
- IV fluids as needed
- Bloods including:
  - Blood cultures
  - FBC
  - Renal function
  - LFTs
  - CRP
- Antibiotics:
  - Same as in non-pregnant population, as per BTS guidelines for CAP, i.e. penicillin-based antibiotic such as amoxicillin ± macrolide
  - Doxycycline, ciprofloxacin, and levofloxacin should be avoided
- VTE prophylaxis
- CXR (as per BTS guidelines) advised for anyone:
  - Admitted to hospital with suspected CAP
  - Where diagnosis is in doubt
  - With unsatisfactory response to treatment for suspected CAP
  - Where an underlying condition such as malignancy is possible

▶ Sputum culture is only indicated in those with underlying lung disease where colonization with organisms such as *Pseudomonas* or *Burkholderia* is a possibility and would alter management if detected (e.g. bronchiectasis, CF).

Fetal considerations
- Monitoring should be provided appropriate to gestational age
- Pneumonia associated with ↑ risk of:
  - Preterm delivery
  - Low birthweight

Rib fracture in pregnancy
- Reported in pregnancy due to bouts of coughing or minimal trauma, thought to be due to opposing muscular forces on the ribs accentuated by changes in thoracic shape from ↑ gravid uterus
- Pain can be severe
- Typical pain does not require radiological confirmation

Treatment
- Analgesia

つ BTS (2009). Guidelines for CAP: ℗ https://www.brit-thoracic.org.uk/standards-of-care/guidelines/bts-guidelines-for-the-management-of-community-acquired-pneumonia-in-adults-update-2009/

Tuberculosis

Background

- *Mycobacterium tuberculosis* is an acid-fast bacillus spread by respiratory droplet transmission
- The organism may be contained within lymph nodes with the immune response generating in granuloma formation
- 1° infection may settle, reactivating years later
- Disseminated disease results if 1° infection is not restricted to the lymph nodes
- ↑ in UK, mostly immunosuppressed ♀ or those born outside the UK
- TB is uncommon in pregnancy but this may reflect under-diagnosis (reluctance to perform imaging or insidious onset of symptoms)
- Resistant strains of TB are ↑, including multidrug-resistant TB (MDR-TB) and extensively drug-resistant TB (XDR-TB)

Clinical features

- Persistent respiratory symptoms (e.g. cough and haemoptysis)
- Underlying systemic features such as weight loss and night sweats
- Extrapulmonary manifestations include:
  - Pericarditis
  - Meningitis
  - Lymphadenitis
  - Abdominal involvement (bowel or peritoneum)

Diagnosis

- DNA PCR if available can be processed within hours
- Sputum microscopy (Ziehl–Nielsen stain) and prolonged culture:
  - Ideally 3 samples at least 8 hrs apart (preferably early morning)
- CXR can be normal even in sputum culture-positive infection
- Biopsy of extrapulmonary site
- Lumbar puncture if tuberculous meningitis suspected
- Bronchoscopy (if no sputum production and no extrapulmonary sites amenable to biopsy) can be performed, but the merits of this vs empirical treatment in later pregnancy should be discussed with a bronchoscopist

Fetal issues

- Untreated TB is associated with fetal growth restriction
- Treated disease is not associated with adverse outcomes
- Transplacental transfer is very rare but blood-borne or amniotic fluid-mediated infection can occur
- Neonatal infection is mostly from exposure to an infected contact
- Isolation is only required if the mother is sputum positive
- After active TB in the neonate is excluded, the baby should be given 6 months of isoniazid preventative treatment then BCG vaccination
- Pyridoxine supplementation should be given to neonates if they are receiving isoniazid, or if the mother is breastfeeding on isoniazid

Who to test for latent TB?
- Suspected recent contact
- Immunosuppression:
  - HIV infection
  - Use of immunosuppressive medication
- Suspicion of active TB
- Recent immigrant, i.e. within 5 years
- Healthcare worker (who has not been screened previously)

Testing for latent TB

1. Tuberculin skin test (TST, also known as Mantoux test)
- Injection of tuberculin purified protein derivative into the inner surface of the forearm to produce a wheal

🌢 Incorrect administration and interpretation yields false results

- False positives can result from:
  - Previous BCG vaccination
  - Non-tuberculous *Mycobacterium* infection
- False negatives can result from:
  - Recent TB infection (within 8–10 wks of exposure)
  - Recent live virus vaccination
  - Some viral illnesses such as measles, overwhelming TB, and cutaneous anergy
  - Only contraindication is previous reaction to a previous TST

2. Interferon-γ release assays (IGRAs)
- Examples include QuantiFERON®-TB Gold and T-SPOT®
- Interferon-γ released from white cells from a person infected with TB when mixed with antigens derived from *M. tuberculosis*
- BCG vaccination does not cause a false-positive result
- Live vaccines may affect these results
- Can be used in place of TST

⊃ WHO. Guidelines on TB: ॐ www.who.int/tb/publications/9789241547833/en/

⊃ UK government guidelines: ॐ www.gov.uk/government/collections/tuberculosis-and-other-mycobacterial-diseases-diagnosis-screening-management-and-data

Treatment of tuberculosis

Pregnancy

The first-line regimen in the non-pregnant setting includes:
- Rifampicin and isoniazid for 6 months
- Ethambutol and pyrazinamide also for the 1st 2 months

See Table 3.2.

Table 3.2 Treatments for TB in pregnancy

Drug	Pregnancy	Notes
Rifampicin	Safe for use in pregnancy	• Liver enzyme inducer • Neonatal haemorrhage has been reported after rifampicin exposure late in pregnancy • PO vitamin K supplementation in the 4 wks before delivery recommended
Isoniazid	Safe for use in pregnancy	• Pyridoxine deficiency (vitamin B_6) can cause peripheral neuropathy • Pyridoxine supplementation (10–25 mg per day) alongside isoniazid is advised • ↑ risk of isoniazid-related hepatitis so regular monitoring of liver function is important
Ethambutol	Safe for use in pregnancy	• Can be used as normal
Pyrazinamide	Safe for use in pregnancy	• Can be used as normal
Streptomycin	Unsafe for use in pregnancy	• Uncommon TB treatment • Causes damage in fetal VIII cranial nerve in ≤10% exposed fetuses

Bronchiectasis

Background
- Localized airway damage
- Can result from recurrent childhood infections
- In ♀ of childbearing age, the most common cause is CF

Management of bronchiectasis in pregnancy

Respiratory
- Lung function if not done pre-pregnancy to assess severity
- Continue chest physiotherapy
- Appropriate and timely treatment of respiratory infections:
  ⚠ Avoid tetracyclines
- Sputum cultures as needed
- Monitor oxygenation, and watch for hypoxia especially in the 3rd trimester

Cardiological
- Echocardiography to look for pulmonary hypertension

Cystic fibrosis

Background

- A multisystem condition, which can affect the:
  - Lungs
  - GI tract
  - Pancreas
  - Liver
  - Reproductive organs
- A common autosomal recessive condition (Table 3.3):
  - Gene frequency of about 1 in 25
  - Most common mutation is F508del (occurs in >88% of CF)
  - Mutations result in abnormal folding and transport of the CF transmembrane conductance regulation (CFTR) chloride channel
- ♂ are often infertile from congenital absence of the vas deferens
- ♀ are often subfertile due to:
  - Anovulation
  - Abnormal cervical mucus
  - Nutritional issues → ↓ BMI
- Improvements in treatment of respiratory infections and maintenance of good pulmonary function means more ♀ are reaching childbearing age and becoming pregnant

Options for high-risk couples include:
- Preimplantation genetic diagnosis
- Prenatal diagnostic testing

Table 3.3 Inheritance pattern if the mother carries CF

Father's CF status	Risk of having an affected child
Unknown	1 in 50
Negative	1 in 500
Carrier	1 in 2

Predictors of poor maternal or fetal outcome in CF

- Hypoxaemia
- Cyanosis
- Pulmonary hypertension
- Poor pre-pregnancy lung function (FEV_1 <50% predicted)
- Pancreatic insufficiency (especially diabetes)
- Malnutrition
- Lung colonization with *Burkholderia cepacia*

MDT management of CF in pregnancy

Respiratory care
- Lung function if not done pre-pregnancy to assess severity
- Continue chest physiotherapy
- Appropriate and timely treatment of respiratory infections (avoid tetracyclines)
- Sputum cultures if infection suspected as these may aid antibiotic choice
- Monitor oxygenation, and watch for hypoxia especially in the 3rd trimester

Cardiological
- Echocardiography to look for pulmonary hypertension

Gastrointestinal
- Vitamin supplementation as at risk of malabsorption
- Monitor liver function for signs of intrahepatic cholestasis of pregnancy
- Appropriate calorie intake
- Pancreatic enzyme supplementation if needed

Endocrine
- Regular assessment of blood glucose:
  - Treatment of hyperglycaemia as needed
  - 8% have pre-existing DM
  - 20% have diabetes by term

Fetal
- Growth scans due to fetal risks:
  - IUGR due to maternal hypoxaemia
  - Preterm labour

Delivery
- Not an indication for a caesarean section
- Aim for a vaginal delivery but consider limitation of the 2nd stage (to ↓ the risk of pneumothorax from repeated Valsalva)
- Avoid general anaesthesia if possible

Postnatal
- No contraindication to breastfeeding, but beneficial to optimize nutrition given the metabolic demands of breastfeeding

Restrictive lung disease

Causes
- Chest wall deformity:
  - Kyphoscoliosis
  - Pectus excavatum
- Neuromuscular weakness:
  - Motor neurone disease
  - Muscular dystrophy
  - Spinal-muscular atrophy
- Morbid obesity
- Interstitial lung disease

Tests
See Table 3.4.

Table 3.4 Lung function test results for restrictive lung diseases

Causes	Lung function results
Chest wall deformity	Extrapulmonary restrictive picture
Neuromuscular weakness	Extrapulmonary restrictive picture
Interstitial lung disease	Intrapulmonary restrictive picture

Management of women with chest wall and neuromuscular abnormalities in pregnancy
- ♀ with these abnormalities can do well in pregnancy
- Oxygen saturations should be regularly monitored at rest and on exertion and supplementary oxygen arranged if needed
- Vigilance for type 2 respiratory failure is required:
  - May require non-invasive positive-pressure ventilation

Interstitial lung disease

Background

- Collective term for a large number of pulmonary conditions that feature inflammation of the interstitium which consists of:
  - Alveolar epithelium
  - Perivascular and perilymphatic tissue
  - Pulmonary capillary endothelium
  - Basement membrane

Causes

See Table 3.4.

Table 3.5 Causes of interstitial lung disease

Known cause	
Drugs	• Antibiotics (e.g. minocycline, nitrofurantoin)
	• Chemotherapeutic agents, (e.g. methotrexate, paclitaxel)
	• Anti-arrhythmics (e.g. amiodarone)
Autoimmune disease	• Rheumatoid arthritis
	• Scleroderma
Granulomatous	
Sarcoidosis	
Other forms	
Lymphangioleiomyomatosis	
Pulmonary Langerhans cell histiocytosis	
Idiopathic interstitial pneumonia	
Chronic fibrosing	• Idiopathic pulmonary fibrosis
	• Idiopathic non-specific interstitial pneumonia
Acute or subacute fibrosing	• Cryptogenic organizing pneumonia
	• Acute interstitial pneumonia
Smoking-related	• Respiratory bronchiolitis interstitial lung disease
	• Desquamatory interstitial pneumonia

Management of interstitial lung disease in pregnancy
- Consideration of underlying cause, e.g. connective tissue disease
- Lung function tests are key for assessment of severity
- ♀ with an FVC ≥1 L should do well in pregnancy:
  - ♀ with lower values can also do well
- Serial transfer factor measurement can be used to assess progression (must be corrected for Hb)
- Regular monitoring of O_2 saturation:
  - May need supplementary O_2 later in pregnancy
- Arterial blood gas if respiratory failure is suspected
- Hb monitoring:
  - Hypoxia may result in polycythaemia (can cause hyperviscosity)
- Assessment for pulmonary hypertension (echocardiography ± right heart catheterization)
- Consider VTE prophylaxis if respiratory symptoms limit mobility

Sarcoidosis

Background

This is a multisystem condition featuring non-caseating granuloma formation.

Clinical features

Respiratory

- 90% of patients have lung involvement, which can include bilateral hilar lymphadenopathy, pulmonary infiltrates, ± lung fibrosis

Extrapulmonary

- There are many extrapulmonary manifestations of sarcoid (Table 3.6)

Management of sarcoidosis in pregnancy

- Remains uncommon in pregnancy
- Improves in many ♀
- Corticosteroids:
  - After exclusion of TB and other differential diagnoses
  - If disease is refractory to corticosteroids, other immunosuppressive agents such as azathioprine can be used
- Treatment of the extrapulmonary manifestations as appropriate
- Cardiac assessment with ECG and echocardiography
- Assessment of bone health including:
  - Vitamin D level and appropriate replacement; monitor calcium during vitamin D replacement
  - DXA scan pre or post pregnancy
- Case series have reported an ↑ incidence of VTE compared to the general population ∴ consider other risk factors ± LMWH
- ↑ risk of preterm delivery and pre-eclampsia
- Postpartum flares are common

Table 3.6 Examples of extrapulmonary manifestations of sarcoidosis

Cardiac (up to 50%)	• Heart block and arrhythmias • Heart failure • Pericardial disease • Sudden cardiac death
Skin	• Erythema nodosum[a] • Subcutaneous nodules • Lupus pernio
Eyes	• Uveitis[b] • Keratoconjunctivitis secca • Eyelid or conjunctival granulomas
Renal	• Calcium deposition and resultant renal failure • Sarcoid interstitial nephritis • Nephrogenic diabetes insipidus • Membranous glomerulonephritis
Lymph notes	• Peripheral lymphadenopathy
Endocrine	• Hypothalamic and pituitary disturbances • Thyroid abnormalities • Central diabetes insipidus
Liver	• Liver granulomas are usually asymptomatic and are not diagnostic when occurring in isolation • Hepatomegaly (20%) • Splenomegaly (less common)
Gastrointestinal	• Rare but any part of GI tract can be involved
Neurological	• Cranial mononeuropathy, e.g. facial nerve palsy[b] • Neurosarcoid • Peripheral neuropathy, e.g. mononeuritis multiplex
Musculoskeletal	• Acute polyarthritis • Migratory polyarthralgia[a]
Electrolytes	• Hypercalcaemia

[a] Lofgren syndrome is the name given to the combination of erythema nodosum, bilateral hilar lymphadenopathy, migratory polyarthralgia, and fever.

[b] Heerfordt's syndrome is an unusual presentation of sarcoid, which features parotid enlargement, anterior uveitis, facial nerve palsy, and fever ('uveoparotid fever').

Pulmonary lymphangioleiomyomatosis

Background
- A rare disorder which features abnormal smooth muscle proliferation and cyst formation
- 1° affects the lungs and lymphatics
- More common ♀ > ♂, particularly in ♀ of childbearing age
- More common in ♀ with the tuberous sclerosis complex
- ♀ can also develop meningiomas and angiomyolipomas:
  - Up to 50% develop angiomyolipomas
- Exacerbated by exogenous oestrogen:
  - Some evidence of a hormonal contribution to development and progression
- Progressive condition
- ⚕ Sirolimus can be used outside pregnancy to slow progression
- Lung transplantation can be considered
- Pulmonary complications include:
  - Pneumothorax
  - Chylothorax
  - Chyloperitoneum

Investigations

Chest radiography
- Can be normal, but may show:
  - Pneumothorax
  - Pleural effusion
  - Interstitial thickening

High-resolution CT
- May be required to make a diagnosis in ♀ not known to have tuberous sclerosis

Lung function tests
- Can show an obstructive picture and a low transfer factor

Management of lymphangioleiomyomatosis in pregnancy
- Complications ↑ when ♀ are pregnant (high rate of pneumothorax reported)
- ♀ should be counselled about risk of accelerated progression in pregnancy and the risk of complications and worsening symptoms

Langerhans cell histiocytosis

Background

Historically, terms such as histiocytosis X were used but now LCH is the preferred term as the abnormal cells resemble Langerhans cells (specialized dendritic cells in the skin and mucosa).

Clinical features

- Most commonly causes focal osteolytic bone lesions with histiocytes visible on biopsy
- Similar histiocytic invasion can be seen in almost all other organs (with the exceptions being the heart and kidney)
- Lung involvement is seen in about 10% of individuals with LCH

Management of LCH in pregnancy

- It appears from small series that pregnancy is generally tolerated well in ♀ with pulmonary LCH
- Important to encourage smoking cessation in all individuals with pulmonary LCH
- Baseline spirometry is useful in case symptoms deteriorate in which case they can be repeated and compared to baseline measurements

Asthma

Background
- Common condition in ♀ of childbearing of age
- Exacerbations seen in up to 45% of pregnant ♀ with asthma
- Meta-analysis shows:
  - 1/3 of pregnant ♀ experience a worsening of symptoms
  - 1/3 improve
  - 1/3 experience no change

Clinical features
- Breathlessness and wheezing with triggers including:
  - Cold exposure
  - Exertion
  - Airborne allergens
- A cough which is often worse at night
- Examination may be normal
- Peak flow can show a diurnal variation (this does not change in pregnancy)
- The features of acute asthma are summarised in Table 3.7.

Eosinophilic asthma
- Eosinophilic, or inflammation-predominant asthma may warrant different treatment to non-eosinophilic, or symptom-predominant asthma

💣 Techniques such as exhaled nitric oxide are being used to guide treatment intervention such as inhaled corticosteroids in non-pregnant individuals. They are likely to be useful in pregnant ♀ also and are ↑ being performed in pregnancy.

Asthma in pregnancy
- If well controlled, not associated with ↑ risk of adverse outcomes
- Poorly controlled or frequent exacerbations are associated with:
  - IUGR and low birthweight
  - Preterm birth
  - Pre-eclampsia
  - Neonatal hypoxia
- ♀ with severe asthma are more likely to experience ↑ in symptoms than those with mild asthma
- Wks 24–36 appear in some studies to be when symptoms are worst
- Aspirin for pre-eclampsia risk ↓ can be used unless there is a history of aspirin sensitivity

Table 3.7 Assessing severity of acute asthma

Moderate acute asthma	• ↑ symptoms • PEF >50–75% best or predicted • No features of acute severe asthma	

Acute severe asthma	• Any one of:
	  • PEF 33–50% best or predicted
	  • Respiratory rate ≥25/min
	  • Heart rate ≥110/min
	  • Inability to complete sentences in 1 breath	

Life-threatening asthma	Any of the following in a ♀ with severe asthma	
	Clinical signs	Measurements
	• Altered conscious level	• PEF <33% best or predicted
	• Exhaustion	• SpO₂ <92%
	• Arrhythmia	• PaO₂ <8 kPa
	• Hypotension	• 'Normal' PaCO₂ (4.6–6.0 kPa)*
	• Cyanosis	
	• Silent chest	
	• Poor respiratory effort	
Near-fatal asthma	Raised PaCO₂ and/or requiring mechanical intubation with raised inflation pressures	

Reproduced from the British Thoracic Society and Scottish Intercollegiate Guidelines Network (2016) *SIGN 153: British guideline on the management of asthma: a national clinical guideline*: Edinburgh with kind permission.

* This is the non-pregnant reference range, we advise using lower reference range in pregnancy

Sub-optimally controlled asthma

Causes of deterioration in pregnancy

- Non-compliance with medications
- Gastro-oesophageal reflux (irritation of bronchi)
- Pregnancy rhinitis
- Aspirin use

Management

Sub-optimally controlled asthma: see Table 3.8.
Acute exacerbation: see Table 3.9.

Table 3.8 Management of sub-optimally controlled asthma

Always an option	40 mg prednisolone for 5–10 days to get quick control[a]
Step 1	↑ dose of inhaled corticosteroid
Step 2	Add in long-acting β agonist or change to combination inhaler, e.g. Fostair® (beclometasone and formoterol)
Step 3	Add in additional therapy • Inhaled long-acting muscarinic antagonists, e.g. ipratropium or tiotropium • Leukotriene receptor antagonist, e.g. montelukast (no reports of fetal effects so should not be withheld in pregnancy if required for asthma control) • Aminophylline—measurement of levels is advised due to ↓ in protein binding in pregnancy, which may result in a lower therapeutic target range • Monoclonal anti-IgE antibody omalizumab is a treatment for moderate to severe persistent allergic asthma 🔊 Safety data from a registry of 191 ♀ exposed in pregnancy showed no ↑ in adverse fetal outcomes

[a] Stress dose steroids at delivery should be considered depending on dose and duration of steroid treatment used in pregnancy.

Management of asthma at delivery

- Exacerbations are relatively rare
- Prostaglandin F2α (carboprost) can cause bronchospasm, so should be used with caution
  🔊 Not absolutely contraindicated as may be life-saving in PPH which has not responded to ergometrine or oxytocin
- Prostaglandin E2 (dinoprostone) and prostaglandin E1 (misoprostol) do not cause bronchoconstriction and can be used as normal in ♀ with asthma
  🔊 Ergometrine can rarely cause bronchospasm but this should not prevent the routine use of Syntometrine® after delivery
- Consider stress-dose steroids
- No contraindications to breastfeeding
- Encourage smoke/dust/animal-free environment

Table 3.9 Treatment of acute exacerbation of asthma or COPD

Immediate treatment	• Maintain O_2 saturations of 94–98% (unless COPD present with evidence of CO_2 retention, in which case O_2 saturation target is 88–92%) • Salbutamol 2.5–5 mg nebulizers (no maximum dose) • Ipratropium bromide 500 mcg nebulizers (max. QDS) • Prednisolone 40 mg orally (or 100–200 mg hydrocortisone IV if unable to take oral medication) • Gestation-appropriate fetal monitoring

Investigations	• CXR
	• Bloods including:
	  • FBC
	  • Renal function
	  • LFTs
	  • CRP
	  • Blood cultures if features of infection
	• Flu swab (seasonal)
	• Arterial blood gas

Additional therapy	• Antibiotics and antivirals depending on clinical history and radiological findings • Magnesium sulfate 2 g IV over 15–30 mins (asthma only) • IV aminophylline (without loading dose if on regular oral therapy)
Treatment escalation	• Refer to intensive care for consideration of respiratory support (nasal high-flow O_2, non-invasive ventilation, or mechanical ventilation) • Senior obstetric input, depending on gestation, about consideration of delivery to aid maternal treatment, if ventilatory support being considered

➔ BTS/SIGN. Asthma guideline: https://www.brit-thoracic.org.uk/standards-of-care/guidelines/btssign-british-guideline-on-the-management-of-asthma/

Chronic obstructive pulmonary disease

Background

- COPD is most commonly the result of smoking in the older population
- Can occur in younger people as the result of inherited defects such as $\alpha 1$ anti-trypsin deficiency
- Patients with COPD lack the hyper-reactivity of the airways seen in patients with asthma but the treatment principles are similar

Management of COPD in pregnancy

- Hypoxaemia is an important determinant of a successful pregnancy outcome so oxygenation should be optimized
- Optimize medical treatment, by continuing:
  - Bronchodilators
  - Inhaled corticosteroids
  - Systemic corticosteroids
  - Mucolytics, e.g. carbocisteine
- Echocardiogram to assess for pulmonary hypertension
- Consider underlying cause and inheritance, e.g. $\alpha 1$ antitrypsin deficiency

Oxygen administration in COPD

⚠ Patients with COPD are at risk of hypercapnia with excessive O_2 administration

- This can also occur in:
  - Severe asthma
  - Patients with obesity hypoventilation
  - Other chronic respiratory conditions

⚠ Patients with COPD optimize their oxygenation by hypoxic vasoconstriction in under-perfused areas of lung, to ↓ V/Q mismatch. O_2 administration ↓ this vasoconstriction and ↑ the mismatch.

⚠ However, in an emergency setting, O_2 administration to a hypoxic, unwell ♀ should never be withheld for fear of hypercapnic respiratory failure.

Lung function tests: spirometry

- Forced expiratory volume in 1 second (FEV_1):
  - Volume of air expired in the 1st second of a forced expiration
- Forced vital capacity (FVC):
  - Total volume exhaled from a maximal inspiration
- FEV_1/FVC ratio:
  - Obstructive picture (ratio <0.7)
  - Restrictive picture (ratio >0.7)

Spirometry results in obstructive lung disease

See Fig. 3.1.
- FEV_1 significantly ↓
- FVC normal or ↓
- FEV_1/FVC <0.7

Causes
- COPD
- Asthma
- Large airway obstruction
- Bronchiectasis
- Obliterative bronchiolitis

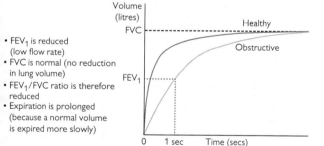

- FEV_1 is reduced (low flow rate)
- FVC is normal (no reduction in lung volume)
- FEV_1/FVC ratio is therefore reduced
- Expiration is prolonged (because a normal volume is expired more slowly)

Fig. 3.1 Spirometry results in obstructive lung disease. Reproduced from Kon O. M. et al. (2008) *Chronic Obstructive Pulmonary Disease* Oxford University Press: Oxford with permission from Oxford University Press.

Spirometry results in restrictive lung disease

- ↓ FEV$_1$
- ↓ FVC
- FEV$_1$/FVC same or >0.7

Causes
- Chest wall deformity:
  - Kyphoscoliosis
  - Pectus excavatum
- Neuromuscular weakness:
  - Motor neurone disease
  - Muscular dystrophy
  - Spinal-muscular atrophy
- Obesity
- Interstitial lung disease

Spirometry in pregnancy

- Can be performed as normal

💣 In ♀ with pre-eclampsia, there is a risk of vascular injury with forced exertion so spirometry is not advised in the presence of significant hypertension, however a relaxed VC measurement can be performed.

Vital capacity monitoring

- Measurement of VC is important in a number of emergency settings where neuromuscular weakness may occur, e.g. Guillain–Barré syndrome or an acute exacerbation of myasthenia gravis
- In these conditions, formal lung function testing may not be possible due to the severity of the illness and the urgency of the test
- Portable VC monitors are now commonplace, and mean that a VC measurement can be obtained in the emergency setting (and should be performed erect and supine)
- Regular measurements are usually advisable so appropriately trained staff are required
- Predicted value is 60–70 mL/kg, and is considered abnormal if ≤80% of predicted

⚠ These should not be confused with peak flow meters and peak flow measurement is **not** a substitute for VC measurement.

Other lung function tests

Flow/volume loop
- For diagnosis of large airway obstruction or neuromuscular weakness

Mouth pressures
- For diagnosis of inspiratory muscle weakness

Lung function tests: static lung volumes

See Fig. 3.2 and Table 3.10.
- Total lung capacity (TLC):
  - Total volume of air in lungs at end of maximal inspiration
- Residual volume (RV):
  - Volume of air left in the lungs at the end of maximal expiration
- Functional residual capacity (FRC):
  - Volume of air remaining in the lungs at the end of tidal expiration

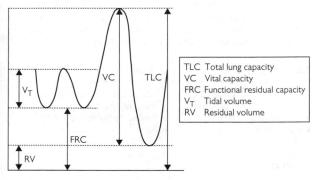

TLC	Total lung capacity
VC	Vital capacity
FRC	Functional residual capacity
V_T	Tidal volume
RV	Residual volume

Fig. 3.2 Lung volumes and capacities. Reproduced from Singer and Webb (2009) *Oxford Handbook of Critical Care* 3rd Ed. Oxford University Press: Oxford with permission from Oxford University Press.

Table 3.10 Static lung volume result interpretation

Result	Interpretation
↓ TLC	• Restrictive defect
↑ TLC	• COPD
	• Transient during asthma exacerbation
↑ RV	• Airways disease
	• Respiratory muscle weakness
↑ FRC	• COPD
↓ FRC	• Fibrotic lung disease (intrapulmonary)
	• Obesity (extrapulmonary)

Lung function tests: diffusion capacity

- Transfer capacity of the lungs for carbon monoxide (TLCO) is the same as diffusion factor for carbon monoxide (DLCO) and reflects the ability to transfer gas from inspired air into circulating haemoglobin
- Transfer coefficient (KCO):
  - Diffusing capacity corrected for lung volume
- Interpretation (Table 3.11)

Diffusion capacity in pregnancy

The levels of carbon monoxide used are very small and of no significant risk to mother or fetus, so these can be performed as normal if required.

△ Predicted DLCO corrects for Hb, so care should be taken to ensure a Hb level from pregnancy is used, otherwise there may be an apparent deterioration in DLCO compared to predicted values.-

Table 3.11 Interpreting patterns of diffusion capacity

Capacity results	Location of defect	Causes
• ↓ TLC • ↓ TLCO • ↓ or normal KCO	Intrapulmonary restrictive defect	• Interstitial lung disease • Cardiac, e.g. pulmonary oedema • Pulmonary vascular disease
• ↑ TLC • ↓ TLCO • ↓ KCO		• Emphysema
• ↓ TLCO • ↑ KCO	Extrapulmonary restrictive defect	• Neuromuscular weakness • Obesity • Pleural disease, e.g. effusion • Skeletal, e.g. ankylosing spondylitis, kyphoscoliosis
• normal or ↑ TLCO • ↑ KCO		• Asthma • Pulmonary haemorrhage, e.g. vasculitis

Respiratory failure: type 1

Definition
Hypoxaemia with normal or ↓ partial pressure of carbon dioxide

Mechanism
- Ongoing perfusion of lung areas that are unable to contribute to effective gas exchange
- Shunting of deoxygenated blood results and causes hypoxaemia that cannot be completely corrected with supplementary oxygen

Causes
- Pneumonia (bacterial, viral, fungal)
- Aspiration pneumonitis
- Pulmonary embolism
- Amniotic fluid embolism
- Transfusion-related lung disease
- Anaphylaxis
- Negative pressure or neurogenic pulmonary oedema
- Drug-related pneumonitis (cocaine, narcotics, nitrofurantoin)
- Sepsis
- Asthma exacerbation

Management of type 1 respiratory failure in pregnancy
⚠ Optimize oxygenation:
- Bedside O_2 administration:
  - Nasal cannulae: provide low and variable levels of oxygen
  - Face mask: provides more O_2 than nasal cannulae
  - Non-rebreathe bag and mask
  - Nasal high-flow O_2
- Non-invasive ventilatory support:
  - Continuous positive airway pressure ventilation
- Tracheal intubation and mechanical ventilation
- Other measures include:
  - High-frequency oscillatory ventilation
  - Prone ventilation
  - Inhaled nitrous oxide can be tried if hypoxaemia persists despite intubation and administration of 100% O_2

⚠ However, if invasive ventilation or other measures are being considered for worsening respiratory function, delivery may be indicated both to aid maternal ventilation and ↓ risk to the fetus of prolonged hypoxia

⚠ Extracorporeal lung support may be used in extreme cases, e.g. extracorporeal membrane oxygenation (ECMO), but this is only available in specialist centres and entails other risks such as thrombosis, haemolysis, and vascular injury (from the very large cannulae required).

➔ Pacheco LD, Saada GR, Hankins GDV. Extracorporeal membrane oxygenation (ECMO) during pregnancy and postpartum. Semin Perinatol 2018;42:21–5.

Acute respiratory distress syndrome

Definition
Acute hypoxaemic respiratory failure is characterized by bilateral diffuse alveolar damage not fully explained by either cardiogenic pulmonary oedema or fluid overload.

- Effectively a final common pathway for a range of pathological processes including:
  - Sepsis
  - Massive haemorrhage
  - Amniotic fluid embolism
  - Aspiration
- The new Berlin definition of the condition divides ARDS on the basis of the ratio of arterial partial pressure of oxygen (PaO_2) to FiO_2 (P/F ratio):
  - Mild (200 < P/F ≤300)
  - Moderate (100 < P/F ≤200)
  - Severe (P/F ≤100)

🔥 Continuous positive airway pressure may be tried as a strategy for avoiding intubation in ARDS that is not severe, but it is important not to delay intubation when this is clearly indicated.

⚠ Avoid volume overload that would exacerbate capillary leak.

Endotracheal intubation in pregnancy
⚠ Failure rate is 10× that occurring in non-pregnant ♀
- Oedema of the upper airways can distort the anatomy, thus restricting the view on direct laryngoscopy
- High risk of aspiration even if fasted due to:
  - Delayed gastric emptying
  - Lower oesophageal sphincter incompetence
⚠ Effective cricoid pressure is essential
- Hypoxaemia develops more rapidly in pregnant ♀
- Desaturation may quickly follow induction of anaesthesia and muscle relaxation

Respiratory failure: type 2

Definition
Hypoxaemia with ↑ partial pressure of carbon dioxide.

Mechanism
- Results from processes which ↓ the amount of air that is breathed in and out
- $PaCO_2$ is inversely related to minute ventilation:
  - Minute ventilation = respiratory rate × tidal volume
  - If ↓ respiratory rate or tidal volume, $PaCO_2$ will ↑

Causes
- Chronic obstructive airways disease
- Respiratory muscle weakness
- Obesity
- Neurological disorders:
  - Motor neurone disease
  - Diaphragmatic weakness
- Severe metabolic acidosis
- Exhaustion

Management
- Caution with high inspired O_2 concentrations as can worsen the respiratory suppression
- Non-invasive positive-pressure ventilation
- Tracheal intubation and mechanical ventilation

Obstructive sleep apnoea
- Sleep-disordered breathing (often but not exclusively related to obesity)
- ↑ problem in the obstetric population
- In non-pregnant adults, obstructive sleep apnoea is associated with:
  - Hypertension
  - Insulin resistance
  - ↑ cardiovascular risk
- In pregnancy, there is ↑ concern regarding possible risks from maternal apnoeic episodes, including:
  - Pre-eclampsia
  - Hypertension
  - Diabetes

⚠ Continuous positive airway pressure may be required in pregnancy when obstructive sleep apnoea complicates an acute respiratory illness such as pneumonia, or limits extubation following general anaesthesia or a period of mechanical ventilation.

Pleural disease

Pleural effusion

Background

This is an accumulation of fluid in the pleural space

- Most commonly is small in size and occurs in the setting of other illness such as infection
- Significant fluid accumulation can occur, resulting in respiratory compromise and necessitating urgent intervention

Causes

- Infection
- Malignancy
- Cardiac failure
- Nephrotic syndrome

Pregnancy-specific causes

- Pre-eclampsia
- Ovarian hyperstimulation
- Oesophageal perforation from hyperemesis

Investigations for a pleural effusion

- Pleural aspiration and fluid sent for:
  - Glucose
  - Protein and LDH (with paired serum samples)
  - Microscopy and culture
  - Alcohol and acid-fast bacilli
  - Cytology
  - pH (can be performed using a blood gas machine or in laboratory, the latter preferred if sample purulent)

Management of a pleural effusion in pregnancy

- Ultrasound-guided pleural aspiration or drain insertion (depending on size of effusion, likely aetiology, and other medical issues)

⚠ ♀ with a chest drain *in situ* must be nursed on a ward where staff are competent in the care of chest drains

---

Pneumomediastinum

- Can occur in pregnancy
- Was reported in association with severe coughing in ♀ during the 2010 swine flu (H1N1) outbreak in the UK
- Can also occur in labour
- Often managed conservatively
- Development of subcutaneous emphysema is an early indicator

Pneumothorax

1° **pneumothorax**

- No underlying lung disease
- Otherwise healthy individuals
- More common in ♂, especially taller ♂
- Smoking ↑ risk
- Recurrence risk up to 54% in the 1st 4 years after an initial episode

2° **pneumothorax**

- Develops in the presence of underlying lung disease such as COPD or interstitial lung disease

In pregnancy
- Spontaneous 1° pneumothorax is uncommon in pregnant ♀
- Pregnancy associated with an ↑ risk of recurrence

Management of pneumothorax in pregnancy

History
- Any indication of underlying lung disease or other cause for the pneumothorax

Examination
⚠ Assessment for signs of tension pneumothorax which can be fatal if untreated
- Hypotension
- Tachycardia
- Respiratory distress
- Hypoxia

Investigations
- CXR (standard PA film in inspiration)

Treatment

1° *pneumothorax*
- Treat as for non-pregnant ♀
- Treatment options (as per BTS guidelines for pleural disease):
  - Not affected by pregnancy
  - If limited symptoms in mother, no fetal concerns and pneumothorax is small (<2 cm), no intervention is required
  - If symptomatic or large pneumothorax, needle aspiration
  - Chest drain insertion if persistent air leak

Recurrent, persistent, or bilateral pneumothorax
- Video-assisted thoracoscopic surgery (VATS) can be performed in pregnancy and is not associated with any adverse pregnancy outcomes

Pregnancy after operative treatment for pneumothorax
- Spontaneous vaginal delivery can proceed as normal

Delivery
- Caesarean section and spontaneous labour are both associated with ↑ risk of recurrence
- Vaginal delivery with regional analgesia is preferred, with:
  - Shortened active 2nd stage
  - Lower threshold for the use of forceps to aid delivery and ↓ the requirements for prolonged Valsalva manoeuvres
- Regional anaesthesia preferred to general anaesthesia

⮕ BTS. Guidelines for the management of pleural diseases: ℅ https://www.brit-thoracic.org.uk/document-library/clinical-information/pleural-disease/pleural-disease-guidelines-2010/pleural-disease-guideline/

Lung transplantation

⚠ Successful pregnancy is possible after a lung transplant, but these are high risk, particularly in ♀ with underlying CF.
- High rates of preterm delivery, low birthweight babies. and maternal mortality have been reported.
- The principles of management of a ♀ with a lung transplant who is considering pregnancy are very similar to those for other solid organ transplants.

Pre-pregnancy recommendations

- Contraception should be planned with every ♀ recipient of a lung transplant who is of childbearing age
- Consider the underlying reason for the transplant
- As with other solid organ transplants, it is advisable to delay conception until ♀ has been in good health for a year (i.e. not necessarily 1 year post procedure)
- ↑ BP should be well controlled
- No episodes of rejection in the preceding year
- The immunosuppressive regimens for lung transplants use similar agents to other solid organ transplants in pregnancy

☙ MMF and sirolimus should be avoided in pregnancy

In pregnancy

Maternal risks
- Acute rejection: the risk appears higher in pregnant ♀ with lung transplants than those with other organ transplants
- Gestational hypertension or pre-eclampsia
- Falling drug levels of immunosuppressive agents: close monitoring required
- Infection

Fetal risks
High incidence of babies who have:
- IUGR
- Been born preterm

General considerations
- Consider the underlying reason for the transplant
- Genetics referral if underlying cause was a condition such as CF
- Review baseline lung function
- Not a contraindication to vaginal delivery or breastfeeding

Gastroenterology

Common symptoms

Constipation

- Very common in normal pregnancies
- Results from:
  - ↓ colonic motility
  - Pressure on the colon from a gravid uterus
  - Poor oral intake in presence of significant nausea
  - Can be worsened by oral iron supplements
- Symptoms often improve with ↑ dietary fibre and regular exercise
- Use of laxatives is often required if conservative measures do not lead to a symptomatic improvement
- Bulk forming and osmotic laxatives should be used 1st line

☞ If these do not work, stimulant laxatives can be considered but care should be taken due to the risk of stimulating uterine contractions.

Gastro-oesophageal reflux

- Common as a result of progesterone-induced relaxation of the lower oesophageal sphincter
- Aluminium-, magnesium-, and calcium-based antacid treatments are all considered safe in pregnancy
- Histamine receptor antagonists (e.g. ranitidine) and proton pump inhibitors (e.g. omeprazole) are appropriate to use if required
- Conventional triple therapy for *Helicobacter pylori* eradication can also be given during pregnancy

Nausea and vomiting

- Common symptoms, particularly in the 1st trimester (when the levels of β-HCG are highest)
- Approximately 50% of pregnant ♀ will experience nausea and vomiting, 25% nausea only, with 25% unaffected
- Classically occurs in the morning but many ♀ will experience symptoms at any time of the day
- Not associated with poor pregnancy outcome
- Usually resolves spontaneously by 16–20 wks

Treatments for nausea and vomiting in pregnancy
- Non-pharmacological:
  - Ginger-containing foods
  - P6 (wrist) acupressure
  - Eating little and often
- Pharmacological:
  - Antihistamines

➲ NICE (updated 2019). Antenatal care for uncomplicated pregnancies (CG62): ♫ https://www.nice.org.uk/guidance/cg62/chapter/1-Guidance#management-of-common-symptoms-of-pregnancy

Hyperemesis gravidarum

- Vomiting severe enough to cause biochemical disturbance:
  - Affects approximately 1% of all pregnancies
  - More likely to occur in multiple or molar pregnancies
- Atypical features include:
  - Haematemesis
  - Epigastric discomfort
  - Weight loss

⚠ If atypical features are present, other pathologies should be considered before a diagnosis of hyperemesis gravidarum is made.

- Management includes:
  - Consideration of inpatient admission
  - Antiemetics (enteral if tolerated, parenteral if not)
  - Fluid supplementation

💢 Wernicke's encephalopathy has been reported in association with hyperemesis gravidarum so care should be taken with fluid and nutritional replacement, in particular avoidance of use of IV glucose without vitamin supplementation, i.e. Pabrinex®.

💢 H. pylori has been associated with hyperemesis gravidarum.

Non-invasive testing for H. pylori (e.g. serology, urease breath testing, or stool antigen testing) should be considered in ♀ with refractory symptoms or symptoms persisting in the 2nd trimester.

First line	H1 receptor antagonist: cyclizine OR promethazine
	Then add in
	Phenothiazine: prochlorperazine OR chlorpromazine
Second line	D2 antagonist: metoclopramide OR domperidone
	(instead of, not in addition to, phenothiazines due to increased risk of side effects in combination)
	Then add in
	5-HT3 receptor antagonist: ondansetron*
Third line	Steroids after discussion with senior obstetrician/obstetric physician

*Recent data suggests a small increase in risk of cleft lip/palate with use in the first trimester, so discussion of the potential risks and benefits to the individual is advised. ⌖ http://www.uktis.org/docs/Ondansetron%202019.pdf

Inflammatory bowel disease

Most common inflammatory bowel conditions are UC and Crohn's disease (Table 4.1).
- In about 5% of ♀ with IBD, the clinical, radiological, and histological findings show mixed results ∴ described as 'IBD—unclassified type'
- 'Indeterminate colitis' is used after colectomy when it is not possible to classify the disease on pathological examination

Extra-intestinal manifestations of IBD

Musculoskeletal
- Monoarthritis
- Sacroiliitis

Dermatological
- Erythema nodosum
- Pyoderma gangrenosum
- Oral ulceration
- Manifestations of nutritional deficiencies, e.g. vitamin B, vitamin C

Liver
- Primary sclerosing cholangitis
- Choledocholithiasis

Ophthalmic
- Anterior uveitis
- Iritis
- Episcleritis

IBD in pregnancy
- Quiescent or well-controlled disease has no impact on fertility or pregnancy outcome
- Features associated with poor outcome include:
  - Active disease at conception
  - 1st presentation in pregnancy
  - Colonic rather than small bowel disease alone
  - Active disease after resection
  - Severe disease treated by surgery
- Risks include:
  - Miscarriage and stillbirth
  - Prematurity
  - Low birthweight
- Pregnancy does not make a relapse more likely if disease is otherwise well controlled

Management of IBD in pregnancy

- Regular MDT review
- Early clinical review if symptoms suggestive of a flare develop
- Discussion of medication and decision about biologic cessation/continuation in 3rd trimester if applicable
- VTE risk assessment and repeated if active disease develops

Mode of delivery

- Decisions should be individualized by MDT
- Caesarean section may be advisable with:
  - Severe perianal Crohn's disease
  - Severe UC in ♀ who may require future pouch formation
- Ileo-anal pouch is not an absolute indication for caesarean section

Table 4.1 Features of UC and Crohn's disease

	UC	Crohn's disease
Population affected	• ♀ predominance	• ♂ predominance
Smoking	• Associated with non- or ex-smokers	• Strong association with smoking, ↑ the risk of severe disease and surgery
Symptoms	• Bloody diarrhoea	• Change in bowel habit • Extra-intestinal manifestations often occur • Malnutrition
Part of GI tract affected	• Colon (sometimes terminal ileum)	• Any part from mouth to anus
Endoscopic findings	• Uniform inflammation, rectum always affected • Thin bowel wall	• Patchy inflammation ('skip lesions') • Thickened bowel wall with deep ulceration ('cobblestone' appearance)
Radiological findings	• Symmetrical inflammation	• Strictures, fissures, and fistulae can occur
Histological findings	• Inflammation of mucosa only • Neutrophil predominance	• Inflammation of mucosa and muscle • Presence of granulomata • Lymphocyte predominance

Management of an IBD flare

⚠ Needs aggressive treatment as flares are associated with adverse fetal outcomes
- Look for other causes of symptoms before diagnosing a flare
- Exclude active infection (send stool culture)

Bloods
- Inflammatory markers
- Consider measuring TPMT activity to guide use of thiopurine drugs

Medications
- The choice of this is determined by:
  - Severity of disease (Table 4.2)
  - Location/extent of disease

Suppositories
- Useful in very distal disease, i.e. proctitis:
  - Mesalazine, 1 g daily

Enemas
- Useful in distal UC (too high for a suppository to reach):
  - Mesalazine, 1 g enema OD
  - Steroid, e.g. prednisolone 20 mg enema OD

Steroids
- Parenteral steroids if severe disease suspected:
  - Hydrocortisone 100 mg QDS IV
- Oral steroids:
  - Prednisolone 40 mg daily

Antibiotics
- Not required in all cases, but indicated if complications suspected

Imaging
⚠ Pregnancy is not an absolute contraindication to abdominal radiography if indicated (e.g. if clinical suspicion of toxic megacolon in acute severe UC)

Other investigations
- Pregnancy is not a contraindication to flexible sigmoidoscopy

Surgery
- Occasionally required when complications occur, e.g.:
  - Bowel obstruction
  - Haemorrhage
  - Perforation
  - Fistula
  - Abscess formation
  - Toxic megacolon

Table 4.2 Severity assessment for UC

	Mild	Moderate	Severe
Bowel frequency	<4 per day	4–6 per day	>6
Blood in stool	No more than small amounts	Between mild and severe	Visible blood
Systemic features			
Temperature >37.6°C	No	No	Yes
Pulse >90 beats per min	No	No	Yes
Anaemia	No	No	Yes
ESR (mm/hr)	≤30	≤30	>30

The diagnosis of severe UC is made with >6 bowel motions per day and the presence of at least 1 systemic feature

Source: data from Truelove S.C. and Witts L.J. (1955) 'Cortisone in Ulcerative Colitis' *Br Med J.* 2(4947): 1041–1048.

Drug treatments for IBD

⚠ Drugs used to treat IBD should be reviewed and evaluated for suitability during pregnancy and lactation.

See Table 4.3.

Table 4.3 Indications and contraindications of IBD drugs

	Pregnancy	Breastfeeding
5-ASA, e.g. mesalazine	• No evidence of teratogenicity	• Transfer into breastmilk can occur, with theoretical risk of watery diarrhoea in the neonate
Steroids	• Can be used as normal • Blood glucose monitoring advised	• Can be used as normal
Sulfasalazine	• Can be continued • High-dose folic acid should be given	• Can be continued
Azathioprine/ 6-mercaptopurine	• Can be continued	• Can be continued
Ciclosporin	• Can be used for steroid-resistant, acute severe UC • Not indicated in the treatment of Crohn's disease	• Can be continued
Methotrexate	• Evidence of teratogenicity • Avoid pregnancy for at least 3 months after cessation	• Lack of evidence but not recommended
Leflunomide	• Not recommended in ♀ considering pregnancy • Stop and follow with cholestyramine washout preconception	• No data so breastfeeding not recommended
Mycophenolate mofetil	• Evidence of teratogenicity • Avoid pregnancy for at least 3 months after cessation	• No data so breastfeeding not recommended

Vedolizumab

- A relatively new monoclonal antibody that binds to the A4B7 integrin
- Results in gut-specific anti-inflammatory activity
- Good results seen in IBD
- Has been described in >90 pregnant ♀, with no association with adverse fetal outcomes
- Animal studies have also been reassuring
- Therefore appropriate to continue this in pregnancy

Pregnancy-specific considerations for the biological agents used in IBD are summarized in ➔ Table 8.11.

Coeliac disease

Definition
Changes in the small bowel mucosa (e.g. inflammation, crypt hyperplasia, and villous atrophy) which develop on exposure to gluten and resolve when gluten is excluded from the diet.

Background
- Often coexists with other autoimmune conditions, e.g. T1DM
- Fat- and water-soluble vitamin malabsorption can occur
- Osteoporosis is also more common in coeliac ♀
- Refractory disease or those with poor compliance to a gluten-free diet are at greatest risk of developing an associated malignancy, most commonly T-cell lymphoma
- Other GI tract malignancies also occur with ↑ frequency

Clinical features
- Abdominal bloating
- Weight loss
- Malabsorption
- Chronic diarrhoea

The diagnosis should be considered when individuals present with:
- Iron deficiency anaemia
- ↓ fertility and/or recurrent fetal loss
- Low birthweight babies
- Abnormal liver function
- Osteoporosis
- Hyposplenism
- Dermatitis herpetiformis:
  - Symmetrical, intensely pruritic rash
  - Characteristically on buttocks, scalp, forearms or knees

◗ For images, see ℬ https://www.dermnetnz.org/topics/dermatitis-herpetiformis/

Coeliac disease in pregnancy
- Untreated disease is associated with:
  - Miscarriage
  - Subfertility
  - Low birthweight

Management of coeliac disease in pregnancy
- Strict adherence to gluten-free diet
- Monitor for malabsorption of:
  - Fat-soluble vitamins such as vitamins A, D, E, and K
  - Fe (transferrin saturation, ferritin)
  - Folate
- Regular assessment of fetal growth (symphysial fundal height measurement)
- Optimization of bone health
- Check pneumococcal vaccination status (hyposplenism)

Antibodies and coeliac disease

Anti-tissue transglutaminase antibodies
- IgA antibodies that are most specific for the diagnosis
- Preferred to anti-endomysial and anti-gliadin antibodies

⚠ False-negative results can occur in IgA-deficient ♀, so an IgA level at the time of antibody testing is recommended

☛ The presence of antibodies in the absence of clinical manifestations is of uncertain significance

Peptic ulcer disease

Background
- Risk factors for the development of peptic ulceration are the same in pregnancy as in the non-pregnant population
- ↑ maternal age has also been associated

Investigation
☛ Historically, there has been a hesitancy to perform upper gastrointestinal endoscopy in pregnancy due to:
  - Concerns about the physical effects on a gravid uterus
  - Use of sedation
- Recent series show no ↑ in adverse fetal outcomes, and that endoscopy should be performed if clinically indicated
- The procedure should be performed by an experienced endoscopist, with the use of the lowest reasonable dose of sedation
- If peptic ulceration is seen, then biopsies can be taken or rapid urease testing (CLO test™) performed

Endoscopy in pregnancy

Oesophagogastroduodenoscopy (OGD)
- This can be performed in pregnancy if indicated
- No ↑ in adverse fetal outcomes
- Advisable to be performed by an experienced endoscopist
- Low-dose sedation can be used
- Fetal monitoring appropriate for gestational age can be performed before and after the procedure

Sigmoidoscopy
- No ↑ in adverse fetal outcomes
- Advisable to be performed by an experienced endoscopist
- Probably preferred to colonoscopy in pregnancy

Colonoscopy
- No evidence for adverse fetal outcomes if performed in the 2nd trimester
- Lack of evidence for outcomes in 1st and 3rd trimesters but can be performed at this time if the alternative, i.e. surgery, would be associated with more risk

Endoscopic retrograde cholangiopancreatography
- One series reported 1st trimester use was associated with preterm birth and low birthweight
- Advisable to be performed by an experienced endoscopist with pulsed rather than continuous fluoroscopy
- Lead shielding to the fetus can be used

Pancreatitis

Background

- The incidence is unchanged by pregnancy
- Complicates approximately 1 in 1000–10,000 pregnancies
- Most common precipitants are the same as those in the non-pregnant population (e.g. gallstones and alcohol)
- Various scoring systems have been used to assess severity in non-pregnant individuals

💎 There are no scoring systems specific to pancreatitis in pregnancy

- Hyperlipidaemia can be a cause in pregnancy:
  - Usually in the setting of an underlying lipid metabolism abnormality, not hypertriglyceridaemia which occurs in normal pregnancy
- Mild pancreatitis—no associated organ failure or complications
- Severe pancreatitis—combination of pancreatic inflammation and organ failure

Clinical features

- Symptoms include:
  - Abdominal pain (epigastric/RUQ but can be poorly localized) that may radiate to the back
  - Nausea and vomiting
  - Those arising from complications such as pleural effusions and ileus
- Signs:
  - Mild pancreatitis—may be minimal
  - Severe pancreatitis—↑ HR, ↓ BP, ↑ RR and fever can occur
  - Features of the underlying cause (e.g. jaundice from gallstones)

Investigations

Blood tests

- Amylase
- Serum lipase (particularly useful in late-presenting patients)
- FBC
- Renal function
- Liver function
- Lactate
- Calcium
- Glucose

Ultrasound

- Pancreas is only identified in 25–50% of ♀ with acute pancreatitis
- Possible to identify abnormalities such as swelling
- Can diagnose contributory pathology (e.g. choledocholithiasis)

CT

- Not essential to confirm the diagnosis (risk of ionizing radiation)
- Can be useful if there is diagnostic uncertainty, or if there is no clinical improvement in the 1st 48–72 hrs

Management of acute pancreatitis in pregnancy
- Assessment of severity (using scoring system such as Ranson or Glasgow)
- Assessment for underlying cause
- May require care on HDU or ITU
- Fetal assessment as guided by gestation
- Supportive care (nil by mouth, IV fluids, analgesia)
- Close observation for development of complications
- Monitor blood glucose and ketones regularly (the latter particularly if nil by mouth)
- Delivery plans depend on gestation and severity of the illness
- Surgical input if required for an underlying cause (e.g. laparoscopic cholecystectomy for gallstones) can usually be delayed until after delivery

→ Calculator for Ranson score: ℘ https://www.mdcalc.com/ransons-criteria-pancreatitis-mortality

→ Calculator for Glasgow score: ℘ http://www.gastrotraining.com/calculators/glasgow-pancreatitis-score-2

Chronic pancreatitis
- Progressive inflammation of the pancreas
- Causes a gradual deterioration in its exocrine and endocrine function
- Pain is often but not always present
- Can be severe, requiring hospitalization
- The underlying cause is not always identified

Management of chronic pancreatitis in pregnancy
- Assessment and monitoring for malabsorption:
  - Symptoms such as steatorrhea
  - Vitamin B_{12} deficiency
  - Fat-soluble vitamin deficiency (vitamins A, D, E, and K)
- Blood glucose monitoring for GDM

Bowel obstruction

Bowel obstruction

- Uncommon occurrence in pregnancy
- Usually related to:
  - Adhesions from previous surgery
  - Volvulus (sigmoid or caecal)

Pseudo-obstruction (Ogilvie's syndrome)

- Recognized complication of caesarean section
- Can result in massive colonic dilatation in the absence of physical obstruction
- Most vulnerable area is the caecum
- Caecal perforation and death have been reported from this complication

Presentation

- Initially painless abdominal distension with normal bowel sounds
- Nausea, vomiting, change in bowel habit, and abdominal pain can develop

Assessment and management

- Initial assessment:
  - Thorough clinical examination
  - Abdominal radiograph, where colonic distension may be demonstrated
- Any potentially contributory medication (e.g. opioid analgesia) should be stopped
- Conservative management includes:
  - Nasogastric tube insertion (Ryles tube rather than fine-bore tube)
  - Keeping the patient nil by mouth
  - Enemas if appropriate
- If conservative measures fail, may require colonic decompression

⚠ If symptoms suggestive of bowel perforation develop, urgent imaging and surgical input are required.

Bariatric procedures

Background
There are several types of bariatric surgical procedure that can be performed including gastric banding, a Roux-en-Y procedure, or sleeve gastrectomy (Fig. 4.1).

Pre-pregnancy
Contraception
- Absorption of oral contraceptives is unreliable after a procedure
- Depo-Provera® injection is associated with weight gain
- Best options include:
  - Barrier contraception
  - Long-acting reversible contraceptives such as an intrauterine device or implant
- Advisable to delay pregnancy for 12–18 months after procedure to allow new eating habits to establish and weight to have stabilized

Management in pregnancy
Obesity-related issues
→ See 'Obesity', p. 118.

Nutritional considerations
- Protein intake can be insufficient soon after a bariatric procedure due to ↓ intake and rapid weight ↓ (if extreme, can be associated with adverse fetal outcomes such as fetal growth restriction)
- Specialist dietetic input to limit weight ↑ and help adherence to post-surgical dietary modifications
- No change to pre-pregnancy diet until 3rd trimester where a calorie ↑ of 200 calories is advised
- Assess Hb, iron status (ferritin, transferrin saturation), folate, vitamin B_{12}, fat-soluble vitamins (A, D, E), calcium every trimester
- Risks of vitamin malabsorption so advisable to take:
  - Folic acid 5 mg OD
  - Ferrous sulfate 200 mg OD
  - Vitamin D—minimum 800 units daily
- Vitamin B_{12} supplementation to continue if taking pre pregnancy
- Pregnancy multivitamin recommended (less vitamin A than normal multivitamin)

Gastric band
- Adjustment of the volume of fluid in the band is not routinely advocated, but can be performed if protracted vomiting occurs
- If symptoms develop, e.g. abdominal pain, vomiting, reflux, then consider band complications such as slippage or erosion

☛ No consensus on whether band should remain inflated (potentially ↑ band complications) or deflated (↑ risk of weight gain and associated complications).

Roux-en-Y bypass and sleeve gastrectomy

- Specialist assessment for potential dumping syndrome at or before conception:
  - Early—abdominal cramps, bloating, nausea, vomiting, diarrhoea
  - Late—also known as postprandial hyperinsulinaemic hypoglycaemia
- Dumping syndrome makes diagnosing GDM difficult with a GTT, so blood glucose monitoring is preferable
- If GI symptoms develop, e.g. abdominal pain or vomiting, then consideration of postoperative complications such as strictures, ulceration, or internal herniation is required

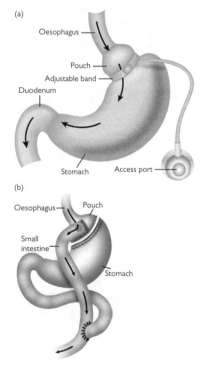

Fig. 4.1 Bariatric procedures. (a) Gastric band. (b) Roux-en-Y procedure. Reproduced from Chaudry M. A. et al. (2014) *Gastric and Oesophageal Surgery* Oxford University Press: Oxford with permission from Oxford University Press.

Liver disease

Pregnancy-related liver changes

- The presence of mildly elevated LFTs is common in pregnancy:
  - 3% of deliveries in one prospective study
- Severe liver dysfunction, however, is much rarer and historically has been associated with high maternal mortality rates
- The normal ranges for liver enzymes in pregnancy differ to that of the non-pregnant population (Table 5.1)
- Transient postpartum derangement of liver transaminases has been observed and requires further investigation if they do not return to normal within 4–8 weeks after delivery

Hyperemesis gravidarum

(\bigodot See p. 141.)

- Transient derangement of liver function occurs in up to 40% of ♀ with hyperemesis gravidarum

HELLP syndrome

(\bigodot See p. 14.)

- Haemolysis, elevated liver enzymes, and low platelets
- Believed to be part of the pre-eclampsia spectrum
- Can sometimes be difficult to differentiate from AFLP

Isolated raised alkaline phosphatase

- Very ↑ alkaline phosphatase levels (>1000 IU/mL) can occasionally be seen in pregnancy
- ♀ is typically very well, with no other signs or symptoms of liver disease or hypertensive conditions
- If isoenzyme analysis is performed, it is usually placental alkaline phosphatase production that is responsible for this ↑
- If the isoenzyme analysis is delayed or not performed, it is appropriate to do a liver USS and liver screen for congenital and acquired abnormalities
- If all test results are reassuring, no intervention is required

---

Liver function tests in pregnancy

See Table 5.1.

Table 5.1 Normal ranges for liver function tests in pregnancy and the changes seen postpartum

	Non-pregnant	1st trimester	2nd trimester	3rd trimester	Postpartum (mean ↑)
Bilirubin (micromol/L)	0–17	4–16	3–13	3–14	37%
Alanine transaminase (IU/L)	0–40	6–32	6–32	6–32	147%
Aspartate transaminase (IU/L)	7–40	10–28	11–29	11–30	88%
γ-Glutamyl transferase (IU/L)	11–50	5–37	5–43	3–41	62%
Alkaline phosphatase (IU/L)	30–130	32–100	43–135	133–418	–
Albumin (g/L)	41–53	31–51	26–45	23–42	–

Adapted from Frise & Williamson (2019) 'Liver Disease in Pregnancy' *Medicine*, 43(11):636–638 with permission from Elsevier.

Causes of jaundice in pregnancy

Causes not specific to pregnancy

- Haemolysis
- Gilbert's syndrome
- Viral hepatitis (hepatitis A, B, C, E; EBV; CMV)
- Autoimmune hepatitis
- Intrahepatic biliary diseases:
  - PBC
  - PSC
- Gallstones
- Cirrhosis
- Drug-induced hepatotoxicity
- Malignancy

Causes specific to pregnancy (10% of cases)

- Hyperemesis gravidarum
- Pre-eclampsia/HELLP syndrome
- AFLP
- Intrahepatic cholestasis of pregnancy (obstetric cholestasis)

Investigations to consider for deranged liver function in pregnancy

Haematology
- FBC
- Coagulation

Biochemistry
- Full liver tests including GGT and AST
- Renal function
- Bile acids
- Glucose
- Lactate

Microbiology
- Hepatitis A IgM
- HBsAg
- Hepatitis C antibody or antigen
- Hepatitis E IgM
- CMV IgM/G
- EBV IgM/G

Immunology
- Anti-nuclear antibodies
- Anti-smooth muscle antibodies
- Anti-liver–kidney–microsome-1 antibodies
- Anti-liver cytosol antibody-1
- Anti-mitochondrial antibodies
- Immunoglobulins

Radiology
- Liver USS ± Doppler of vessels
- Clinical situation determines need for further imaging, e.g. MRCP

Acute fatty liver of pregnancy

This is a rare condition, which typically occurs in the 3rd trimester, and is associated with a significant maternal and fetal mortality.

Risk factors
- ♂ fetus
- Multiple pregnancy

Clinical features
- Prodrome of non-specific, flu-like symptoms often reported
- Symptoms include:
  - Vomiting
  - Abdominal pain
  - Polyuria and polydipsia (transient diabetes insipidus)
- Clinical findings include:
  - Encephalopathy
  - Abdominal tenderness

Diagnosis
- Haematological abnormalities include:
  - Leucocytosis
  - Disseminated intravascular haemolysis
- Biochemical abnormalities include:
  - Acute kidney injury
  - Liver function test abnormalities (↑ transaminases, ↑ bilirubin)
  - Hyperuricaemia
  - Hypoglycaemia (can be profound)
- Hypertension and proteinuria may be present but are usually mild

> **Management of AFLP**
> - Location: HDU or ITU
> - Delivery when patient stable
>
> *Treatment of complications*
> - Hypoglycaemia
> - Coagulopathy—blood products (red blood cells, fresh frozen plasma, cryoprecipitate, platelets as needed)
> - BP control
> - Acetylcysteine can be considered
> - Transfer to liver unit if acute liver failure develops

Mechanism of transient diabetes insipidus in AFLP
- Placenta produces vasopressinase, which metabolizes ADH and can cause gestational diabetes insipidus (➲ see p. 410)
- In AFLP, hepatic metabolism of vasopressinase is thought to be ↓, thereby ↑ circulating vasopressinase → further ↓ in ADH

Features that may aid distinction of AFLP from HELLP

(For details of HELLP, → see p. 14.)
- See the Swansea diagnostic criteria (Table 5.2)
- In AFLP:
  - Hypertension and proteinuria are normally mild
  - Hypoglycaemia can be profound
  - Marked hyperuricaemia
  - Early coagulopathy
  - Bright liver on USS

Table 5.2 Swansea diagnostic criteria for acute fatty liver of pregnancy

The presence of 6 or more features from the following list are consistent with the diagnosis, in the absence of another cause

- Vomiting
- Abdominal pain
- Polydipsia/polyuria
- Encephalopathy
- Elevated bilirubin
- Hypoglycaemia
- Elevated urate
- Leucocytosis
- Elevated transaminases
- Elevated ammonia
- Renal impairment
- Coagulopathy
- Ascites or bright liver on ultrasound
- Microvesicular steatosis on liver biopsy

Source: data from Knight et al. (2008) 'A prospective national study of acute fatty liver of pregnancy in the UK' *Gut* 57(7):951–6.

Consideration of liver transplantation

⚠ Criteria used to judge severity of liver disease in non-pregnant ♀ and whether liver transplant referral should be made does **not** apply in pregnancy. If in doubt about an unwell pregnant ♀ with acute liver failure, contact a liver centre early.

Intrahepatic cholestasis of pregnancy

Background

- ICP is also known as obstetric cholestasis (OC)
- Defined as pruritus and ↑ bile acids with no alternative diagnosis
- Affects 0.7% of pregnancies in the UK
- More common in ♀ of Asian ethnicity and there is geographical variation in prevalence
- 1/3 of ♀ have a family history of the condition
- Usually occurs in the 3rd trimester but has been reported as early as 8 wks
- Resolves spontaneously after delivery

Clinical features

- May be a family history of ICP or gallstones
- May be a personal history of pruritus when taking the combined oral contraceptive pill
- Pruritus of the trunk and limbs, without a skin rash (often worst at night)—may occur before LFTs become abnormal
- Anorexia and malaise
- Steatorrhoea and dark urine (less common)
- Jaundice occurs in <5%
- ↑ transaminases is more common than ↑ alkaline phosphatase

Diagnosis

- Send LFTs and bile acids for all ♀ itching, without a rash:
  - If normal, they should be repeated every 1–2 weeks if symptoms persist, as itching can predate abnormal LFTs
- Exclude other causes of pruritus and liver dysfunction

Maternal risks

- Vitamin K deficiency

Fetal risks

- Preterm labour (spontaneous but also iatrogenic)
- Stillbirth (associated with bile acids >100 micromol/L)
- ↑ risk of meconium (delivery in an obstetric unit is recommended)

Management of ICP

Medications

- Oral vitamin K should be considered at diagnosis
- Symptoms may be ↓ by topical emollients
- Antihistamines cause sedation but often do not improve pruritus
- Ursodeoxycholic acid:
  - 8–12 mg/kg daily in 2 divided doses
  - ↓ pruritus between 1 and 7 days after starting
  - No proven reduction in fetal adverse effects
- Rifampicin:
  - 150 mg BD, up to a maximum of 300 mg BD
  - Can be used if bile acids and/or ALT are continuing to ↑ on maximum dose of UDCA
  - May cause abnormal liver function so are not advisable when ALT is greatly ↑
  - Turns secretions including urine and tears orange so ♀ who wear contact lenses should be warned about the potential for discolouration

Fetus

- Fetal surveillance with ultrasound and CTG monitoring are commonly used but of no proven benefit

Postnatally

- Resolution of symptoms and LFTs should be established

Recurrence

- Risk in subsequent pregnancy is 45–70%
- It can also recur with the combined contraceptive pill

⚠ Intrauterine death is usually sudden and cannot be predicted by biochemical results, CTG findings, or on USS.

💣 Timing of delivery (to avoid stillbirth) is controversial as there is an ↑ risk of perinatal and maternal morbidity with early intervention. Stillbirth risk appears to be ↑ when bile acids >100 micromol/L (3.4% compared to 0.4% of normal population), so earlier delivery (35–37 wks) of these ♀ is suggested. Early delivery is not supported by this data for those with bile acids below this level.

🔗 RCOG (2011). Obstetric cholestasis (green-top guideline no. 43): 🔗 https://www.rcog.org.uk/en/guidelines-research-services/guidelines/gtg43/

Hepatitis B

Background
- DNA virus
- Spread by infected blood, blood products, or sexual contact
- Incubation 2–6 mths
- Incidence of carrier status in UK ♀ is ~1:100

Clinical features
- Acute infection has a prodrome of non-specific systemic and GI symptoms followed by an episode of jaundice
- Those with chronic infection are usually asymptomatic

Diagnosis
Based on clinical picture and serology (Table 5.3).

Maternal risks
Pregnancy does not alter the course of acute infection, and so prognosis is similar to that of non-pregnant individuals:

- 65% subclinical disease with full recovery
- 25% develop acute hepatitis
- 10% become chronic carriers
- <0.5% fulminant hepatitis (associated with significant mortality)

Fetal risks
Severe acute infection may → miscarriage or preterm labour, but no related congenital defects have been identified.

> #### Management of chronic hepatitis B in pregnancy
> ▶ In the UK, all ♀ should be screened at booking as detection of infection has important consequences for ↓ of mother-to-child transmission (MTCT).
> - Nucleoside analogues (i.e. entecavir/tenofovir) are advised in highly viraemic ♀ (viral load >1,000,000 IU/mL) to ↓ MTCT (usually started in the 2nd/3rd trimester)
> - No evidence that caesarean section prevents vertical transmission
> - Breastfeeding is not contraindicated

Neonatal risks

- Transmission usually occurs at delivery, but <5% may be due to transplacental bleeding *in utero*
- Neonatal infection may be fatal, and usually results in chronic carrier status with significant lifelong risks of cirrhosis and hepatocellular carcinoma
- The carrier status of the mother at delivery determines the risk of vertical transmission:
  - HBsAg and HBeAg +ve: ~95% risk
  - HBsAg +ve and HBeAg –ve and viral load <100,000: <15% risk

⚠ Babies whose mothers have acute or chronic HBV should receive HBV vaccination within 24 hrs of delivery, and some require HBV IgG (as per Health Protection Agency guidelines in the UK). This is up to 95% effective at preventing HBV infection.

Diagnostic tests for hepatitis B infection

HBsAg	Hepatitis B surface antigen
HBeAg	Hepatitis B e antigen
HBV DNA	Hepatitis B virus DNA
Anti-HBs	Antibody to hepatitis B surface antigen
Anti-HBe	Antibody to hepatitis B e protein
Anti-HBc	Antibody to hepatitis B core antigen

Table 5.3 Interpreting test results for hepatitis B infection

Diagnosis	Positive	May be positive or negative
Vaccination	• Anti-HBs	
Incubation period		• HBsAg
		• HBeAg
		• HBV DNA
Acute infection	• HBsAg	
	• HBeAg	
	• HBV DNA	
	• Anti-HBc IgM	
Past infection	• Anti-HBs	• HBV DNA
	• Anti-HBc	• Anti-HBe
Chronic infection	• HBsAg	• HBeAg
	• HBV DNA	• Anti-HBe

Hepatitis C

Background

- RNA virus
- Main method of transmission is IV drug abuse
- In the last decade there have been advances in treatment hence the ↓ risk of complications such as cirrhosis and hepatocellular carcinoma
- Older treatments were of limited benefit and associated with adverse effects (pegylated interferon α and ribavirin)
- Oral direct antiviral agents were introduced after 2011 and have transformed the treatment of hepatitis C with shorter treatment duration (8–16 wks) and they are much better tolerated with a 95% cure rate
- Drug regimens are available that work across all genotypes

Clinical features

- Acute infection is normally asymptomatic
- Chronic infection is identified either through screening or when cirrhosis is diagnosed
- Up to 30% clear the virus spontaneously after the acute episode
- Cirrhosis and liver failure can occur
- Many extra-hepatic manifestations have been described including membranoproliferative glomerulonephritis, cryoglobulinaemia, and thyroid disease

Diagnosis

- Serological testing for anti-hepatitis C antibody (remains positive after successful treatment)
- Positive viral RNA confirms infection:
  - If RNA positive, then genotyping should be performed
- LFTs are of limited value as can be normal even in the presence of significant cirrhosis
- Liver USS may identify abnormal liver appearance, and/or the presence of complications such as splenomegaly
- Liver biopsy can be performed to assess fibrosis, but non-invasive tests are preferred (Fibroscan®, or transient elastography; not usually used in pregnancy)

New identification of hepatitis C antibody positivity in pregnancy

- Thorough history for potential source
- Send blood for viral RNA level
- If negative:
  - Likely to have spontaneously cleared infection or been treated
- If positive:
  - Ensure also tested for HIV and hepatitis B
  - Arrange liver USS (for cirrhosis, portal hypertension)
- Refer to hepatology for review with respect to treatment

Management of hepatitis C in pregnancy

- Anti-hepatitis C antibodies are not routinely screened for but should be measured in ♀ assessed to be at risk (see later in this topic)
- Hepatitis C infection is not a contraindication to vaginal delivery or breastfeeding, although ♀ with high viral loads have greater vertical transmission rates
- Invasive fetal monitoring and prolonged labour should be avoided
- Infected ♀ should be referred for treatment after delivery
- The newer treatments are not currently recommended in pregnancy due to a lack of safety and efficacy data

---

♀ who warrant screening for hepatitis C

- History of IV drug use
- Recipient of blood products before 1992
- Haemophilia carriers who received factor concentrates before 1987
- History of haemodialysis
- Unexplained elevated ALT
- HIV-positive ♀

Other viruses that cause hepatitis in pregnancy

Hepatitis A

- Pregnancy does not alter the course or outcome

Hepatitis E

- Acute self-limiting illness in the non-pregnant population
- Can cause severe infection with fulminant liver failure in pregnant ♀
- Treatment is supportive and there is no evidence for efficacy of specific antiviral therapy

Other viruses

- Abnormal liver function can be seen in ♀ with:
  - HSV
  - CMV
  - EBV

Cirrhosis

Background

- Commonest cause of cirrhosis in ♀ of childbearing age is alcohol
- Can be quite advanced yet have no symptoms and minimal/no change in LFTs
- Low platelets suggest cirrhosis
- Fertility is often ↓ but pregnancy can still occur so contraception should be considered in all ♀ with cirrhosis

Pre-pregnancy counselling

- Assess synthetic function (INR)
- Endoscopy—screen for varices and treat if possible
- Propranolol for prophylaxis for variceal bleeding can be continued
- USS—in particular looking for splenic artery aneurysm
- Calculate MELD/UKELD score

Maternal risks

- Worsening of synthetic function
- Hepatic decompensation (10% of cirrhotic ♀ with 20% mortality rate)
- Gestational hypertension

Fetal risks

- ↑ rate of spontaneous pregnancy loss (27% compared to 7% in ♀ without cirrhosis)
- Preterm labour and perinatal death
- Placental abruption

Management of cirrhosis in pregnancy

⚠ Maternal mortality rate of 3.4% with deaths reported in the year postpartum.

- Management by an MDT with high-risk pregnancy experience is essential
- Calculating severity score may be useful to predict risk of hepatic decompensation (♀ with MELD score <6 or UKELD score <42 are likely to do well)
- Regular review for development of complications and hypertension
- Regular bloods including FBC, LFTs, and coagulation
- Endoscopy for oesophageal or gastric varices in the 2nd trimester
- Paracentesis can be performed in pregnancy if required, no ↑ in complications has been reported
- Amiloride and/or furosemide can be used for managing ascites

Delivery options

- Significant varices may warrant caesarean or assisted vaginal delivery
- Risks include bleeding from abdominal wall varices (may require MRI to assess presence of these), ascites, and poor wound healing

Causes of cirrhosis

- Alcohol
- NAFLD
- Chronic hepatitis B infection
- Chronic hepatitis C infection
- PBC
- Autoimmune hepatitis
- PSC
- Wilson's disease
- Hereditary haemochromatosis
- α1-antitrypsin deficiency

Consequences of cirrhosis

- Thrombocytopenia
- Coagulopathy
- Hypoalbuminaemia
- Variceal bleed
- Decompensation:
  - Ascites
  - Encephalopathy
  - Coagulopathy
  - Acute kidney injury
- Hepatocellular carcinoma

Scoring systems to assess severity of end-stage liver disease

- Model for end-stage liver disease (MELD): https://www.mdcalc.com/meld-score-model-end-stage-liver-disease-12-older
- MELD with sodium (MELD-Na): https://www.mdcalc.com/meldna-meld-na-score-liver-cirrhosis
- UK end-stage liver disease model (UKELD): https://qxmd.com/calculate/calculator_442/ukeld-score

Portal hypertension

Background

- Hepatic venous pressure gradient is an estimate of the difference in pressure between the hepatic portal vein and the IVC:
  - ≥5 mmHg defines portal hypertension
  - >10 mmHg is significant portal hypertension
  - At >12 mmHg variceal haemorrhage is more likely to occur

Clinical features

- Ascites
- Splenomegaly and thrombocytopenia
- Varices:
  - Oesophageal
  - Gastric
  - Anterior abdominal wall

Causes

See Table 5.4.

Table 5.4 Causes of portal hypertension

Cirrhosis	
Non-cirrhotic causes	
Pre-hepatic	• Portal vein thrombosis • Splenic vein thrombosis
Pre-sinusoidal	• Idiopathic • PBC • PSC • Sarcoid
Sinusoidal	• Chronic viral hepatitis • NAFLD • Alcohol-related liver disease
Post-sinusoidal	• Budd–Chiari syndrome • Veno-occlusive disease
Post-hepatic	• IVC obstruction • Right heart failure

⚠ **Management of variceal bleed in pregnancy**
- Resuscitation
- Antibiotic prophylaxis
- Endoscopy
- Treatment with banding ligation (1st line for oesophageal varices), and cyanoacrylate glue (gastric varices)
- Avoid vasopressin/terlipressin (risk of uterine ischaemia due to vasoconstriction)
- Post banding: proton pump inhibitors
- Terlipressin contraindicated
- Somatostatin/octreotide preferred if available
- Transjugular intrahepatic portosystemic shunt/surgical shunts have been performed in pregnancy

Splenic artery aneurysm
- Most common visceral artery aneurysm
- Rupture is associated with fetal and maternal mortality

⚠ Screening should be performed in all pregnant ♀ with portal hypertension.

Non-alcoholic fatty liver disease

Background

- Non-alcoholic fatty liver disease (NAFLD) is the commonest cause of abnormal LFTs in developed countries (prevalence up to 30%, up to 70% of people with T2DM)
- Reflects excessive accumulation of hepatic triglyceride in the absence of significant alcohol intake, viral infection or drug-related causes
- Features macrovesicular steatosis (very different to the microvesicular steatosis seen in AFLP), inflammation and fibrosis
- Risk factors for progression include
  - Insulin resistance (diabetes)
  - Older age
  - Obesity
  - Smoking
- Commonly seen in ♀ with other features of metabolic syndrome such as DM, hypertension, and obesity
- May be associated with cirrhosis but in morbidly obese ♀ there is some reversibility in hepatic fibrosis with weight loss
- This is a spectrum of conditions:
  - Steatosis → steatohepatitis (NASH) → fibrosis → cirrhosis

Clinical features

- Normal LFTs do not exclude the diagnosis and can be seen even in advanced disease
- Presentation in pregnancy is often asymptomatic abnormal LFTs

Diagnosis

- In non-pregnant individuals, scoring systems such as FIB-4 help to stratify the likelihood of the condition (based on age, platelet count, AST and ALT)
- Non-invasive testing such as Fibroscan® (transient elastography) can be used to assess the level of fibrosis
- Abdominal ultrasound may show coarse or irregular echotexture, which in combination with splenomegaly is strongly predictive of cirrhosis
- To make the diagnosis, the individual must consume alcohol below a certain level (1 standard drink or 15 g per day in ♀)

Management of NAFLD in pregnancy

- Despite the ↑ frequency of this condition, there is little published to guide practice
- It is important to address the other associated abnormalities in these ♀ such as obesity, risk of GDM and VTE
- LFTs in isolation are not helpful in the diagnosis or the management
- Fibroscan® cannot be used as liver stiffness is increased in pregnancy (rapidly reverses after delivery)
- See page 170 for cirrhosis-specific considerations if cirrhosis is present
- Ensure postnatal follow-up with Hepatology is arranged

Hepatic adenomas

Background
- Type of benign liver lesion that is ↑ in incidence
- ↑ incidence may be due to oral contraceptive pill usage, but are also ↑ identified on imaging performed for other reasons
- Range in size and can be very large (up to 30 cm)
- Symptoms such as pain being more common at larger sizes
- Associated with malignant change, rupture, and spontaneous haemorrhage

Clinical features
- LFTs are usually normal
- α-fetoprotein is only abnormal in the setting of malignant transformation

Issues in pregnancy
- Thought to be more common in pregnancy due to the ↑ levels of circulating oestrogen
- Main risk is spontaneous haemorrhage, which can be life-threatening
- Prior to pregnancy, surgical resection should be performed if indicated (e.g. single lesion >5 cm)
- Treatment in pregnancy can be considered for those with large lesions or associated with significant symptoms

Liver haemangiomata
- Benign liver lesions that are similar to adenomas
- Likely that ↑ circulating oestrogen in pregnancy results in ↑ growth
- Symptoms are related to size
- Small risk of rupture causing intra-abdominal haemorrhage which ↑ in pregnancy
- Treatment options should be discussed before pregnancy, but intervention (embolization) in pregnancy has been reported

Budd–Chiari syndrome

Background
- Hepatic venous outflow obstruction which can involve:
  - Hepatic venules (hepatic veno-occlusive disease)
  - Large hepatic veins
  - IVC
  - Right atrium
- 1° (venous thrombosis) or 2° (external compression) can occur
- Can be acute, subacute, or chronic
- Life-threatening liver failure may result
- Often associated with an underlying thrombophilia or a myeloproliferative disorder such as polycythaemia rubra vera

Clinical features
- The most common features at presentation are:
  - Ascites
  - Jaundice
  - RUQ pain
- Hepatomegaly
- LFTs can be very abnormal

New presentation in pregnancy
- Consider with newly deranged LFTs and symptoms described previously
- USS is the key initial investigation, but needs to include flow in the portal and hepatic veins
- Treatment is anticoagulation with LMWH
- Careful assessment of liver synthetic function is required
- Early discussion with a liver unit if the ♀ is unwell with significant liver dysfunction

⚠ Management of acute severe Budd–Chiari syndrome in non-pregnant ♀ may include the insertion of a transjugular intrahepatic portosystemic shunt, but thrombolysis, percutaneous angioplasty, and liver transplantation have all been used.

💊 In pregnancy, decisions about interventions would need to be individualized, depending on factors including severity of the disease and gestational age.

> #### Management of Budd–Chiari syndrome in pregnancy
> ▶ Occurs more commonly in pregnancy, but most are present before pregnancy
>
> *Pre-existing Budd–Chiari syndrome*
> - Likely good outcome but risk of preterm birth may be >50%
> - Anticoagulation should be reviewed and therapeutic LMWH substituted for warfarin
> - A recent USS is required to assess for portal hypertension
> - A recent OGD is useful to assess for the presence of varices

Autoimmune liver disease

Background

- Autoimmune, progressive liver inflammation → fibrosis and cirrhosis
- More common in ♀ than ♂
- Can overlap with PBC (➲ see p. 180) and PSC (➲ see p. 181)

Clinical features

- These are variable
- Individuals may be asymptomatic and the presence of abnormal LFTs (↑ ALT/AST ± hyperbilirubinaemia) is the only feature
- Symptoms such as abdominal discomfort, pruritus, and small joint pain are also reported
- Up to 25% can present with acute liver impairment
- Up to 33% can present with cirrhosis and the associated sequelae
- Other autoimmune conditions often coexist, including thyroid disease, UC, T1DM, SLE, and coeliac disease

Diagnosis

- LFTs may show a very ↑ ALT/AST
- Alkaline phosphatase can be ↑ but this may be mild
- ↑ IgG (with normal IgA and IgM)
- Autoantibodies are present in most cases (Box 5.1).
- Histological analysis of liver tissue is needed to confirm the diagnosis (shows abundant plasma cells and provides information on the degree of fibrosis)

Box 5.1 Antibodies found in autoimmune liver disease

- Anti-nuclear antibodies
- Anti-smooth muscle antibodies
- Anti-liver–kidney microsome-1 antibodies (ALKM-1)
- Anti-liver cytosol antibody-1 (ALC-1)

► Previously autoimmune liver disease was categorized into types 1 and 2, based on the antibody results; however, this categorization is no longer used.

Management of autoimmune liver disease in pregnancy

- Induction of remission involves steroid treatment ± azathioprine, which can be used in pregnancy as needed
- Budesonide, ciclosporin, and tacrolimus can also be used in pregnancy if needed

⚠ MMF is teratogenic and should be changed to an alternative agent in ♀ considering pregnancy

- Flares in pregnancy are more common in ♀:
  - Not on immunosuppression
  - Who had a flare in the year before conception
  - More commonly occur postpartum
- The presence of cirrhosis is associated with:
  - ↓ live birth rate
  - ↑ rates of special care baby unit admission
  - ↑ risk of serious maternal complications including decompensation, death, or need for transplantation

Biliary atresia

Background
- Progressive obliteration of the extra-hepatic biliary tree
- Can be congenital (and often associated with other malformations) or acquired
- It usually presents in the neonatal period
- Surgical intervention (hepatoportal enterostomy 'Kasai procedure') is more successful the earlier it is performed
- Portal hypertension and recurrent cholangitis can develop in adulthood following a Kasai procedure in childhood
- The majority of individuals with biliary atresia require liver transplant when young
- UDCA may be of benefit when used long term

Management of biliary atresia in pregnancy
- Liver transplant: see 'Liver transplantation', p. 184
- Assessment for portal hypertension:
  - Including bloods and USS for splenomegaly
- MDT management
- Regular LFTs
- Close monitoring for infection and cholestasis
- Continue UDCA if taking prior to conception; low threshold for starting UDCA in pregnancy

Cholecystitis
- Gallstones are common in ♀ of childbearing age
- Complications of gallstone disease occur in a small number of pregnancies
- Conservative management often sufficient
- ERCP can be performed if indicated
- Elective surgical intervention can be performed but preferably in the 2nd trimester

Primary biliary cholangitis

Background
- Progressive destruction of bile ducts → cholestasis, cirrhosis, and liver failure
- Previously known as primary biliary cirrhosis
- 95% of cases occur in ♀

Clinical features
- May present with cholestasis (dark urine, pale stool) ± pruritus
- Progression to cirrhosis and liver failure can then occur over many years
- Features of other autoimmune conditions may also be present e.g.:
  - Hypothyroidism (up to 20% of individuals with PBC)
  - Sjögren's syndrome
- Iron deficiency anaemia may be present (from occult bleeding if cirrhotic or coexistent coeliac disease)
- Osteoporosis is also common

Diagnosis
- This is usually made when >1 of the following features is present:
  - Biochemistry consistent with intrahepatic cholestasis
  - Positive anti-mitochondrial antibodies (present in 95%)
  - Liver biopsy showing features consistent with the condition
- Other laboratory tests that may aid diagnosis include:
  - ANA: positive in up to 50%
  - Sp100 and gp210 antibodies: can confirm diagnosis in anti-mitochondrial antibody-negative PBC
  - Elevated serum IgM: often seen but not specific to PBC

Management of PBC in pregnancy
- Check FBC, ferritin, TFTs
- Malabsorption with risk of fat-soluble vitamin deficiencies:
  - Consider vitamin K replacement if malabsorption prominent
  - Vitamin D should be appropriately supplemented during pregnancy and while breastfeeding
- UDCA is 1st-line treatment (obeticholic acid and bezafibrate are also used as 2nd-line therapies):
  - Good pregnancy outcomes have been seen after 1 year of UDCA treatment prior to conception
  - In one study, all the ♀ stopped UDCA and although they remained well during pregnancy, liver function deteriorated postpartum

Primary sclerosing cholangitis

Background

- Progressive inflammation and fibrosis of the intra- and extra-hepatic bile ducts
- Cirrhosis and liver failure eventually results
- More common in ♂ than ♀
- Associated with IBD, mainly UC:
  - UC occurs in 70% of cases of PSC
  - PSC occurs in up to 10% of cases of UC
- Cholangiocarcinoma is seen in 10–15%
- Often need transplantation but the condition can recur in the graft

Clinical features

- Symptoms include those of cholestasis (jaundice, pruritus, dark urine, pale stool)
- Weight loss and RUQ pain can also be seen

Diagnosis

- LFTs are consistent with cholestasis (high alkaline phosphatase)
- Imaging shows irregular structuring:
  - ERCP
  - MRCP (is the diagnostic imaging of choice because of the risks of pancreatitis after ERCP)

⚠ It is important to exclude IgG4 sclerosing cholangitis which can present in a similar way but has a different treatment regimen and prognosis.

Management of PSC in pregnancy

- Very few reported cases of PSC in pregnancy
- UDCA is used with limited benefit in non-pregnant ♀ and can be used in pregnancy if required
- As in PBC, malabsorption may be seen and therefore fat-soluble vitamin deficiency is a risk:
  - Vitamin K replacement should be considered if malabsorption is prominent
  - Vitamin D should be appropriately supplemented during pregnancy and while breastfeeding

Hereditary haemochromatosis

Background
- An autosomal recessive condition (mutations in the *HFE* gene)
- Iron overload results from ↑ intestinal iron absorption
- Excess iron is deposited in tissues, impairing their function
- Regular blood loss from menstruation is thought to explain why ♀ usually have a less severe phenotype than ♂
- Rare to have cirrhosis in ♀ of childbearing age

Clinical features
- Often asymptomatic initially but as iron deposition ↑, symptoms arise from the end-organ dysfunction that results:
  - Impaired LV systolic function and arrhythmias if an associated cardiomyopathy is present
  - Cirrhosis, portal hypertension, and the associated risk of variceal bleeding
  - Pancreatic deposition resulting in DM
  - Endocrine dysfunction including anterior pituitary and adrenals
  - Joint deposition
- Blood test abnormalities include an elevated ferritin and transferrin saturation (≥45% in ♀)
- *HFE* gene and non-*HFE* gene panels help with diagnosis
- Ferritin <1000 micromol/L is a negative predictor for liver fibrosis and a liver biopsy is only needed if >1000 micromol/L

Management of haemochromatosis in pregnancy
- The risks associated with pregnancy depend on end-organ damage and include:
  - GDM
  - Cirrhosis
  - Cardiomyopathy
- Maintenance phlebotomy can continue in pregnancy
- If cirrhosis is present; ➜ see 'Cirrhosis', p. 170 for management
- Genetic counselling should be considered

Wilson's disease

Background

- Rare autosomal recessive condition
- Results in copper accumulation in tissues such as the liver
- Caused by a mutation in the gene that encodes a transporter of copper into the bile from hepatocytes
- Progressive and fatal if not treated

Clinical features

- Can present with:
  - Acute liver failure (with haemolytic anaemia)
  - Renal failure
  - Neurological symptoms such as tremor or ataxia, or psychiatric symptoms develop later and may be the 1st feature in up to 50% of individuals
  - Infertility, menstrual abnormalities, or miscarriage
- Slit lamp examination may reveal Kayser–Fleischer rings and sunflower cataracts

Diagnosis

- Low caeruloplasmin (<0.2 g/L; normal range 0.2–0.5 g/L) is diagnostic in an individual with Kayser–Fleischer rings; however, as it is an acute phase reactant it may be normal in affected individuals with decompensated liver disease
- Elevated urinary copper (>1.6 micromol/24 hrs) is suggestive but not diagnostic of Wilson's disease
- LFTs often show a low alkaline phosphatase (an alkaline phosphatase:bilirubin ratio of <2 in acute liver failure suggests Wilson's disease)
- A liver biopsy can also be useful if a large enough sample is taken, as an elevated copper concentration of liver by dry weight is the best biochemical test for Wilson's disease
- Mutational analysis (>300 mutations) can help

Management of Wilson's disease in pregnancy

- Treatment is with copper chelation, e.g. penicillamine, trientine, or zinc
- Dietary modification to avoid copper-rich foods such as chocolate, mushrooms, shellfish, and nuts is also advised
- ♀ with Wilson's should be encouraged to continue treatment during pregnancy and breastfeeding as abrupt cessation has been associated with maternal morbidity and mortality
- Penicillamine at high doses used in cystinuria has been associated with adverse outcomes, but the lower maintenance dose in Wilson's disease has been associated with good outcomes in the majority of reported pregnancies
- Penicillamine inactivates pyridoxine (vitamin B_6), so supplements should be prescribed to any ♀ on this drug
- Referral to a genetics counsellor should also be considered

Liver transplantation

Background
- Many ♀ have successful pregnancies following liver transplantation
- Pregnancy does not appear to affect graft survival or outcome
- Liver transplantation may rarely be required for acute liver failure resulting from pregnancy-specific liver disorders such as AFLP

Maternal risks
- Gestational hypertension or pre-eclampsia
- Toxicity from immunosuppressive agents
- Infection

Fetal risks
- IUGR
- Preterm delivery

Management of liver transplantation in pregnancy
⚠ Immunosuppressive treatment must be continued.

Prior to pregnancy
- Consider the underlying reason for the transplant
- Genetics referral if underlying cause was genetic
- Review medications and convert to alternative agent if on MMF
- Advisable to delay conception until ♀ has been in good health for at least 1 year (i.e. not necessarily 1 year post procedure)
- ↑ BP should be well controlled
- No episodes of acute rejection in the preceding year
- If undergoing IVF, advise single embryo transfer

In pregnancy
- Regular antenatal review for renal and liver function, symptoms or signs of pre-eclampsia, and therapeutic drug monitoring
- Early treatment of anaemia (avoid blood transfusion if possible)
- Urgent review if any changes in liver or renal function
- Regular fetal growth scans from 24 wks
- Screen for GDM (if on steroids/tacrolimus)
- Breastfeeding is not contraindicated in ♀ taking medications such as steroids, tacrolimus, azathioprine, and ciclosporin

Delivery
- Aim for vaginal delivery (caesarean section for obstetric indications)
- Parenteral hydrocortisone if on maintenance oral steroids

Renal disease

Physiological changes

Normal changes in pregnancy
- ↑ blood flow → 50% ↑ in GFR → ↓ urea and ↓ creatinine
- ↑ renal size
- ↑ proteinuria (up to 300 mg/24 hrs)
- ↑ in erythropoietin production
- Changes in tubular function:
  - ↑ glycosuria
  - ↑ bicarbonaturia
  - Hypercalciuria
- Physiological hydronephrosis can be seen:
  - Often right > left, as size of the gravid uterus ↑
  - Does not cause symptoms or renal impairment so if either are present another cause should be sought

Renal disease and antenatal screening tests
⚠ HCG and PAPP-A are vital components of antenatal screening tests for trisomies and fetal growth restriction.

These can both be elevated in renal disease:
- ↑ HCG—risk of false positive
- ↑ PAPP-A—risk of false negative

A high trisomy risk based on bloods in ♀ with renal disease needs expert interpretation and consideration of screening using cell-free DNA if available.

Glomerular filtration rate

- Creatinine is a poor marker for renal function as it is affected by multiple variables including age, weight, sex, and muscle mass
- The CKD-EPI (Chronic Kidney Disease Epidemiology Collaboration) calculation is preferred to creatinine clearance estimates such as the Cockcroft–Gault equation and calculations such as MDRD (Modification of diet in renal disease), as CKD-EPI provides greater accuracy at higher filtration values
- Therefore the 'estimated GFR' is often reported alongside creatinine (Table 6.1)

Estimated GFR

- Aims to ↑ identification of renal disease at an earlier stage
- Calculation based on the patient's age, sex, ethnicity, and serum creatinine
- Given the limited number of variables included, the results in non-pregnant adults should be interpreted with caution and further investigation undertaken before labelling an individual with CKD

⚠ Physiological changes to creatinine in pregnancy mean that eGFR calculations are not valid in pregnancy, so renal function should be interpreted by using serum creatinine only.

Table 6.1 Interpreting eGFR

Stage	eGFR (mL/min)	
1	90+	Urine or structural abnormality but no impairment of function
2	60–89	Mildly ↓ function
3a/b	30–59	Moderately ↓ function
4	15–29	Severely ↓ function
5	<15	Very severe/end-stage kidney failure

Proteinuria

Background

- Urinary protein can be glomerular, tubular, or overflow of pathological circulating proteins such as light chains
- Vast majority of filtered albumin is reabsorbed
- Pregnancy ↑ proteinuria (hence higher threshold compared to non-pregnant) up to 300 mg/24 hrs (or PCR <30 mg/mmol)
- Proteinuria may be the 1st sign of pre-eclampsia, and in some ♀ can be the only abnormality prior to eclampsia/HELLP developing
- Persistent proteinuria is a risk factor for renal disease progression and cardiovascular disease in non-pregnant adults

Differential diagnosis of proteinuria

- Physiological (upright posture, exercise, infection, pregnancy)
- Discontinued ACE-I (can ↑ by 20–200%)
- Renal disease
- Pre-eclampsia (after 20 wks)

Methods

See Table 6.2.

Table 6.2 Methods for assessing proteinuria

Urine dipstick		
1+ protein	Minority have significant proteinuria	Proteinuria on dipstick correlates poorly with protein quantified in other ways
2+ protein	Many have significant proteinuria	
≥3+ protein	Majority have significant proteinuria	
24 hr urine collection		
Normal (non-pregnant)	<150 mg/day	50% collections are inadequate
Normal (pregnant)	<300 mg/day	Volume should be >900 mL or >15 mg/kg creatinine (non-pregnant adults)
Spot protein:creatinine ratio (PCR)		
Normal (pregnant)	<30 mg/mmol	30 mg/mmol is ~ equivalent to 300 mg/day (replaced 24 hr collection in clinical practice)
Spot albumin:creatinine ratio (ACR)		
Normal (non-pregnant)	<3.5 mg/mmol	More sensitive test than PCR
Normal (pregnant)	<8 mg/mmol	

Management of new-onset proteinuria in pregnancy

Assessment

- Careful history including:
  - History of conditions associated with renal disease
  - Symptoms of renal disease or complications of renal disease
  - Symptoms of pre-eclampsia
- Examination including:
  - BP
  - Fluid balance
- Urine:
  - PCR
  - Urine culture
  - Microscopy for red cell casts if renal disease suspected or microscopic haematuria on dipstick
- Bloods including:
  - Renal function
  - ANA, ANCA, anti-dsDNA, immunoglobulins, C3/4
  - HbA1c if risk factors for T2DM
  - Antiphospholipase A2 receptor antibodies
- Renal tract USS

Ongoing management

- Consistent with pre-eclampsia (onset >20 wks):
  - Management as per local and national guidelines
- Consistent with renal disease (onset <20 wks, associated renal impairment, presence of antibodies, background of associated conditions such as T1DM):
  - Nephrology opinion: consider renal biopsy if clinical suspicion of vasculitis or inflammatory disease and if diagnosis would inform decisions on treatment (dependent on gestation, history, and presentation)
- Not consistent with pre-eclampsia or renal disease:
  - Regular review of BP and quantification of proteinuria
  - Awareness of symptoms of pre-eclampsia and the need for urgent review if these develop
  - Some centres advocate early induction (i.e. 40 wks rather than the usual 41–42 wks) in view of proteinuria even in absence of ↑ BP or other abnormalities, but no guidelines are available to aid this decision-making
- VTE prophylaxis:
  - Required for all ♀ with proteinuria >3 g/day (threshold for benefit not known; a lower threshold may be reasonable if other risk factors present)

Postnatal management

- Need repeat quantification of proteinuria after delivery to ensure resolution
- Renal referral if proteinuria persists >3 mths after delivery

Haematuria in pregnancy

Visible (macroscopic) haematuria
⚠ Not normal for pregnancy.

Investigations
- USS of the kidneys, ureters, and bladder
- Investigation of choice is a cystoscopy:
  - May be difficult to perform in 3rd trimester due to the gravid uterus
- Further cross-sectional imaging in pregnancy should be determined by the individual history and abnormalities identified on USS

Non-visible (microscopic) haematuria
- False-positive results on urine dipstick can occur as a result of:
  - Contamination with vaginal secretions or haemorrhoids
  - Haemoglobinuria
  - Myoglobinuria
  - Strenuous exercise

Investigations
- Microscopy for red cells
- Renal function assessment
- Urine culture
- USS of the kidneys, ureters, and bladder
- Further investigation of confirmed haematuria depends on:
  - History (other features and/or presence of disorders associated with renal dysfunction)
  - Coexistent proteinuria and ↑ BP
- In a well ♀ with no other abnormalities on bloods, urine testing, or USS, it is reasonable to reassess after delivery and refer for further investigation if haematuria persists (it will resolve in the majority of ♀)

Urinary tract infection

Background

- ↑ risk of infection because of urinary stasis and dilation of the upper renal tract
- Asymptomatic bacteriuria (the growth of a pathogenic organism from 2 consecutive samples in the absence of infective symptoms) occurs in 2–7% of pregnant ♀
- Untreated asymptomatic bacteriuria is associated with an ↑ risk of ascending infection
- In contrast to other patient groups, treatment for asymptomatic bacteriuria is recommended in pregnancy because of the ↑ risk of pyelonephritis, and the potential obstetric complications, most notably preterm labour

Clinical features

- Symptoms of infection include:
  - Dysuria
  - Frequency
  - Urgency
  - Suprapubic pain
- Symptoms of upper urinary tract infection (pyelonephritis) include:
  - Loin pain
  - Fever
  - Rigors
- Examination should include looking for markers of sepsis, e.g.:
  - Pulse
  - BP
  - RR
  - Temperature
- Abdominal examination is often normal but may reveal:
  - Suprapubic tenderness in UTI
  - Renal angle tenderness in pyelonephritis

⚠ Exclude a diagnosis of pyelonephritis in ♀ with apparent hyperemesis gravidarum or threatened preterm labour.

Diagnosis

- Bloods may show ↑ CRP and/or ↑ WCC
- Urine culture (➔ see Table 6.3)

⚠ Renal impairment does not occur as a result of unilateral pyelonephritis so if present, may represent sepsis or an alternative diagnosis.

Management of UTI in pregnancy

Testing
- Urine culture should be sent at 1st antenatal visit for screening for asymptomatic bacteriuria
- In ♀ with symptoms of UTI, a midstream specimen of urine should be sent for culture and empirical antibiotics commenced while awaiting sensitivity
- Use of urine dipstick as a screening tool for infection is **not recommended** due to the low sensitivity and specificity
- Mixed growth, 'equivocal' growth, or significant growth of a single organism that is a likely contaminant should not be treated routinely (➔ see Table 6.3)
- If there is significant growth of a pathogenic organism in an asymptomatic ♀, the culture should be repeated and treatment initiated if this culture confirms asymptomatic bacteriuria, i.e. the same organism is grown from both samples

Treatment
- **Asymptomatic AND urine culture positive** for significant growth of pathogenic organism:
  - Repeat culture
  - Treat if 2nd culture confirms growth of the same organism
  - Repeat culture 1 wk after cessation of antibiotics to ensure clearance
- **Symptomatic BUT NO culture results available yet:**
  - Empirical antibiotics (nitrofurantoin, trimethoprim, or cefalexin; ➔ see Table 6.4 for contraindications) after urine sample taken
  - Analgesia if required
  - Review antibiotic choice when culture results available
- **Symptomatic AND urine culture positive** for significant growth of pathogenic organism:
  - Oral antibiotics (amoxicillin 1st line if sensitive)
  - Repeat culture after 1 wk after cessation of antibiotics to ensure clearance
  - Analgesia if required
- **Persistent bacteriuria despite antibiotic course:**
  - Further course of antibiotics to which the organism is sensitive should be prescribed
- **Symptomatic despite treatment and negative culture:**
  - Consider alternative cause (urethral syndrome, interstitial cystitis, painful bladder syndrome, vaginitis)
  - Get specialist advice

Complications of bacteriuria

Pyelonephritis

- Pyelonephritis complicates 1–2% of all pregnancies
- 20% of pregnant ♀ with pyelonephritis have structural abnormalities including renal stones

Management of pyelonephritis in pregnancy

- Hospital admission due to risk of obstetric complications
- Blood tests including FBC, renal function, CRP, and blood cultures
- Urine cultures
- IV antibiotics (as per local guidelines)
- Appropriate fetal monitoring depending on gestation
- Renal USS

Recurrent urinary tract infections

- Prophylactic antibiotics should only be considered in the setting of recurrent infections with the same organism **after confirmation of clearance** of the infection (➔ see Table 6.4)
- Advice about adequate daily fluid intake and perineal hygiene (such as voiding after sexual intercourse) may be of benefit
- It is also useful to provide a clean specimen container to these ♀ so that a timely specimen can be collected if symptoms develop
- Renal USS and prophylactic antibiotics if:
  - ≥3 culture-positive episodes of infection in 1 year (or 2 in 6 mths)

  And
  - A recent culture has confirmed clearance

Antibiotic prophylaxis

- Can be considered in:
  - Recurrent infection (as previously described)
  - Single infection in individual who is immunosuppressed
  - Single infection in setting of congenitally abnormal urinary tract
  - Single episode of pyelonephritis
- Potential prophylactic antibiotic regimens include:
  - Trimethoprim 100 mg at night (not in 1st trimester)
  - Nitrofurantoin (immediate release not MR) 50–100 mg at night (if eGFR >45 mL/min)
  - Cefalexin 125 mg OD

Group B *Streptococcus* in urine

If GBS is isolated in a urine sample at any gestation:
- ♀ should be treated according to sensitivities at the time of diagnosis
- Intrapartum prophylaxis should be administered as per local guidelines

◆ The threshold for treatment differs in international guidelines.

In the USA, treatment of any level of growth is advocated (>10^4 CFU/mL) but in the UK, treatment of growth above >10^5 CFU/mL is advised (RCOG guidelines)[1].

1 RCOG green-top guideline on GBS in pregnancy: ✆ https://obgyn.onlinelibrary.wiley.com/doi/epdf/10.1111/1471-0528.14821

Risk factors for urine infection

♀ *more at risk of infection*
- An abnormal urinary tract, e.g.:
  - Congenital anomalies of the renal tract
  - Renal calculi
  - Vesicoureteric reflux
  - Neurogenic bladder
  - Urinary obstruction
- Recent instrumentation
- Recurrent urine infection prior to or during pregnancy
- Confirmed asymptomatic bacteriuria in pregnancy

♀ *more at risk of complications of infection*
- Immunosuppressive medications, e.g.:
  - Long-term steroids
  - Anti-rejection medications post transplantation
- Poorly controlled DM

Interpreting urine culture results

See Table 6.3.

Table 6.3 Definitions: urine culture results

Significant growth	Growth of a single organism at >10^5 CFU/mL
Equivocal growth	Growth of a single organism, but 10^4—10^5 CFU/mL
Mixed growth	One or more organisms grown on culture with no single predominant organism
Recurrent infection	Further growth of a pathogenic organism after treatment has resulted in clearance (confirmed on negative culture)
Persistent infection	Growth of the same organism on repeated samples with no negatives samples in between
Pathogenic organism	Likely to be the cause of symptoms, e.g. *Escherichia coli*
Contaminant	Organism grown as a result of suboptimal collection technique, which is unlikely to be the cause of urine infection, e.g. *Staphylococcus epidermidis*

⚠ If an organism is reported that is unfamiliar, it is advisable to check that this is not a probable contaminant before prescribing treatment.

Antibiotics for urinary tract infection

See Table 6.4.

Table 6.4 Antibiotics commonly used to treat UTI in pregnancy

Agent	Dose	Side effects	Specific pregnancy concerns	Contraindications
Cefalexin	500 mg BD PO for 3–5 days	• Diarrhoea • Vomiting • Abnormal LFTs • 0.5–6.5% of penicillin sensitive patients will get hypersensitivity	• None	• Cephalosporin hypersensitivity
Nitrofurantoin	50 mg QDS PO for 3–5 days	• Diarrhoea • Vomiting • Abnormal LFTs • Peripheral neuropathy	• Haemolytic anaemia in the neonate (avoid after 37+0 wks or earlier if risk factors for preterm delivery)	• Renal impairment (eGFR <45 mL/min) • G6PD deficiency
Amoxicillin	500 mg TDS PO for 3–5 days	• Diarrhoea • Vomiting • Abnormal LFTs • Rash	• 1st choice antibiotic if sensitivities known, but not for empirical treatment	• Penicillin allergy
Co-amoxiclav (amoxicillin and clavulanic acid)	625 mg TDS PO for 3–5 days	• Cholestasis • Jaundice	• Avoid in ♀ at risk of preterm labour (20–36/40) ↑ risk of necrotizing enterocolitis in neonate	• Penicillin allergy • Liver/biliary disease

| Trimethoprim | 200 mg BD PO for 3–5 days | • Diarrhoea
• Vomiting
• Abnormal LFTs
• Rash | • Avoid in 1st trimester (folate antagonist) | • Blood dyscrasias (depression of haematopoiesis) |
| Gentamicin | Depends on severity of UTI | • Theoretical discussion about ototoxicity in fetus not supported by small studies | • Balance of risk (maternal sepsis, preterm delivery, etc.)
• Dose depends on renal function
• If repeated doses required, gentamicin trough levels should be monitored | |

Acute kidney injury

Definition

An acute change in renal function detected by a change in blood creatinine
($\pm$ urea) or $\downarrow$ urine output as well as abnormalities in fluid balance.

▶ 'Acute kidney injury' (AKI) has replaced the term 'acute renal failure'.

Pregnancy

- AKI in pregnancy is most commonly caused by pre-eclampsia but is
  often multifactorial
- Renal recovery is usually good
- Look for contributory factors and treat them
- Control complications

⚠ Various criteria are used to categorize AKI, e.g. the RIFLE or the AKIN
(Acute Kidney Injury Network) criteria; however, the normal physiological changes seen in pregnancy mean that these scores are not valid in
pregnant ♀.

Investigations

Urine
- Dipstick testing is useful 1st-line test, but the low specificity and
  sensitivity should be borne in mind and a negative result should not
  prevent other tests being sent
- PCR

Bloods to consider
- Haematology:
  - FBC, coagulation
- Biochemistry:
  - U&Es, LFTs, calcium, phosphate, glucose, CRP
- Immunology:
  - ANA, ANCA, anti-glomerular basement membrane antibodies, anti-
    dsDNA antibodies, C3, C4, serum electrophoresis

Infection screening
- Midstream specimen of urine
- High vaginal swab
- Blood cultures

Imaging
- Renal USS in all AKI with unclear aetiology, or not responding to initial
  treatment

ECG
- If K^+ >5.5 mmol/L

Assessment of fetal well-being
- USS or CTG depending on gestation

Causes

See Box 6.1.

Box 6.1 Causes of acute kidney injury in pregnancy

Early pregnancy
- Hyperemesis gravidarum
- Septic abortion/miscarriage
- Acute retention (retroverted uterus)

Mid–late pregnancy
- Pre-eclampsia and HELLP
- Ureteric obstruction (especially if single kidney)
- Placental abruption
- AFLP
- HUS/TTP

Peripartum
- Chorioamnionitis
- Postpartum haemorrhage
- Ureteric injury related to operative delivery
- NSAIDs

Any time
- Intravascular volume depletion (e.g. sepsis, vomiting)
- Lupus nephritis
- Glomerulonephritis
- Interstitial nephritis (i.e. drug-related)
- Renal stone disease

Source: data from Wiles K and Banerjee A (2016) 'Acute kidney injury in pregnancy and the use of non-steroidal and anti-inflammatory drugs' *The Obstetrician and Gynaecologist* 18:127–35.

Chronic kidney disease

- Abnormal kidney structure or function, present for >3 mths
- Can be caused by a wide range of conditions
- Divided into stages based on the eGFR (Table 6.5).

CKD and subfertility

A number of mechanisms are responsible for the subfertility seen in ♀ with CKD:

- Impaired cyclical release of LH by the pituitary
- Cyclical variation in oestradiol may be absent
- ↑ prolactin
- Absence of progesterone effect on endometrium from anovulation
- Peritoneal dialysis-associated peritonitis may cause tubal damage
- Manifestations of this include menstrual irregularities and sexual dysfunction

Maternal risks

- Depends on the degree of renal impairment, the underlying cause, and the presence of complications (e.g. ↑ BP)

Obstetric

- ↑ risk of gestational hypertension
- ↑ risk of pre-eclampsia
- ↑ risk operative delivery/lower segment caesarean section

Renal

- Risk of deterioration in function that does not recover after delivery

Other

- VTE (with significant proteinuria)
- UTI (if congenital anomaly of the renal tract or vesicoureteral reflux is present, or if individual is immunosuppressed)

Fetal risks

- Prematurity (spontaneous or iatrogenic)
- Low birthweight
- ↑ neonatal mortality

Management of CKD in pregnancy

Pre-conception
- Pre-pregnancy counselling regarding risks (Table 6.5)
- Baseline investigations including assessment of proteinuria
- Optimize treatment of complications, e.g. ↑ BP and anaemia
- Optimize glycaemic control in ♀ with diabetes

Optimize medication
- Review the choice of antihypertensive and convert to pregnancy-appropriate medication if necessary
- Statins should be stopped in advance of conception
- Discuss timing of cessation of agents such as ACE-Is:
  - If for ↑ BP treatment, often stopped in advance of conception
  - If for proteinuria, can be continued while trying to conceive if early confirmation of pregnancy is possible, and stopped on 1st positive pregnancy test, i.e. not if cycles irregular or pregnancy test unreliable (e.g. CKD 5)

When pregnant
- Aspirin 75 mg OD from 12 wks
- Close monitoring for complications such as:
  - ↑ BP
  - Anaemia (may need iron and erythropoietin supplementation)
  - Disorders in calcium and phosphate balance
  - UTI (if congenital anomaly of tract or vesicoureteral reflux is present, or ♀ is immunosuppressed)
- Regular fetal assessment from 24 wks
- VTE risk assessment

Table 6.5 Complications by severity of CKD

Stage	Preterm delivery <37/40	Preterm delivery <34/40	SGA <5 centile	NICU	Pre-eclampsia	Fall in CKD stage postpartum
1	Up to 25%	5%	5%	10%	5–10%	0–8%
2	25–50%	10–20%	10–25%	10–20%	10–20%	10%
3	50–75%	25–50%	25–40%	20%	~50%	15–20%
4–5	75–100%	~50%	~50%	70%	50–75%	20–50%

Data obtained from Piccoli *et al*, *J Am Soc Nephrol* 2015; 26: 2011–22 and Bramham *et al Kidney International* 2016; 89: 874–85.

Hyperkalaemia

⚠ Potassium >6.5 mmol/L is an emergency and needs urgent assessment.

Principles of treatment

- Verify results if result unexpected and ♀ is well
- Assess severity according to local or national guidance
- Use blood gas machine for analysis of venous sample to aid rapid decision-making

Causes

- Oliguric renal failure
- Rhabdomyolysis
- Metabolic acidosis
- Excess K⁺ therapy
- Addison's disease
- Massive blood transfusion
- Burns
- Drugs, e.g. K⁺-sparing diuretics, ACE-I, suxamethonium
- Artefactual result (e.g. haemolysis)

Cardiac arrhythmias

⚠ Hyperkalaemia can result in life-threatening cardiac arrhythmias
- ECG changes seen with hyperkalaemia include (Figs. 6.1 and 6.2):
  - Tall, 'tented' T waves
  - Small P waves
  - Broad QRS complexes (eventually becoming sinusoidal)
  - Ventricular fibrillation

⚠ If any changes of hyperkalaemia are demonstrated on ECG, or K⁺ >6.5 mmol/L:
- Treat as a medical emergency and get senior help
- Set up continuous cardiac monitoring
- Give 10 mL 10% calcium chloride or 30 mL 10% calcium gluconate IV immediately
- Repeat dose if ECG changes persist after 5 mins

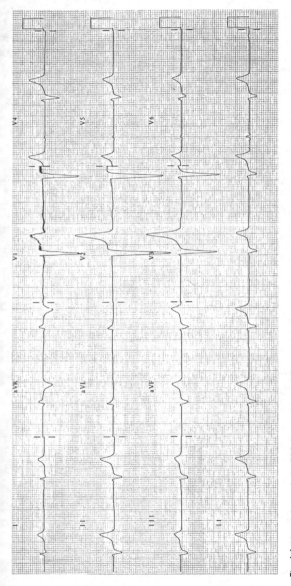

Fig. 6.1 Hyperkalaemia 1: this ECG shows tall 'tented' T waves (which can occur in isolation as the first sign of hyperkalaemia), loss of P waves, and widening of the QRS complexes.

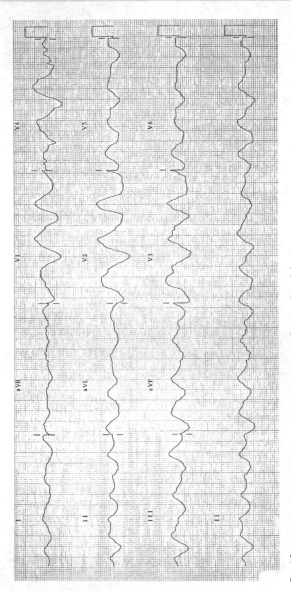

Fig. 6.2 Hyperkalaemia 2: this ECG shows the 'sine wave' pattern of extreme hyperkalaemia.

Treatment of hyperkalaemia

See Table 6.6.

Table 6.6 Treatments for hyperkalaemia

Treatment	Mechanism of action	Notes
Calcium gluconate (10–30 mL of 10%) Or Calcium chloride (10 mL of 10%)	Cardioprotection	• Short-acting, so may need repeat dose/s
Short-acting insulin 10 units and glucose (100 mL of 20% preferred to a smaller volume of the more irritable 50%)	↑ K⁺ uptake into cells Prevents hypogycaemia with insulin	• Always give with glucose • Monitor blood glucose for 8–12 hrs after doses • Does not ↓ K but must be given with insulin to prevent hypoglycaemia
Nebulized salbutamol (repeated doses of 2.5–5 mg)	↑ K⁺ uptake into cells	• Maternal side effects limit the therapeutic use of this; not to be used as monotherapy
Calcium polystyrene sulfonate (15 g QDS PO or 30 mg BD PR)	Ion exchange resin—binds K and prevents absorption	• Not useful for acute hyperkalaemia

Dialysis

Haemodialysis

- Removal of blood via an arterial port → bathed in dialysate → fluid and electrolytes are removed by diffusion across a semi-permeable membrane → returned via the venous port
- A typical non-pregnant individual on maintenance HD in a hospital setting will undergo HD 3 times a week for 3–5 hrs at a time
- Can be performed via a variety of vascular access routes (➔ see p. 208)

⚠ Contraception should always be discussed with ♀ on HD as although subfertility is common, pregnancy is still possible and high risk

Peritoneal dialysis

- Performed via a Tenckhoff peritoneal catheter (tube inserted into the peritoneal space through the abdominal wall)
- Dialysis fluid is introduced into the peritoneal space
- Fluid and electrolytes then diffuse across the peritoneum then the fluid is drained out (each cycle of draining/filling is an 'exchange')
- Various regimens are commonly used including solely overnight and intermittent exchanges throughout the day
- Better for individuals with some residual renal function
- Complications include:
  - PD peritonitis (signs include abdominal pain, fever, cloudy fluid draining off), can be treated with intraperitoneal or IV antibiotics
  - Sclerosing peritonitis (may develop after several years of PD)

PD and pregnancy

- Use depends on access, so can be used in pregnancy if available and acceptable
- Practical challenges arise from performing PD with adequate volumes in advancing gestation
- Higher risk of adverse pregnancy outcomes including miscarriage, infection, low birthweight babies, and preterm delivery compared to HD

Haemofiltration

- Similar to HD but uses convection to remove fluid and electrolytes as the blood passes through the machine and then replaces the fluid removed
- Used in the emergency setting as the fluid shifts are ↓ compared to HD, but this is a continuous process
- Can add filtration techniques to intermittent dialysis to provide haemodiafiltration (common in the UK)

Haemodialysis in pregnancy

Management of HD in pregnancy

- If no fistula, then a Tesio® line is used (or vascular catheters in an emergency setting)

⚠ Fistula formation usually not performed in pregnancy as takes several weeks to mature and post-pregnancy dialysis requirements will not be known

- Intensive HD regimens (36 hrs/wk or more), in ♀ on HD pre-pregnancy, are associated with improved pregnancy outcomes (?due to ↓ variability in biochemistry and ↑ similarity to normal physiological state)
- ♀ on HD are advised to undergo ↑ hours of HD from early in pregnancy (titrated gradually to ↑ tolerability of fluid shifts)
- Target fluid removal on HD is guided by dry weight, which changes in pregnancy ∴ allowances should be made for this
- Thromboprophylaxis is required
- No dietary changes routinely required, but discussion with specialist dietician advised
- Additional phosphate may be required
- Post-HD bloods can be taken from the arterial port at the end of HD to assess the success of the HD in improving biochemistry
- Regular fetal growth assessment from 24 wks
- Monitor for pre-eclampsia (can be challenging if ♀ anuric)
- Anticipate significant ↑ in erythropoietin requirement
- Not a contraindication to vaginal delivery

☀ Threshold for starting HD in pregnancy is not known, and the ideal target for post-HD biochemistry is also unclear.

⚠ It is important to review the reason for the underlying renal impairment in ♀ on HD as it may have implications for the pregnancy (e.g. lupus, diabetes).

If new to HD in pregnancy (i.e. HD performed to ↓ risks of high urea to fetus), duration should be titrated to renal function as intensive regimens show no evidence of benefit and some risk of harm (faster loss of residual renal function).

Vascular access for HD

Vascular catheter ('central line')
- Multiple lumen, non-tunnelled, large-bore central venous catheter into either internal jugular or femoral vein
- Can be inserted in an emergency setting and used immediately
- For temporary use only

Tesio® line
- 2 separate large-bore lines (1 'arterial' with red port, 1 'venous' with blue port), inserted into the internal jugular vein (both on the same side, positioned so their opening ports open at different levels in the superior vena cava) and then each is tunnelled under the skin over the clavicle to emerge on the anterior chest wall
- Can be inserted in a semi-elective setting and used immediately, providing intermediate-term use until fistula created and useable

Arteriovenous fistula
- Connection between an artery and vein in the arm, formed surgically, as an elective procedure
- Requires 4–6 wks for vein to arterialize before it is ready to use

Indications for renal replacement therapy

- Risk of fetal toxicity from ↑ maternal urea
- Uraemic complications:
  - Pericarditis
  - Encephalopathy
- Poisoning with dialysable drug, e.g. ethylene glycol
- If refractory to medical therapy:
  - Fluid overload
  - Hyperkalaemia
  - Metabolic acidosis

Renal transplantation

Pre-conception

- Consider the underlying reason for the transplant
- Assess the associated comorbidities
- Advisable to delay conception until the ♀ has been in good health for 1 year (i.e. may be >1 year post procedure, if episodes of rejection have complicated post-transplantation course)
- Best outcomes are achieved 1 to 5 years post-transplantation with:
  - Well-controlled BP
  - No/minimal proteinuria and good renal function
  - No recent episodes of rejection
- Immunosuppressive regimens in pregnancy for renal transplantations use similar agents to other solid organ transplantations

⚠ MMF and sirolimus should not be used in pregnancy.

Maternal risks

- GH or pre-eclampsia
- Complications from immunosuppressive agents (e.g. hyperglycaemia)
- UTI
- Graft rejection risk unchanged from non-pregnant ♀
- Permanent ↓ in graft function can occur in some ♀, but this depends on pre-pregnancy graft function, hypertension, and proteinuria

Fetal risks

- Low birthweight babies
- Preterm delivery

Simultaneous pancreas–kidney transplant recipients

- If the pancreas is well functioning, expect normal glucose control
- Assess for complications of diabetes before pregnancy (e.g. retinopathy)
- May be ↑ HCO_3 loss if pancreas draining to bladder, so advisable to monitor HCO_3 levels throughout pregnancy in this setting

Pregnancy in renal transplant donor

- ♀ who have donated a kidney may be at ↑ risk of pre-eclampsia
- Offer aspirin 75 mg OD from 12 wks
- ↑ monitoring for pre-eclampsia throughout pregnancy

Management of renal transplantation in pregnancy

▶ Transplanted kidneys have a normal physiological response to pregnancy

Pre-pregnancy
- Consider the underlying reason for the transplantation
- Genetics referral if underlying cause was genetic such as polycystic kidney disease
- Review medications and convert to alternative agent if on MMF
- All ♀ must continue immunosuppressive medication
- If undergoing IVF, advise single embryo transfer

In pregnancy
- Regular antenatal review for renal function, symptoms or signs of pre-eclampsia, and therapeutic drug monitoring
- Early treatment of anaemia (avoid blood transfusion if possible)
- Urgent review if renal function ↓
- Regular fetal growth scans from 24 wks
- Screen for GDM (if on steroids/tacrolimus)
- Breastfeeding is not contraindicated in ♀ taking medications such as steroids, tacrolimus, azathioprine, and ciclosporin

Delivery
- Aim for vaginal delivery (caesarean section for obstetric indications)
- Parenteral hydrocortisone if on maintenance oral steroids

Transplant rejection
- Consider this diagnosis in any ♀ whose renal function is worsening (i.e. creatinine ↑ beyond pre-pregnancy values)

Transplantation medications

See Table 6.7.

Table 6.7 Transplantation medications and their use in pregnancy and breastfeeding

	Recommendations in pregnancy	Recommendations in breastfeeding

Steroids	• *Fluorinated steroids* (betamethasone, dexamethasone):
	  • Cross placenta readily thus preferred for fetal treatment (e.g. lung maturation prior to preterm delivery)
	• *Non-fluorinated steroids* (hydrocortisone, prednisolone):
	  • Do not cross placenta readily so fetal dose much smaller than maternal dose
	• *All steroids:*
	  • Can predispose to hyperglycaemia so glucose monitoring advised (either daily monitoring or GTT, depending on other risk factors and gestational age)
	  • If on for over 3 wks, then requires stress-dose steroids at delivery
		• Can be used as normal

Azathioprine	• Can be continued throughout pregnancy • TPMT genotype and enzyme activity level is advised in all individuals starting azathioprine	• Can be used as normal

Ciclosporin	• Can be continued throughout pregnancy:
	  • Can predispose to hyperglycaemia so glucose monitoring advised
	  • Levels may ↓ particularly in the 1st trimester so monitoring of trough levels is advised
		• Can be used as normal

Continued

Table 6.7 (Contd.)

	Recommendations in pregnancy	Recommendations in breastfeeding

Tacrolimus	• Can be continued throughout pregnancy:
	  • Can predispose to hyperglycaemia so glucose monitoring advised
	  • Levels may ↓ particularly in the 1st trimester so monitoring of trough levels is advised
		• Can be used in breastfeeding
		• Levels may ↑ after delivery so monitoring of trough levels should continue

Sirolimus	• Current advice is to avoid in pregnancy (based on animal studies)	• No data available so alternative agent preferred
Mycophenolate mofetil	• This is associated with miscarriage and congenital malformations so use in pregnancy is not advised (ideally stop 6–12 wks pre-conception and ensure stable disease prior to conception)	• Very limited information available so alternative agent preferred
Cyclophosphamide	• Causes an embryopathy if used in 1st trimester, but can be used later in pregnancy if required (under expert guidance)	• Very limited information available so alternative agent preferred if possible • Neutropenia reported in 2 infants whose mothers received cyclophosphamide postnatally

ACE-I	• ♀ with renal indication for treatment:
	  • If cycles regular and able to perform regular pregnancy tests (e.g. fortnightly), can be continued until a positive pregnancy test
	• ♀ with condition such as hypertension as only indication for use, where other alternatives are equally appropriate:
	  • Change to alternative agent if pregnancy planned
		• Enalapril and captopril can be used in breastfeeding

ARBs	• Less evidence available than for ACE-Is, but similar cautions advised	• Not recommended during breastfeeding

Renal biopsy in pregnancy

Background

- Rarely performed in pregnancy
- ↑ rate of complications in pregnancy compared to postnatally
- Bleeding complications occur most commonly if performed at 22–28 wks
- Only undertaken if the results will alter management

Examples of when renal biopsy may be appropriate in pregnancy

1st and 2nd trimester

- Early in pregnancy: diagnostic information would inform discussion about continuation of pregnancy and treatment
- Later in pregnancy: histological clarification of diagnosis which may alter immediate management prior to delivery
- Kidneys confirmed to be normal size on USS

Examples

- New diagnosis of nephrotic syndrome presenting at <20 wks
- Renal impairment and proteinuria in setting of systemic disease (excluding diabetes)/positive autoimmune serology

3rd trimester

- In most situations, delivery then postpartum renal biopsy is preferable

Nephrolithiasis (renal stones)

Background
- Common with ↑ age
- Often asymptomatic
- 80% consist of calcium, but can also be uric acid, struvite, or cystine
- Pregnancy does not alter the incidence, but the ↑ size of the gravid uterus can make it harder to pass stones later in pregnancy

Clinical features
- Can cause severe pain (loin pain) and other symptoms such as vomiting, dysuria, or frequency
- Can act as a nidus for infection so pyelonephritis is more common
- Urine dipstick often reveals non-visible (microscopic) haematuria

Management of renal stones in pregnancy

Imaging
- USS is preferred, however, small stones may be missed and physiological ureteric dilatation can be hard to distinguish from pathological obstruction
- Intravenous urogram (IVU) is infrequently performed in non-pregnant ♀ now due to the superiority of CT urogram, but a 'limited' IVU may be of use in pregnancy
- If further imaging is required, MRI is commonly used but can also miss small stones

⚠ CT urogram is usually not performed in pregnancy.

Infection
- Infection in an individual with renal stones should prompt urgent USS to check that the stone is not causing obstruction (an infected obstructed kidney requires emergency intervention, i.e. nephrostomy)

Treatment
- Depends on size and location:
  - Analgesia (NSAIDs are an option in 1st and 2nd trimester)
  - Encourage hydration—IV fluids if oral intake insufficient
  - Small stones are likely to be passed spontaneously but sometimes medication is given to aid this, such as nifedipine

Interventions
⚠ Usually only performed in pregnancy for infected, obstructed kidney.
- Ureteroscopic stone retrieval is preferred ± stone fragmentation with YAG laser (no ↑ in complications if performed in pregnancy)
- Percutaneous nephrostomy can be performed:
  - Ideally by experienced operator to minimize radiation exposure
- Ureteric stent can be considered (anterograde stent inserted via renal puncture, i.e. at time of nephrostomy; retrograde stent is inserted via cystoscopy)

⚠ Extra-corporeal lithotripsy is contraindicated in pregnancy due to concerning fetal effects in animal models.

Polycystic kidney disease

Background
- Autosomal dominant (ADPKD) or autosomal recessive condition
- Large cysts in the kidneys occur in association with a variety of extra-renal manifestations

Clinical features
- Renal manifestations include:
  - Mild concentrating defect
  - Nephrolithiasis in up to 25%
  - Haematuria
  - ↑ BP
  - Flank pain (can be related to size of cyst/s)
- Proteinuria is uncommon
- Cerebral aneurysms occur in:
  - ~5% of younger patients
  - ~10% of older patients
  - Those who have a family history at greatest risk

⚠ Aneurysm rupture is more common in ♀ with ADPKD than those with intracranial aneurysms and no ADPKD.

- Other extrarenal manifestations include:
  - Hepatic and pancreatic cysts
  - Cardiac valve lesions (most commonly aortic regurgitation and mitral valve prolapse)
  - Bowel diverticula (colon or duodenum)

Management of ADPKD in pregnancy
- Offer genetics counselling regarding risk of inheritance
- Aspirin 75 mg OD from 12 wks
- Close monitoring for UTI
- Close monitoring for development of pre-eclampsia
- Imaging of the fetal kidneys is not indicated

Nephrotic syndrome

Nephrotic syndrome
This is defined as proteinuria >3 g/day and hypoalbuminaemia.

Causes

1°
- Minimal change disease
- Focal segmental glomerulonephritis (1° or 2°, e.g. associated with HIV, IV drugs, obesity, infections such as parvovirus)
- Membranous glomerulonephritis

2°
- Diabetic nephropathy
- Amyloid
- SLE
- Pre-eclampsia

Complications
- VTE
- Hyperlipidaemia
- Infection
- Intravascular depletion

Management of nephrotic syndrome in pregnancy

In remission
- Regular assessment of proteinuria to ensure no relapse
- Continue immunosuppressive medication, e.g. steroids or tacrolimus

Ongoing/new nephrotic syndrome
- Assessment of proteinuria (new-onset proteinuria before 20 wks or significant ↑)
- Investigate for underlying cause:
  - Consider renal biopsy depending on gestation
- VTE prophylaxis if proteinuria >3 g/day (or PCR >300 mg/mmol)
- Treatment of underlying cause, e.g. steroids for minimal change disease

Other renal conditions

Reflux nephropathy

- Typically diagnosed and treated in childhood
- ↑ risk of asymptomatic and symptomatic bacteriuria
- ~50% chance of offspring developing the same condition:
  - Infant needs paediatric review if develops signs of infection
- ↑ risk of pre-eclampsia and low birthweight babies
- Aspirin 75 mg OD from 12 wks

Lupus nephritis

- Associated with significant morbidity
- Close monitoring to ensure early treatment if flare occurs
- Features overlap with those of pre-eclampsia making diagnosis in pregnancy more challenging
- Active nephritis is associated with poorer pregnancy outcomes
- Risk of a flare is not ↑ by pregnancy
- Renal biopsy may be warranted as early diagnosis and institution of correct treatment is important

Diabetic nephropathy

- Complication of poorly controlled and longstanding DM
- In ♀ of childbearing age the vast majority have T1DM
- Combination of T1DM and renal disease is associated with worse maternal and fetal outcomes, compared to ♀ with T1DM and no renal complications
- Pregnancy is associated with ↑ maternal anaemia:
  - Likely due to failure to ↑ production of erythropoietin, profound anaemia can ensue in the absence of iron or folate deficiency
  - Erythropoietin supplementation may be of benefit
- Pregnancy is associated with ↑ proteinuria:
  - Can be exacerbated by stopping ACE-I

IgA nephropathy

- Most common glomerulonephritis worldwide, causing slowly progressive CKD over decades
- Characterized by IgA deposits in the glomerulus
- Peak incidence in the 2nd and 3rd decades of life
- Most common cause of unexplained microscopic haematuria in pregnancy
- In ♀ with abnormal renal function there is an ↑ rate of pre-eclampsia, stillbirth, and risk of a decline in baseline function
- Aspirin 75 mg OD from 12 wks should be recommended to all ♀ with IgA nephropathy, irrespective of CKD stage

⚠ In rare cases of significant, resistant ↑ BP or renal decline, biopsy and treatment with immunosuppressive agents may be required in pregnancy, but otherwise a renal biopsy can be performed postnatally if renal function is abnormal or there is persistent proteinuria.

Renal tubular acidosis

Type 1 (distal) RTA

Causes
- Inherited
- Acquired:
  - Autoimmune
  - Toxins (e.g. amphotericin)
  - Nephrocalcinosis (1° hyperparathyroidism)
  - Obstructive nephropathy

Clinical features
- Hydrogen ion excretion in distal tubule is ↓:
  - Metabolic acidosis with normal anion gap
  - Can be associated with renal stone formation
- Bloods show:
  - Hyperchloraemia
  - HCO_3 <15 mmol/L
  - Normal or ↓ K^+
- Urine pH remains >5.5 in presence of acidaemia

> **Management of type 1 RTA in pregnancy**
> - Treatment is $NaHCO_3$ or sodium citrate
> - Potassium citrate can also be used for hypokalaemia
> - Citrate binds urinary Ca^{2+} and ↓ renal stone formation
> - Assess regularly for renal insufficiency and hypertension

Type 2 (proximal) RTA

Causes
- Inherited
- Fanconi syndrome:
  - Inherited/idiopathic
  - 2° to amyloid
- Renal disease associated with proximal tubule injury (cystinosis, medullary cystic disease)

Clinical features
- ↓ reabsorption of HCO_3 in proximal tubule:
  - Metabolic acidosis with normal anion gap
- Bloods show:
  - Hyperchloraemia
  - Hypophosphataemia
  - Hypokalaemia (normal or ↓)
  - HCO_3 >15 mmol/L
- Urine pH is inappropriately ↑ in presence of acidaemia

Management of type 2 RTA in pregnancy

- May worsen in pregnancy
- Symptoms relate to severe hypokalaemia
- May have complete biochemical resolution after delivery
- Treatment includes:
  - Addressing the underlying cause
  - $NaHCO_3$ and K^+ supplementation
  - Thiazide diuretic can also be used to ↑ HCO_3 reabsorption

Type 4 (hyperkalaemic) RTA

Causes

- Aldosterone deficiency:
  - 1° (causes: 1° adrenal insufficiency, congenital adrenal hyperplasia, aldosterone synthase deficiency)
  - 2° (causes: 2° adrenal insufficiency, diseases of the pituitary or hypothalamus)
- Aldosterone resistance:
  - Drugs including NSAIDs, mineralocorticoid receptor antagonists (eplerenone, spironolactone)
  - Pseudohypoaldosteronism

Clinical features

- ↓ secretion of K^+ and H^+ resulting from defective cation exchange in distal tubule:
  - Metabolic acidosis with a normal anion gap
- Bloods show:
  - Hyperchloraemia
  - HCO_3 >15 mmol/L
  - Hyperkalaemia
- Urine pH <5.5

Management of type 4 RTA in pregnancy

- $NaHCO_3$
- Fludrocortisone may also be required if aldosterone deficient
- Needs ↑ $NaHCO_3$ towards end of pregnancy (possibly due to progesterone opposing aldosterone activity)

Neurology

Epilepsy

Background

- One of the commonest medical conditions in ♀ of childbearing age
- Structural causes (space-occupying lesions, head injury, etc.) can result in epilepsy, however most cases are idiopathic
- Remains a significant cause of maternal mortality, mainly because of SUDEP (sudden unexpected death in epilepsy)
- Different types are outlined in Table 7.1

Table 7.1 Types of epilepsy

Generalized	
Absence (previously 'petit mal')	• Sudden ↓ in communication and impaired consciousness
Tonic–clonic (previously 'grand mal')	• Sudden impaired consciousness, muscle stiffening, and rhythmic muscle contractions, followed by postictal phase
Tonic	• Sudden muscle stiffening and impaired consciousness
Clonic	• Rhythmic jerking muscle contractions
Atonic	• Sudden loss of muscle control
Myoclonic	• Muscle contractions of any muscle group/s
Focal	
Focal seizures with awareness maintained (previously 'simple partial')	• Manifestations depend on the brain region affected
Focal seizures with impaired awareness (previously 'complex partial')	• Manifestations depend on the brain region affected, but this is associated with impaired responses and sometimes 'automatisms', e.g. chewing, lip smacking
Other	
Status epilepticus	• Repeated seizures without complete recovery in between, or 1 seizure of duration >5 mins
Non-epileptiform	• Episodes that lack the above features, often associated with no postictal phase or involuntary behaviours (tongue biting, urinary incontinence)

Management of a seizure

- Call for help
- Initial assessment (ABC)
- Left lateral tilt if antenatal and >18 wks
- Medical assessment to confirm suspicion of seizure
- Check blood glucose
- If eclampsia is suspected:
  - 4 g IV magnesium sulfate by slow IV bolus (5–10 mins) then maintenance infusion (if anuric, give loading dose only)
  - Control BP
- Seizure in ♀ with epilepsy without evidence of eclampsia:
  - Benzodiazepine: lorazepam 4 mg IV (1st line), or if not available, diazepam 5 mg IV or 5–10 mg rectally
  - Repeat dose after 10–20 mins if seizure ongoing
  - If this fails, IV agent such as phenytoin or levetiracetam
  - If refractory to treatment, needs general anaesthesia and consideration of delivery

Differential diagnosis of 1st seizure in pregnancy

- Eclampsia
- Epilepsy
- Metabolic (e.g. alcohol withdrawal)
- Hypoglycaemia
- Hyponatraemia
- Hypocalcaemia (e.g. Mg^{2+} therapy)
- Cerebral venous sinus thrombosis
- Thrombotic thrombocytopenic purpura
- Ischaemic stroke
- Intracranial haemorrhage
- Space-occupying lesion
- Infection:
  - Viral encephalitis, most commonly HSV
  - Bacterial meningitis
  - Intracranial abscess

➔ Useful resources:
🔗 https://www.womenwithepilepsy.co.uk and
🔗 https://www.epilepsyandpregnancy.co.uk

➔ MBRRACE-UK. 2017 report: 🔗 https://www.npeu.ox.ac.uk/mbrrace-uk/reports/confidential-enquiry-into-maternal-deaths

Antiepileptic drugs

- AEDs are associated with teratogenicity, which varies with:
  - Type of AED (Table 7.2)
  - Number of AEDs being taken
  - Doses of each AED
- Newer agents such as lamotrigine and levetiracetam are preferred to older agents such as valproate and phenytoin:
  - Better maternal side effect profile
  - ↓ rates of teratogenicity
- Typical malformations include:
  - Neural tube defects
  - Genitourinary abnormalities
  - Cardiac anomalies (especially phenytoin and phenobarbitone)
  - Facial clefts (phenytoin, carbamazepine)
- Developmental delay and behavioural problems can also occur:

▶ This may be ↓ by folic acid 5 mg OD prior to conception and antenatally

Table 7.2 Antiepileptic drugs

Enzyme-inducing AEDs	
Carbamazepine Oxcarbamazepine Primidone Phenytoin Topiramate	• No evidence supporting routine prescription of vitamin K to mothers in 3rd trimester • Neonates should be offered 1 mg IM vitamin K at birth • Potentially ↓ efficacy of oral contraceptives, including the emergency contraceptive; copper IUD preferred
Non-enzyme-inducing AEDs	
Lamotrigine	• Levels can fall dramatically during pregnancy, but this can also occur when taken alongside an oestrogen-containing contraceptive
Levetiracetam	• Levels may ↓ in pregnancy but to a lesser extent than lamotrigine
Gabapentin	• No specific issues
Pregabalin	• No specific issues
Sodium valproate	• Avoid if possible in ♀ of childbearing age • If no alternative, consider MR preparation, in divided doses to ↓ peak blood concentration
Clobazam/clonazepam	• Not teratogenic • Can be sedating for mother and also neonate, potentially contributing to respiratory depression, if taken in large doses while mother is in labour or breastfeeding

Epilepsy in pregnancy

- Pregnancy can → ↑ seizures as a result of:
  - Cessation of AEDs because of concern about safety of medication in pregnancy
  - Vomiting → ↓ absorption of AEDs
  - Pregnancy-related changes in pharmacokinetics → ↓ circulating levels of AEDs
  - Sleep deprivation
- ↑ seizure frequency most likely in ♀:
  - Who had seizures in the year prior to conception
  - Who were poorly controlled prior to pregnancy
  - Who stop their AEDs
- Focal seizures, or tonic–clonic seizures of short duration, are unlikely to result in significant placental under-perfusion
- 2/3 of ♀ will **not** have ↑ seizure frequency
- 1–2% incidence of seizures in labour

Epilepsy management: pre-pregnancy

- Confirm diagnosis with neurologist
- Use lowest effective dose of the most appropriate AED
- Consider ↓ number of AEDs (↑ risk of congenital anomalies with polytherapy)
- Start folic acid 5 mg OD:
  - ↑ cognitive outcomes in offspring exposed to AEDs
  - ↓ in neural tube defects

Valproate and pregnancy

⚠ All ♀ of childbearing age taking valproate should be made aware of the complications that can result from valproate use in pregnancy.
- Consideration of switching to an alternative AED should occur in all ♀ on valproate
- Only if no alternative is appropriate, should valproate be continued and in that case, divided doses may → a ↓ in peak blood levels

---

➲ Advice for women with epilepsy: ℜ https://www.epilepsy.org.uk/sites/epilepsy/files/Looking_after_baby_or_small_child_when_you_have_epilepsy.pdf

➲ NICE (2012, updated 2018). Epilepsies: diagnosis and management (CG137): ℜ https://www.nice.org.uk/guidance/cg137

➲ RCOG (2016). Epilepsy in pregnancy (green-top guideline no. 68): ℜ https://www.rcog.org.uk/en/guidelines-research-services/guidelines/gtg68/

Epilepsy management: antenatal

- Folic acid 5 mg OD until at least 12 wks
- General safety advice (e.g. showers rather than baths)
- Continue AEDs and review doses regularly:
  - Lamotrigine levels ↓ significantly so a dose ↑ is often needed
  - Levetiracetam does not usually need to be ↑
- Routine drug level monitoring is **not** recommended but may help:
  - If ↑ seizure frequency
  - To ensure no toxicity after a dose ↑
- Serial fetal scans are advocated looking for growth restriction
- Insufficient evidence to support routine maternal vitamin K before delivery to ↓ haemorrhagic disease of the newborn or maternal PPH
⚠ Be aware of the potential for other medication to alter AED levels, e.g. some antibiotics
- Anaesthetic referral is warranted for all ♀ with epilepsy
- Delivery in a consultant-led unit is advised

Epilepsy management: delivery

▶ Not an indication for induction of labour or elective caesarean section
- No need to change the corticosteroid dose for fetal lung maturation even if taking enzyme-inducing AEDs
- Risk of a seizure at delivery is low, but measures to ↓ precipitants, e.g. avoidance of sleep deprivation, are sensible
- Not to be in a single room unsupervised
- All babies born to ♀ on enzyme-inducing AEDs should be offered 1 mg IM vitamin K
- If deemed at very high risk for a seizure at delivery, clobazam can be given, e.g. 5–10 mg one-off dose in labour, or 5–10 mg pre and post delivery

⚠ Pethidine should be avoided as this may ↓ seizure threshold.

Epilepsy management: postpartum

- Breastfeeding is encouraged
- Doses of AEDs need ↓ to pre-pregnancy doses
- Discussion about contraception:
  - Potential ↓ efficacy of hormonal contraceptives if on enzyme-inducing AEDs
  - All methods of contraception can be used with non-enzyme-inducing AEDs
- Advice about safety at home and caring for newborn includes:
  - Nappy changing on the floor rather than a high table
  - Co-sleeping discouraged
  - Bathing baby in shallow water with supervision available

➔ Advice for women with epilepsy: ⌖ https://www.epilepsy.org.uk/sites/epilepsy/files/Looking_after_baby_or_small_child_when_you_have_epilepsy.pdf

Ischaemic stroke

Background

- Impairment of blood supply to a specific region of the brain, resulting in sudden abnormal neurological symptoms and signs
- Ischaemic stroke occurs most commonly as a result of a thromboembolic event in ♀ of childbearing age, but can also occur as a result of stenosis or small vessel disease
- Rare in ♀ of reproductive age
- ↑ risk if vascular risk factors present (smoking, DM, ↑ BP, hypercholesterolaemia, family history of vascular disease)
- The younger the stroke, the more likely it is to be 'cryptogenic' (no cause found) or occur in the presence of an underlying condition
- Typical presentation is an abrupt onset of neurological symptoms including speech disturbance, weakness, or sensory disturbance in a pattern that fits with a central rather than peripheral lesion
- 'Transient ischaemic attack' (TIA) is used to describe symptoms consistent with ischaemia that resolve rapidly and completely
- Ischaemic changes may be evident on a plain CT, but MRI, in particular MRI using diffusion-weighted sequences, is more sensitive for acute ischaemic changes

---

Pregnant ♀ with a previous ischaemic stroke

- Risk of recurrence in pregnancy is very low, even if the previous stroke occurred in pregnancy
- 75 mg aspirin OD is advisable
- Anticoagulation is not required unless other indications

Pregnant ♀ with an ischaemic stroke in pregnancy

- Antiplatelet therapy is recommended as outside pregnancy:
  - Aspirin 300 mg OD for 2 wks (advised in NICE guidelines)
  - Followed by a lower-dose antiplatelet agent (often clopidogrel)

⚠ In the 3rd trimester, use of high-dose aspirin (i.e. 300 mg OD) can cause premature closure of the ductus arteriosus, so clopidogrel can be used as an alternative in the event of an acute stroke.

Investigations

- ECG
- Echocardiogram
- Consider a bubble study to look for a PFO
- Autoantibodies (including antiphospholipid and ANA) if vasculitis or other inflammatory condition is suspected

⚠ ↑ risk of ischaemic stroke persists for several weeks postpartum so antiplatelets should be continued for at least 3 months after delivery

⚠ Prophylactic LMWH is not advised in the 1st 2 wks following an ischaemic stroke so mechanical measures such as compression stockings or Flowtron® boots should be used.

Interventions for acute stroke

Systemic thrombolysis

- Alteplase can be used for thrombolysis of acute ischaemic stroke if strict criteria are met, including:
  - Time of onset <3 hrs
  - The patient does not have any of the standard exclusion criteria
- Small case series show no ↑ in intracranial haemorrhage compared to a non-pregnant population.
- The decision to thrombolyse for an acute ischaemic stroke in the 1st few days postpartum is difficult and should be individualized, based on the nature of delivery and pre-existing complications.

⚠ Pregnancy is a 'relative exclusion criterion' in 2016 American Heart Association guidelines, where they advise thrombolysis for moderate to severe ischaemic stroke when the benefit justifies the potential risk to the fetus and potential risk of uterine bleeding.

Thrombectomy

In many large centres this is now a treatment option for acute stroke. Pregnancy is not a contraindication for this procedure but only a small number of cases of mechanical clot retrieval in pregnancy have been reported.

Causes of ischaemic stroke in pregnancy

- Pre-eclampsia/eclampsia
- Central nervous system vasculitis
- Carotid artery dissection
- Emboli:
  - Mitral stenosis
  - Peripartum cardiomyopathy
  - Endocarditis
  - Paradoxical emboli, i.e. from PFO or ASD
  - Arrhythmia
- Coagulopathies:
  - Thrombophilia
  - Antiphospholipid syndrome
  - Myeloproliferative disorders
- TTP
- Venous infarct 2° to venous sinus thrombosis
- Sickle cell disease

⊃ Charity for younger stroke survivors: ℘ https://differentstrokes.co.uk/

⊃ The Stroke Association: ℘ https://www.stroke.org.uk/

Transient ischaemic attack

- Careful history and examination
- Consideration of other causes of transient abnormal neurology (Box 7.1)
- Highest risk period for recurrence is the 2 wks after the 1st episode
- Neuroimaging should be performed urgently, ideally an MRI:
  - Frequency of MRI abnormalities varies with duration of the episode and anatomical location
  - Normal imaging does not exclude an ischaemic cause of the symptoms
- Treatment with antiplatelet therapy should be commenced:
  - Before imaging if symptoms have resolved
  - As soon as a haemorrhage is excluded by imaging if symptoms not resolved before imaging can be performed

---

Box 7.1 Differential diagnosis for transient abnormal neurology
- Syncope (vasovagal or cardiogenic)
- Migraine
- Transient ischaemic attack
- Seizure
- Non-epileptic attack
- Anxiety and hyperventilation

Intracranial haemorrhage

Intracranial haemorrhage includes bleeding in several anatomical locations. The term 'haemorrhagic stroke' is often used in the presence of bleeding and neurological sequelae; however, this can be confusing, so for clarity, the anatomical classification will be used.

Extradural

- Most commonly the result of trauma, usually in association with a skull fracture, and classically involves the middle meningeal artery
- Appears as a lentiform or biconvex haemorrhage on CT or MRI
- Is often associated with mass effect, but is limited by cranial sutures
- Surgical decompression is often required

⚠ Pregnancy should not alter investigation or management.

Subdural

- In young people, acute subdural haemorrhage usually results from trauma (compared to an older population where chronic subdural haematoma can occur for other reasons)
- Typically crescentic in shape
- Not limited by cranial sutures
- Has been associated with epidural and spinal anaesthesia, thought to be caused by low CSF pressures which stretch and damage bridging vessels between the cerebral cortex and venous sinuses

⚠ Pregnancy should not alter investigation or management.

Intracerebral

- Intracerebral haemorrhage involves the cerebral cortex and can be caused by both traumatic and non-traumatic causes

Causes of a non-traumatic intracerebral haemorrhage

- Hypertension and hypertensive disorders of pregnancy
- Arteriovenous malformations
- Haemorrhagic infarction (e.g. from venous sinus thrombosis)
- Brain tumours
- Drugs (cocaine, amphetamines)
- Bleeding diatheses
- Vasculitis
- Moyamoya
- Cerebral amyloid angiopathy (in older population)

Subarachnoid haemorrhage

- Typically presents with a 'thunderclap' headache which may be associated with vomiting
- Focal neurological symptoms may be present if intracerebral haemorrhage is also present
- Commonest cause is the rupture of an intracranial aneurysm
- Non-aneurysmal SAH can occur in other conditions including RCVS (➔ see p. 234)
- Blood is seen in the subarachnoid space on CT scan
- CT is sensitive for the presence of acute SAH (98% within 12 hrs, but only 50% 1 wk later)
- To exclude the diagnosis, a LP is recommended to look for presence of blood degradation products (➔ see 'Lumbar puncture for the diagnosis of SAH', p. 232)

Management of a SAH

If diagnosis is proven on CT ± LP:
- Maintain good hydration status
- Nimodipine 60 mg every 4 hrs (to prevent vasospasm)
- Intracranial angiogram (to identify aneurysm)
- Curative procedure directed at the identified cause, e.g. aneurysm clipping or coiling

▶ This may involve fetal exposure to radiation but pregnancy is not a contraindication to this being performed if indicated.

Management of a pregnant ♀ with a history of SAH

- If coiled/clipped and there is no associated underlying condition, they can be treated as normal
- No need for routine imaging unless an underlying condition is present which would predispose to further aneurysm formation
- Untreated aneurysm identified before or in pregnancy, the decision to intervene would depend on factors such as location, size, etc.
- It is advisable to avoid:
  - Home birth
  - Prolonged labour
  - Repeated Valsalva manoeuvres (e.g. pushing)

▶ This is not an absolute indication for caesarean section.

Pregnant ♀ with conditions associated with intracranial aneurysms (but no personal history of SAH)

- Screening not routinely indicated in pregnancy but if deemed at very high risk this can be performed

Lumbar puncture for the diagnosis of SAH

- Xanthochromia is bilirubin from lysed red blood cells:
  - ∴ LP should only be performed >12 hrs after onset of the headache or can be falsely negative
  - Can remain positive for up to 14 days after an SAH

Interpreting the results

- Raised oxyhaemoglobin and bilirubin: diagnostic of SAH
- Raised bilirubin only: not certain diagnosis of SAH as can occur with ↑ CSF protein or ↑ serum bilirubin
- False positives can occur with:
  - Repeated LP sampling alone
  - ↑ CSF protein
  - ↑ serum bilirubin in combination with traumatic LP
- False negatives can occur if:
  - LP is <12 hrs after onset of symptoms
  - Sample is exposed to light
  - There is a delay in processing of the sample

Arteriovenous malformations

- AVMs make up a greater proportion of the cases of intracranial haemorrhage in pregnant compared to non-pregnant ♀
- May be the result of hormonal changes, ↑ vasodilation, and ↑ tendency to bleed
- In some cases, an underlying condition is identified, e.g. hereditary haemorrhagic telangiectasia

Management with known AVM and no evidence of bleeding

- Previously treated AVM: It is advisable to avoid prolonged labour and home birth but can otherwise be treated as normal

Bleed from AVM in pregnancy

- Pregnancy is not a contraindication to embolization but stereotactic surgery should wait until after delivery
- Tight BP control
- Mode of delivery depends on the individual and their pregnancy history, but either a vaginal delivery with a passive descent or a caesarean section would be appropriate

Screening in asymptomatic ♀ with a related condition (e.g. hereditary haemorrhagic telangiectasia)

- Routine screening in asymptomatic ♀ is not required
- These ♀ often have MRI of their spine to assess for AVMs before regional anaesthesia so cranial imaging can be performed at the same time

Reversible cerebral vasoconstriction syndromes

Background
- Group of conditions characterized by reversible multifocal cerebral arterial narrowing which can cause a variety of symptoms including thunderclap headache and focal neurological deficits
- SAH occurs in about 30%
- These include conditions previously known as:
  - Migrainous vasospasm
  - Postpartum cerebral angiopathy
  - Drug-induced arteritis
- Features may overlap with that of SAH resulting from an aneurysm rupture, but the vasoconstriction in RCVS tends to be widespread and symmetrical, which may aid diagnosis
- It can also be challenging in some cases to distinguish RCVS from a 1° cerebral vasculitis, however the following criteria are highly specific and helpful for distinguishing from vasculitis:
  - Recurrent thunderclap headache, **or**
  - Single thunderclap headache with either a normal MRI or evidence of border zone infarcts or vasogenic oedema, **or**
  - No thunderclap headache but abnormal angiography and no brain lesions

Pregnancy-associated RCVS
- The majority of the ♀ who develop this, develop it in the 1st wk postpartum and then the changes resolve within 12 wks
- Recurrence is very rare

Management of RCVS in pregnancy
There is no proven treatment for this, so treatment is generally supportive:
- Avoidance of dehydration
- Analgesia
- Ca^{2+} channel blockers such as nimodipine (may ↓ symptoms but do not appear to influence resolution of the angiographic abnormalities)

Cervical artery dissection

Background

- This refers to any dissection affecting the intracranial or extracranial carotid arteries, or vertebral arteries
- Disruption of the arterial wall → dissection, and this can result in under-perfusion of tissues supplied by that vessel or distant thromboembolism
- In addition, dissection of intracranial vessels can result in vessel rupture causing a SAH
- Neurological symptoms can develop, which depend on the anatomical location of the lesion, e.g.:
  - Horner's syndrome (sympathetic pathway damage which results in a small pupil, partial ptosis, and anhidrosis on the side of the lesion) from an extracranial carotid artery dissection
  - Hypoglossal nerve palsy and other brainstem signs from a vertebral artery dissection

---

Causes of cervical artery dissection

- Minor trauma is thought to be the cause in many cases with different sports being associated
- Underlying connective tissue disease or vascular disorder:
  - Fibromuscular dysplasia
  - Ehlers–Danlos syndrome type IV
  - Marfan syndrome
  - Loeys–Dietz syndrome
  - RCVS

Management of a pregnant ♀ with previous cervical artery dissection

- Ensure aware of signs and symptoms of vascular dissection
- Ensure knows to seek medical advice urgently if any concerns
- Single antiplatelet agent throughout pregnancy
- Good BP control

Management of cervical artery dissection in pregnancy

- Pregnancy ↑ the risk of vessel dissection. This risk persists for several weeks postnatally
- Acute ischaemic symptoms and **extracranial** dissection:
  - Antiplatelet therapy is advised
  - Anticoagulation with LMWH may be advised
- Acute ischaemic symptoms and **intracranial** dissection:
  - Antiplatelet therapy is advised
  - Anticoagulation is often avoided due to the risk of SAH
- No ischaemic symptoms and **extracranial** dissection:
  - Antiplatelet therapy is advised
- If SAH is present, to be managed as per SAH advice (➔ see p. 231)

⚠ Dissection is not a contraindication to thrombolysis for an acute ischaemic stroke if otherwise indicated

💣 There is no consensus on the optimum antiplatelet regimen

⚠ It is not an indication for caesarean section

⚠ Ensure optimal BP control throughout pregnancy and the postpartum period to avoid worsening of the dissection

Cerebral venous sinus thrombosis

Background
- As with other types of VTE, changes in coagulation parameters seen in pregnancy and postpartum ↑ the risk of CVST
- Incidence in pregnancy and postnatally ranges from 1:2500 to 1:10,000 pregnancies
- Can present in a variety of ways and can be difficult to diagnose
- Thromboprophylaxis should be given to all pregnant ♀ with a previous CVST

Clinical features

Symptoms
- Headache which can be:
  - Gradual in onset
  - Sudden 'thunderclap'
  - Like migraine with aura
- Symptoms of ↑ intracranial pressure:
  - Headache worse on bending over
  - Headache worse in the mornings
- Confusion
- Focal neurological symptoms
- Seizures

Signs
- Papilloedema on fundoscopy
- Focal neurological deficits

Management of CVST in pregnancy
- This condition requires therapeutic anticoagulation with LMWH, even if there is associated haemorrhage
- Requires MDT care with neurosurgical input for those ♀ with progressive deterioration despite pharmacological treatment

Moyamoya

Background

- A progressive cerebral vasculopathy, which results in stenosis and occlusion of the vessels of the circle of Willis, and development of collaterals
- More common in Japan and Asia than in Europe and the USA
- 'Moyamoya' means 'puff of smoke' in Japanese and describes the appearance of the tangle of tiny vessels formed to compensate
- Can result in ischaemia or intracranial haemorrhage
- 4 types have been defined by the Ministry of Health and Welfare in Japan:
  - Ischaemic
  - Haemorrhagic
  - Epileptic
  - Other
- Some ♀ undergo extracranial–intracranial bypass
- If diagnosed before pregnancy, it appears to be associated with good outcomes
- If diagnosed in pregnancy, e.g. in the setting of pre-eclampsia or eclampsia, there appears to be ↑ maternal morbidity and mortality
- These ♀ are likely to be sensitive to changes in BP (both ↑ and ↓) as cerebral autoregulation may be impaired, particularly in ♀ with previous bypass surgery

Management of moyamoya in pregnancy

- Good BP control
- Aspirin 75 mg OD
- Caesarean section is frequently chosen in published case reports but vaginal delivery has also been described
- Maintenance of haemodynamic stability (avoidance of ↓ BP, ↑ BP, and hypocapnia) by good pain control, cautious use of fluids, and avoidance of Valsalva
- Epidural anaesthesia preferred to general anaesthesia

➥ Information for healthcare professionals regarding moyamoya: ℛ https://rarediseases.org/rare-diseases/moyamoya-disease/

➥ Information for people diagnosed with moyamoya: ℛ http://www.moyamoya.com/

Myasthenia gravis

Background

- Antibody-mediated condition, where antibodies to the nicotinic acetylcholine receptors (nAChR) or, less commonly, other post-synaptic antigens including muscle-specific receptor kinase (MuSK) at the neuromuscular junction cause dysfunction
- Results in weakness and fatigability
- Affects more ♀ than ♂ (occurs at a younger average age in ♀)
- 75% present with ocular features, which then progress to involve bulbar muscles, then proximal limbs then respiratory muscles
- 75% then develop generalized disease
- AChR antibodies are present in 80–90% of patients with myasthenia
- 40–70% of the remainder have MuSK antibodies
- 'Seronegative' myasthenia gravis has been associated with:
  - LRP4 antibodies (a receptor which is part of the MuSK complex)
  - Cortactin antibodies (a protein involved in AChR clustering at the neuromuscular junction)

Treatment options

- Anticholinesterases:
  - Pyridostigmine
  - Neostigmine (used in the now rarely performed Tensilon® test)
- Immunosuppression:
  - Corticosteroids
  - Azathioprine
  - MMF (not in pregnancy)
  - Methotrexate (not in pregnancy)
- Thymectomy is often advised if AChR antibody positive
- IVIg
- Plasma exchange:
  - Benefit within days
  - Effect only lasts for 6–8 wks

Medications that can worsen myasthenia gravis

Anaesthetic agents
- Neuromuscular blockers

Antibiotics
- Aminoglycosides such as gentamicin
- Clindamycin
- Fluoroquinolones such as ciprofloxacin, levofloxacin
- Vancomycin

Cardiac
- β blockers such as labetalol and metoprolol
- Procainamide
- Quinidine

Other
- Magnesium
- Hydroxychloroquine
- Penicillamine
- Quinine

⚠ Magnesium for seizure prophylaxis in pre-eclampsia should be avoided, but can be used with close monitoring if an eclamptic seizure occurs

● Information for patients on myasthenia and pregnancy: ℅ https://www.myaware.org/myasthenia-and-pregnancy

● Norwood F, Dhanjal M, Hill M, et al. Myasthenia in pregnancy: best practice guidelines from a UK multispecialty working group. *J Neurol Neurosurg Psychiatry* 2014;85:538–43.

Myasthenia gravis: pregnancy

Pregnancy

- Good outcomes if disease is well controlled, and no modification to medications is required
- Previous thymectomy associated with a ↓ in complications in pregnancy so if indicated, should be performed before conception
- MDT involvement is very important in these ♀
- May be stable or improve during pregnancy but may worsen after delivery

Management of myasthenia gravis in pregnancy

⚠ Do not make changes to medications without specialist input.

- Coexistent autoimmune conditions should be looked for especially thyroid disease
- Avoid medications such as labetalol that can worsen MG
- ♀ should be advised to monitor fetal movements after 24 wks
- Fetal growth scans are advised
- If on steroid treatment, an oral GTT or blood glucose monitoring is advised
- Careful monitoring for infection
- ↑ doses of anticholinesterases may be required, guided by symptoms

Delivery

- Aim is to facilitate spontaneous labour and vaginal delivery at term
- Should be in hospital with access to critical care support for both mother and infant
- Paediatrician present at time of delivery
- Epidural analgesia and anaesthesia may ↓ maternal fatigue
- Stress-dose steroids if indicated
- Patients should be aware of the potential need for respiratory support on intensive care after delivery
- Breastfeeding should be encouraged
- Period of neonatal monitoring for at least 2 days, longer may be advisable

Anaesthesia in myasthenia

- Normal medication should be continued
- Entonox® can be used as normal
- Opioids may worsen respiratory depression so should be avoided

⚠ General anaesthesia should be avoided if at all possible because of the sensitivity to muscle relaxants

Myasthenia gravis: neonatal effects

Transient neonatal myasthenia gravis
- Occurs in up to 30% of babies of mothers with myasthenia gravis
- Results from transplacental transfer of the IgG antibodies
- Poor correlation between maternal disease activity and likelihood of neonatal myasthenia gravis
- Can present from hours to a week after delivery
- If anti-AChR antibodies are present the neonate can present with:
  - Ptosis
  - Generalized weakness
  - ↓ tone
  - Respiratory compromise
- Anti-MuSK antibodies are associated with a more severe form, but this is less common
- May be self-limiting, but can require treatment including:
  - Pyridostigmine
  - IVIg
  - Plasma exchange

Arthrogryposis multiplex congenita
- Congenital condition resulting in multiple joint contractures
- Can occur with a high level of maternal antibodies to a specific fetal subunit of the AChR
- Mothers may have few or no symptoms of myasthenia gravis and in some cases are only diagnosed after the fetal abnormalities occur

Fetal acetylcholine receptor inactivation syndrome
- Recently described
- Milder phenotype of congenital abnormalities than arthrogryposis
- Compatible with life but may leave the child with residual deficits such as velopharyngeal myopathy
- Thought to result from antibodies against the fetal AChR causing receptor blockade at a specific point in fetal development

Myotonic dystrophy

Background

- Muscle disorder featuring impaired muscle relaxation, also known as dystrophia myotonica
- Autosomal dominant
- 2 types known as DM1 and DM2
- Involving expansion of:
  - CTG triplet repeats in the dystrophia myotonica protein kinase (*DMPK*) gene on chromosome 19 (DM1)
  - CCTG repeats in the *CNBP* gene on chromosome 3 (DM2—milder phenotype)
  - The manifestation depends on the number of triplet repeats

Clinical features

- Diagnosis is made on:
  - Typical clinical features
    And
  - Confirmatory genetic testing
- Electromyography may be of use if features overlap with other muscle disorders

---

Typical clinical features of myotonic dystrophy

Neurological/ophthalmological

- Myotonia
- Muscle weakness:
  - DM1—typically involves facial muscles → a typical facial appearance, forearms
  - DM2—typically involves fingers and neck
- Cataracts
- Cognitive impairment

Cardiac

- Cardiomyopathy
- Arrhythmias

Respiratory

- Type 2 respiratory failure from muscle weakness (DM1, rare in DM2)
- Can be worsened by sedatives

Gastrointestinal

- Dysphagia (aspiration risk)
- Gallstones

Management of myotonic dystrophy in pregnancy
Pre-pregnancy
- Genetic counselling about the autosomal dominant inheritance, with consideration of pre-implantation genetic diagnosis with IVF
- Cardiac assessment:
  - Echocardiogram
  - ECG
- Respiratory assessment:
  - Lung function tests
- Metabolic:
  - GTT/HbA1c
- Assess functional limitations

During pregnancy
- Genetic counselling about the autosomal dominant inheritance, with consideration of cell-free fetal DNA testing
- Cardiac assessment:
  - Echocardiogram
  - ECG
- Respiratory assessment:
  - Lung function tests
- Early GTT
- Assess functional limitations (contractures, deformity, etc.) and consideration of supportive intervention such as physiotherapy
- Regular review to monitor cardiac and respiratory function
- Uterine contraction can be affected, which can manifest as:
  - Preterm delivery
  - 2nd trimester pregnancy loss
  - PPH
  - Failure to progress in labour, resulting in caesarean section or instrumental delivery
- Case series have reported an ↑ miscarriage rate
- Polyhydramnios occurs in up to 25% and may be suggestive of an affected fetus
- Anaesthetic review given issues with medications used in general anaesthesia and opioid sensitivity; MRI may be required if skeletal deformity

⚠ Pregnancy is associated with a worsening of maternal symptoms, which do not always return to pre-pregnancy levels after delivery

⚠ Risk of more severe disease in offspring even if maternal disease is mild due to anticipation (↑ number of triplet repeats)

⮕ Information for patients and healthcare professionals: ℅ https://www.mda.org/disease/myotonic-dystrophy

Multiple sclerosis

Background
- Common demyelinating inflammatory condition affecting the brain and spinal cord
- Most cases are diagnosed between the ages of 20 and 45 yrs
- More ♀ are affected than ♂

Clinical features
- Diagnosis is based on clinical events or imaging changes consistent with demyelination that are disseminated in space and/or time
- History and examination consistent with demyelination-specific neurological symptoms such as numbness or weakness in limbs, with examination findings of an upper motor neuron pattern
- Imaging, i.e. with MRI evidence of lesion/s
- LP for oligoclonal bands may aid diagnosis but is rarely required
- Somatosensory and visual evoked potentials (SSEPs/VEPs) may also be useful

Pregnancy
- Does not ↑ the chances of future long-term disability
- Pregnancy does not ↑ the risk of a relapse
- Tends to improve, but 25% will deteriorate postnatally
- Association of ↓ birth weight and ↑ incidence of operative delivery
- Treatment should not be delayed until a woman has completed her family

Management of MS in pregnancy
- See Table 7.3
- Vitamin D supplements are advised
- Relapse can be treated with methylprednisolone as normal (after infection excluded), may need plasma exchange if very severe
- Epidural or diazepam in labour may help with spasticity
- MS is not a contraindication to vaginal delivery
- Elective caesarean section may be warranted in the minority who are functionally very limited
- Vigilance for development of UTI as this can worsen symptoms
- ♀ with sensory loss below T11 may not experience labour pain, so other signs of labour should be discussed
- Autonomic dysreflexia may mimic pre-eclampsia in ♀ with severe spinal cord disease
- Awareness of the ↑ incidence of postpartum depression in these ♀

➲ Dobson R, Dassan P, Roberts M, et al. UK consensus on pregnancy in multiple sclerosis: 'Association of British Neurologists' guidelines. *Pract Neurol* 2019;19:106–14. ➲ Source of information including advice regarding pregnancy: ℘ https://www.mssociety.org.uk/

Table 7.3 Treatments for MS in pregnancy

Drug	Issues
Interferon β	• Often discontinued in pregnancy • No adverse outcomes associated, continue if required • Safe with breastfeeding
Glatiramer	• No association with adverse fetal outcomes • No information about use in breastfeeding
Natalizumab	• High risk of rebound if stopped • Can be used in pregnancy until about 34 wks • Some advocate administration every 8 wks in pregnancy • Continue routine monitoring for JC virus (with LPs) and progressive multifocal leucoencephalopathy (with MRI) during pregnancy
Alemtuzumab	• No clear association with teratogenicity or adverse fetal outcomes, but some advocate a 4 mth washout prior to conception • Irradiated blood products advised for ♀ who have received alemtuzumab • Monitor for autoimmune disease in pregnancy • Not to be used while breastfeeding
Fingolimod	• Possible association with developmental abnormalities so effective contraception is advised while on fingolimod and for 2 mths after cessation • Breastfeeding contraindicated
Teriflunomide	• Teratogenic in animal models at human equivalent doses • Very long enterohepatic circulation time, so ♀ planning to conceive should undergo an 'accelerated elimination procedure' or use effective contraception for 2 years • Breastfeeding contraindicated
Dimethyl fumarate	• GI side effects on commencing treatment may affect absorption of oral contraceptive agents • Use in pregnancy and lactation not advised (lack of data)
Ocrelizumab	• Humanized monoclonal IgG antibody • No data about B-cell depletion in neonates so contraception advised while taking ocrelizumab and for 12 mths after cessation • Breastfeeding not advised
Cladribine	• Inhibits DNA synthesis and repair and is embryotoxic and teratogenic in animal studies • Barrier contraception advised during treatment and for at least 4 wks after the last dose • Advised to avoid pregnancy for at least 6 months after a treatment course • Avoidance of breastfeeding advised during treatment and for 1 wk after the last dose • Irradiated blood products advised

Neuromyelitis optica

Background

- Results from antibodies to aquaporin 4 water channel proteins, which are mainly expressed in the optic nerve and spinal cord
- Mean age of onset is about 40 yrs
- Affects more ♀ than ♂
- Up to 60% have other autoantibodies
- Treatment options include immunosuppressive agents such as:
  - Rituximab
  - Azathioprine
  - Immunoglobulins

Clinical features

- Characterized by:
  - Optic neuritis (unilateral or bilateral pain and/or visual deficit)
  - Transverse myelitis (inflammation of the spinal cord that can be partial or complete, and results in severe pain and neurological deficit)
- Up to 30% have other autoimmune disease
- 25% have several autoimmune diseases, e.g. Sjögren's syndrome, SLE

Management of NMO in pregnancy

- Can present for the 1st time in pregnancy
- The risk of relapse ↓ during pregnancy, but ↑ towards term
- High risk of relapse after delivery
- Annual relapse rate appears to be ↑ by a pregnancy
- NMO appears to ↑ miscarriage rate if conception soon after disease onset or higher disease activity
- An ↑ risk of pre-eclampsia, which is strongly associated with the presence of other autoimmune conditions

⊋ Information for patients and healthcare professionals: ℕ https://myelitis.org/

Headaches

Background
- One of the commonest symptoms pregnant ♀ encounter (Table 7.4)
- Vast majority are benign in nature
- Most important part of the assessment is the taking of a careful medical history and thorough examination

Thunderclap headaches
- Headache of very sudden onset
- Reaches the maximum intensity in <1 min

Causes of thunderclap headaches
- Common:
  - SAH
  - RCVS
- Rare:
  - Intracerebral haemorrhage
  - Acute ↑ BP
  - Cervical artery dissection
  - Pituitary apoplexy
  - 1° thunderclap headache

Assessment of a pregnant ♀ with a headache

History
- Needs to be careful and thorough
- Any previous headache history
- Features of this headache
- Any concerning features (adapted from SIGN Guideline 107):
  - Worse in the morning
  - Pattern of onset (e.g. thunderclap or waking from sleep)
  - Exacerbating factors (e.g. posture, exertion, coughing)
  - Associated focal neurological symptoms (e.g. weakness, aura) or non-focal symptoms (e.g. cognitive change)
- Fever
- History of HIV, immunosuppression, or malignancy
- Risk factors for VTE

Examination
- BP
- Urine dipstick
- Full examination including careful neurological examination
- Fundoscopy
- Concerning features include:
  - Any abnormal neurology
  - Fever
  - Neck stiffness/photophobia

➲ SIGN. Diagnosis and management of headache in adults: ℘ https://www.sign.ac.uk/assets/sign107.pdf

Table 7.4 Common types of headache

Type	Clinical features	Management
Migraine	See p. 252	

Tension headache	• Typical description is of a tight band around head that is often dull, can be pulsating in a minority
	• Can be associated with muscle tenderness
	• Common precipitants include stress and certain head and neck movements
	• Can be episodic or chronic
		• Non-pharmacological:
		  • Avoidance of precipitants
		  • Rest
		  • Acupuncture
		• Pharmacological:
		  • Paracetamol
		  • Ibuprofen or aspirin (less commonly used for this indication in pregnancy)

Cluster headache	• Frequent, sudden headaches lasting up to 3 hrs and occurring in clusters, i.e. several a day for a few days then settling
	• Typically described as a stabbing pain around the orbit or temple
	• May feature symptoms that overlap with migraine
	• Autonomic symptoms may be present
		• Abortive treatments include:
		  • Oxygen (excellent)
		  • Triptans
		• Preventative treatments:
		  • Verapamil

Trigeminal neuralgia	• Rarely affects ♀ of childbearing age • Recurrent, paroxysmal, unilateral sharp pain affecting the area supplied by the trigeminal nerve • Pain on chewing or brushing teeth sometimes mean a dental cause is investigated prior to a neurological cause being suspected	• Common treatments include carbamazepine, lamotrigine, or botulinum toxin

Table 7.4 Continued

Type	Clinical features	Management
Meningitis	• Typical symptoms include severe headache, associated nausea and vomiting, photophobia, and fever • Can be bacterial or viral • Bacterial meningitis can occur in the absence of systemic sepsis, so an absence of a typical meningococcal rash does not exclude the diagnosis • Systemic markers of infection may not be raised at presentation • If symptoms of confusion, ↓ Glasgow Coma Scale score or seizures, consider the diagnosis of viral encephalitis and add in IV aciclovir	• Urgent LP for Gram stain and culture; rapid tests for PCR are ↑ also used to hasten diagnosis • Urgent antibiotics—typically ceftriaxone 2 g BD • Dexamethasone 10 mg QDS IV also indicated as some survival benefit in pneumococcal infection • Add amoxicillin 2 g 4-hourly in pregnancy for *Listeria* cover • CT is not mandated prior to LP unless there are signs suggestive of raised intracranial pressure or other issues that may complicate LP
SAH	⊕ See p. 231	
IIH	⊕ See p. 260	
Post-dural puncture headache	• Frontal or occipital headache that occurs after dural puncture • Classically worse on sitting or standing and relieved by lying flat • Develops in the first 1–3 days after the procedure • 10–30% of procedures can be complicated by this; no association with volume of fluid removed or operator performing procedure	• Conservative measures: • Analgesia • Adequate hydration • Anecdotally, caffeine-containing drinks can help • Occasional severe cases require an epidural blood patch, which sometimes need to be repeated for a second time

Type	Clinical features	Management
Arterial dissection	→ See p. 235	
Hypertensive crisis		
Pituitary apoplexy	• Acute headache, often in association with other symptoms such as diplopia, ophthalmoplegia, change in mental status, but examination can be normal • Biochemical features of glucocorticoid deficiency may be present (→ see p. 405) but an absence at time of initial presentation does not exclude the diagnosis	• MRI pituitary is more sensitive than CT • Urgent glucocorticoid replacement • Glucose monitoring (risk of hypoglycaemia)

Migraine

- Typically a unilateral headache
- May be preceded by a visual aura (e.g. flashing lights or zigzag lines)
- Can be associated with photophobia and vomiting

Migraine in pregnancy

- May → a ↓ in migraine frequency, but can also ↑ frequency or change the nature of the headache
- Aura can occur without headache
- Migraine can present for the 1st time in pregnancy
- Findings of typical migraine features with the presence of 'positive phenomena' such as flashing lights or zigzag lines (fortification spectra) mean a clinical diagnosis can be made and no imaging is required

---

Treatment of acute episode of migraine

Non-pharmacological methods
- Relaxation techniques, e.g. mindfulness
- Avoidance of known triggers (e.g. ensuring regular sleep hours, regular meals)

Analgesia
- Paracetamol 1 g QDS
- Avoid codeine if possible
- Ibuprofen (should be avoided due to risk of premature closure of the fetal ductus arteriosus but can be considered <28 wks)

Antiemetic
- Prochlorperazine 3 mg buccally
- Metoclopramide 10 mg orally

Abortive measures
- Triptans:
  - Sumatriptan and rizatriptan used most commonly
  - Consider non-oral options such as intranasal sumatriptan or buccal rizatriptan

---

Prevention of migraine in pregnancy

Consider if:
- >2 disabling headaches per month
- Use of abortive treatment >2× per week
- Migraine with neurological sequelae
- Ineffective symptomatic treatment

Prophylactic options
- β blockers, i.e. propranolol 40 mg BD (↑ to maximum of 160 mg per day)
- Amitriptyline (10 mg daily ↑ gradually to 70–100 mg daily depending on response)
- Greater occipital nerve block
- Low-dose aspirin (75 mg OD)

⚠ *Treatments that are advised against*
- Ibuprofen after 28 wks (regular use of ibuprofen in 3rd trimester associated with premature closure of the ductus arteriosus and fetal pulmonary hypertension)
- Ergotamine (risk of hypertonic uterine contractions and vasospasm)
- High-dose aspirin (>75 mg OD)
- Antiepileptic medication such as topiramate or valproate:
  - Associated with teratogenicity
  - Only prescribed in severe cases in conjunction with a neurologist

Guillain–Barré syndrome

Background

- Immune-mediated, acute polyneuropathy which often, but not always, follows an acute infection (most commonly *Campylobacter jejuni* gastroenteritis, but also reported with CMV, EBV, and Zika infection)
- The weakness is usually ascending and associated with loss of tendon reflexes
- Back pain can be severe and predate the weakness
- Sensory abnormalities are not usually a prominent feature
- A significant proportion develop respiratory muscle weakness severe enough to warrant invasive ventilation
- Autonomic instability is seen in many patients and can manifest as:
  - ↑ HR
  - Postural ↓ BP
  - ↑ BP
  - Urinary retention

Pregnancy in a ♀ with a history of GBS

Pregnancy does not ↑ the risk of recurrence and no changes to routine obstetric care are required.

Management of GBS in pregnancy

- Initial assessment includes:
  - Observations including BP and pulse (due to the risk of autonomic instability and arrhythmias)
  - Full neurological examination
  - FVC—requires a specific meter, a peak flow reading is not a substitute for this
- Neck imaging only required if doubt about diagnosis, not routinely required prior to starting treatment
- Admission to a location where close monitoring can be provided including regular FVC measurement
- Treatment options:
  - IVIg **or**
  - Plasma exchange

Inherited neuropathies

Hereditary motor sensory neuropathy (Charcot–Marie–Tooth disease)

- Refers to a collection of conditions resulting from a variety of aberrations in genes including those for myelin
- Majority are autosomal dominant, but other inheritance patterns have also been identified
- There are 7 types, of which HMSN 1 and 2 are the most common and typically present in the 1st or 2nd decade of life
- Symptoms include:
  - Leg weakness
  - Deformity (such as pes cavus and hammer toes)

Management of hereditary motor sensory neuropathy in pregnancy

- Genetic counselling about inheritance
- Vigilance for the development of worsening neurological symptoms (can occur in pregnancy and improve after delivery; recurs in subsequent pregnancies)
- Active management of 3rd stage of labour and delivery in an appropriate setting due to ↑ risk of uterine atony and PPH

Friedreich's ataxia

- Autosomal recessive condition with varying numbers of triplet repeats in the *FXN* gene encoding for the mitochondrial protein frataxin
- Results in progressive neurological disability
- Symptoms and signs most commonly include:
  - Ataxia
  - Leg weakness
  - Dysarthria
  - Dysphagia
- Associated with hypertrophic cardiomyopathy which can result in heart failure and arrhythmias
- Impaired glucose tolerance is common

Management of Friedreich's ataxia in pregnancy

- Genetic counselling about inheritance
- Oral GTT
- Echocardiogram to assess for cardiomyopathy
- Not an indication for induction of labour or caesarean section

Acquired neuropathies

Carpal tunnel syndrome

- Results from compression of the median nerve in the carpal tunnel
- More common in pregnancy due to fluid accumulation
- Symptoms include numbness and paraesthesia in the median nerve distribution (lateral half of hand and the 1st 3 digits), which can be worse at night
- Management in pregnancy is conservative, i.e. the use of splints
- Surgical intervention is rarely required as improves after pregnancy

Meralgia paraesthetica

- Results from compression of the lateral cutaneous nerve of the thigh
- Symptoms include pain, numbness, and paraesthesia of the outer region of the upper thigh, which may be worse on standing and relieved by sitting or lying down
- No intervention is required as gradually improves after pregnancy

Postpartum compression neuropathies

- Most commonly affect the obturator, femoral, or peroneal nerves and result from vaginal delivery or the positions adopted during labour and delivery
- Resolution is seen in the majority of cases within weeks to months after delivery.

Bell's palsy

- Isolated palsy of the facial nerve which results in asymmetric facial weakness and unilateral weakness of eye closure
- More common in pregnancy and the early postpartum period
- The differential diagnosis is shown in Table 7.5.

Clinical features

- Neurological examination for any other neurological signs
- Confirm the pattern of abnormality:
  - **Lower** motor neuron pattern (involves the forehead)
  - **Upper** motor neuron (spares forehead)
- Assessment of severity
- Examination of ear and ear canal for vesicles (Ramsay Hunt syndrome; VZV reactivation)

Management of Bell's palsy in pregnancy

- If incomplete eye closure, ensure eye care provided, including:
  - Lubricating ointment and artificial tears eye drops as needed
  - Tape for use overnight
- If <72 hrs from the onset of symptoms and no evidence of aural vesicles, start prednisolone 60 mg OD for a week
- If severe or complete (House–Brackmann criteria severity of grade IV or above) consider antiviral treatment (e.g. valaciclovir 1000 mg TDS for a week) in addition to steroid treatment

Differential diagnosis of lower motor neuron facial weakness

- Herpes zoster infection (Ramsay Hunt syndrome)
- Otitis media
- Sarcoidosis
- Lyme disease
- Guillain–Barré syndrome
- HIV infection
- Space-occupying lesion including:
  - Vestibular schwannomas
  - Parotid gland tumours
- Ischaemic stroke affecting the pons and facial nerve nucleus

Table 7.5 House–Brackmann criteria for the assessment of facial nerve dysfunction

	Gross function	At rest	Forehead	Eye	Mouth
I Normal	Normal	Normal	Normal	Normal	Normal
II Mild	Slight weakness on close inspection	Normal symmetry and tone	Moderate to good function	Complete closure with minimal effort	Slight asymmetry
III Moderate	Obvious but not disfiguring difference; noticeable but not severe synkinesis, contracture or hemifacial spasm	Normal symmetry and tone	Slight to moderate movement	Complete closure with effort	Slightly weak with maximal effort
IV Moderately severe	Obvious weakness and/ or disfiguring asymmetry	Normal symmetry and tone	None	Incomplete closure	Asymmetric with maximal effort
V Severe	Only barely perceptible motion	Asymmetry	None	Incomplete closure	Slight movement
VI Total paralysis	No movement	Asymmetry	None	No movement	No movement

Source: data from House, J.W., Brackmann, D.E. (1985) 'Facial nerve grading system' *Otolaryngol Head Neck Surg*, 93:146–147.

Posterior reversible encephalopathy syndrome

Background

- Also known as reversible posterior leucoencephalopathy syndrome
- Can present with a variety of symptoms including:
  - Headache
  - Reduced level of consciousness
  - Visual disturbance
  - Seizures
- The diagnosis is made when posterior white matter changes reflective of vasogenic oedema are identified on MRI, which are usually, but not always, reversible
- Causes include:
  - ↑ BP
  - Drugs such as ciclosporin

Management of PRES in pregnancy

- Associated with hypertensive disorders of pregnancy
- No specific treatment, aside from:
  - Treatment of the underlying condition
  - Tight BP control
- Magnesium sulfate as seizure prophylaxis should be administered, as development of PRES can be a marker of severe pre-eclampsia

Idiopathic intracranial hypertension

Background
- The symptoms and signs of ↑ intracranial pressure are present, with no other cause found for this and normal CSF constituents
- Symptoms include:
  - Headache
  - Visual impairment
  - Pulsatile tinnitus
- Signs include:
  - Papilloedema
- LP demonstrates ↑ opening pressure
- Most commonly affects overweight ♀ of childbearing age

Causes of ↑ intracranial pressure
- IIH
- Intracranial mass or abscess
- Venous outflow obstruction, e.g. cerebral venous thrombosis
- Obstructive hydrocephalus
- ↑ CSF production, e.g. choroid plexus papilloma

Pregnancy
- Can worsen the symptoms and signs
- Can present for the 1st time in pregnancy, typically during or after the 2nd trimester

Investigation
- Cranial CT or MRI to investigate cause
- LP for opening pressure and biochemical analysis

Management of IIH in pregnancy
- Should have vision tested regularly (acuity and fields)
- Acetazolamide can be used in the 2nd and 3rd trimester (regular monitoring of bicarbonate and U&E required)
- Thiazides can also be used
- Acute visual loss is an indication for a short course of IV steroids prior to surgical intervention (optic nerve sheath fenestration or insertion of a CSF shunt)

💧 LP can be performed as a therapeutic measure in pregnancy, with the aim to remove CSF until a ↓ in opening pressure is seen.

Ventriculoperitoneal shunt

Background

This is a shunt from the ventricle into the peritoneal space, and is used as a permanent treatment for hydrocephalus, e.g. after meningitis infection or for congenital hydrocephalus.

Management of a VP shunt in pregnancy

- As uterine size ↑, it can cause shunt occlusion which may manifest as signs of ↑ intracranial haemorrhage including headaches and vomiting
- If a caesarean section is performed, awareness of the location of the shunt tip is required to ensure avoidance of inadvertent manipulation during the procedure
- Prophylactic antibiotics at the time of delivery are not routinely recommended

⚠ Presence of a VP shunt does not preclude the use of regional analgesia and is not an indication for caesarean section

Rheumatology

Rheumatoid arthritis

Background
- A symmetrical, deforming polyarthropathy
- More common in ♀ than ♂
- Early treatment with DMARDs important to prevent permanent joint damage

Clinical features
- Most often in small joints of the hands
- Usually symmetrical
- Many possible extra-articular features (Table 8.1)

Rheumatoid factor
- Autoantibody against Fc portion of IgG:
  - +ve in 70–80% of individuals
  - Can also occur in unaffected individuals and those with other rheumatic conditions
- Anti-cyclic citrullinated peptide (anti-CCP) is more specific for RA

Management of RA in pregnancy
- Pre-pregnancy counselling is important to optimize disease control and amend medication
- Often improves with pregnancy
- ≤90% suffer postpartum exacerbation:
  - T cell immunity ↓ in pregnancy then returns to normal
- Screen for anti-Ro/La antibodies:
  - If +ve requires regular fetal heart auscultation from 16 wks and fetal echocardiography
- Review medications (➔ see Table 8.10)
- Refer to obstetric anaesthetist:
  - Risk of atlantoaxial dislocation (very rare) and limitation of hip abduction
- Aspirin 75 mg OD from 12 wks
- Assess VTE risk (active inflammatory disease causes ↑ VTE risk)
- Hydrocortisone replacement at delivery if on long-term steroids (➔ see p. 429)

Table 8.1 Extra-articular features of rheumatoid arthritis

Lung	• Rheumatoid lung nodules
	• Interstitial lung disease
	• Pleural effusion
Haematological	• Anaemia of chronic disease
	• Felty's syndrome (seropositive RA + splenomegaly + neutropenia)
	• Thrombocytosis
Dermatological	• Rheumatoid nodules
	• Raynaud's phenomenon
	• Peripheral ulcers
	• Cutaneous vasculitis
Vascular	• Vasculitis
Ophthalmic	• Scleritis
	• Episcleritis
	• Keratoconjunctivitis sicca
Renal	• Glomerulonephritis
	• (Secondary) amyloidosis

Raynaud's phenomenon
- Usually improves in pregnancy:
  - ↑ skin blood flow and vasodilatation
- Can occur solely on the nipple

Treatment
- Heated gloves
- Heated compresses in bra for Raynaud's of nipple
- Nifedipine sustained release starting at 10 mg BD
- Can be exacerbated by β blockers so they should be avoided
- Warm delivery room

Systemic lupus erythematosus

Background
- A multisystem, autoimmune, inflammatory condition
- More common in ♀ than ♂ (9:1)
- Onset is commonly in childbearing years
- More common in Afro-Caribbean ♀ and certain other ethnic groups, compared to Caucasian populations

Clinical features
- Diagnosis is based on clinical criteria (Box 8.1)
- Features of a flare are not changed by pregnancy but can overlap with both normal pregnancy symptoms and features of pre-eclampsia (Table 8.2)

Diagnosis of SLE in pregnancy
- Mainly clinical
- Likely that as sFlt-1/PLGF ratio testing is introduced to clinical practice this will help (ratio ↑ in pre-eclampsia but not in SLE)
- Renal biopsy is not often required but can aid diagnosis.

Box 8.1 Diagnosis of SLE

4 or more of the following features are required (simultaneously or following each other):
- Malar rash ('butterfly' rash on face)
- Discoid rash
- Serositis, e.g. pleuritis or pericarditis
- Oral or nasopharyngeal ulceration
- Arthritis:
  - Non-erosive, migratory of 2 or more joints
- Photosensitivity
- Neurological features, e.g. seizures, psychosis
- Haematological features:
  - Haemolytic anaemia
  - Leucopenia ($<4 \times 10^9$/L)
  - Lymphopenia ($<1.5 \times 10^9$/L)
  - Thrombocytopenia ($<100 \times 10^9$/L)
- Immunological features, e.g. anti-dsDNA antibodies, antinuclear antibodies

Table 8.2 Differentiating a flare of SLE from pre-eclampsia

Both	• Hypertension
	• Proteinuria
	• Thrombocytopenia
	• Renal impairment
SLE only	• Rising anti-dsDNA titre
	• RBCs or casts in urine
	• Relative fall in C3/4 compared to 1st trimester baseline, even if still in normal range
	• No ↑ in uric acid
	• No abnormal LFTs
Pre-eclampsia only	• ↑ sFLT1/PLGF ratio

Fertility treatment in SLE

- 1° infertility rates similar to general population
- Advisable to:
  - Review immunosuppression prior to cycle
  - Ensure Ro/La status known
  - Avoid stimulation for 6–12 mths after a flare
  - Use lowest possible dose of oestradiol
  - Undergo embryo implantation via frozen cycle preferred to fresh cycle to ↓ risk of ovarian hyperstimulation syndrome
  - Undergo single embryo transfer
  - Consider a 'natural cycle' for egg collection may be possible and ↓ the effects of hormones
  - Ensure VTE assessment performed and low threshold for prophylactic LMWH

Systemic lupus erythematosus and pregnancy

Maternal risks
- Risk of flare not ↑ if disease quiescent for 4–6 mths prior to conception
- ↑ risk of hypertensive disorders and placental abruption

⚠ Cessation of hydroxychloroquine can precipitate a flare so do not stop

Fetal risks
- Miscarriage
- Preterm delivery
- Preterm rupture of membranes
- Fetal growth restriction
- Stillbirth

💣 ↑ risk of these complications if active disease at conception or renal involvement
- Risks of anti-Ro/La positivity (Box 8.2)

Management of SLE in pregnancy
- Pre-pregnancy counselling is important
- Aim to delay conception until >6 mths free of active disease
- Assessment of:
  - Disease severity and activity
  - Antiphospholipid antibody status
  - Anti-Ro/La antibody status
- Review medication
- Optimize BP control
- Aspirin 75 mg OD from 12 wks
- Baseline bloods including FBC, U&Es, LFTs
- Baseline urinary PCR (i.e. off ACE-I)
- Fetal growth scans
- Stress-dose steroids at delivery if on long-term steroids (➲ see p. 429)

Box 8.2 Anti-Ro and anti-La antibodies

▶ Found in ~30% of ♀ with SLE as well as in other autoimmune conditions.

Congenital heart block
- Occurs in 2–3% of all anti-Ro/La +ve ♀:
  - ≤25% of anti-Ro/La positive ♀ who have had a previously affected infant
- Can occur from 18–20 wks
- Fetal bradycardia can be preceded by 1st- or 2nd-degree heart block so fetal heart auscultation every 1–2 wks from 16/40 advised
- Fetal echocardiography mandated for all ♀ even if fetal heart rate normal when measured, normally performed at 20/40 and 28/40
- Survival in complete heart block depends on how early it develops, but is often fatal
- 50–60% of those who survive need a permanent pacemaker in infancy (others need it in their teenage years)
- Conducting system inflammation and fibrosis, pancarditis, and myocarditis can also be associated
- No treatment options (dexamethasone/IVIg previously used but of no benefit in complete heart block or 1st/2nd-degree heart block respectively)
- Hydroxychloroquine ↓ the risk of complete heart block in pregnancies following a pregnancy affected by anti-Ro/La-related complete heart block, but is not universally advocated for 1° prevention at present
- 50% of asymptomatic mothers who have an affected infant may develop connective tissue disease within the next 15 yrs

Neonatal cutaneous lupus
- Occurs in 5% of infants born to anti-Ro/La+ve mothers
- Often develops at 2–3 wks and can occur after sun exposure
- Most commonly seen on face and scalp
- Can occur anywhere on body
- Rash resolves spontaneously and requires no treatment
- Does not result in scarring

Antiphospholipid syndrome

Background
- APS is a multisystem disorder characterized by thromboembolic events and/or obstetric complications
- Thromboembolic event in the setting of APS ↑ lifetime recurrence rate → long-term anticoagulation advised
- Associated with the presence of antiphospholipid antibodies

⚠ Diagnosis is **not** made on the presence of antibodies alone (criteria outlined in Box 8.3)

Clinical features
- Diagnosis of APS requires both clinical features and laboratory abnormalities
- Catastrophic APS is rare occurrence **but** associated with significant mortality so a high index of suspicion is required
- Other features that may be seen in APS include:
  - Thrombocytopenia
  - Haemolytic anaemia
  - Transverse myelopathy/myelitis
  - Livedo reticularis
  - Endocardial valve disease (mitral > aortic)
  - Chorea
  - Migraine
  - Epilepsy

1° *APS*
- No features of underlying connective tissue disease

2° *APS*
- Established connective tissue disease present

Maternal risks
- Include placental abruption, pre-eclampsia, and arterial or venous thrombosis

Fetal risks
- Include miscarriage, stillbirth, and fetal growth restriction

---

Management of APS in pregnancy
- Review medications
- Aspirin 75 mg OD from 12 wks
- Anticoagulation—therapeutic- or prophylactic-dose LMWH depending on clinical features and previous history of thrombosis
- Anaesthetic referral
- Postpartum avoid combined oral contraceptive pill

Box 8.3 Diagnostic criteria for APS

Clinical
- Arterial thrombosis (e.g. intracranial, retinal, coronary, mesenteric, peripheral)
  Or
- Venous thrombosis (e.g. intracranial, ocular, renal, hepatic, or IVC)
  Or
- Renal thrombotic microangiopathy

  And/or

Obstetric complications
- 3 or more consecutive miscarriages (<10 wks with normal parental chromosomes, maternal anatomy, and hormones)
  Or
- 1 or more fetal death (>10 wks)
  Or
- 1 or more preterm delivery (34 wks or earlier) due to pre-eclampsia or placental insufficiency

  AND the presence of one or more of:
- IgG and/or IgM anticardiolipin antibody at medium/high titre on 2 or more occasions (≥12 wks apart)
- IgG and/or IgM anti-beta2-glycoprotein antibody at high titre on 2 or more occasions (≥12 wks apart)
- Lupus anticoagulant activity on 2 or more occasions (6 wks or more apart), e.g. measured by the direct Russell viper venom test (DRVVT)

Catastrophic APS

- Multiorgan failure resulting from widespread thromboses
- Usually affects small vessels rather than large vessels
⚠ Mortality ≤50% even when anticoagulant and immunosuppressive treatment is used

The diagnosis is suggested by:
- Presence of antiphospholipid antibodies
- ≥3 new organ thromboses within a 7-day period
- Biopsy confirming microthrombus
- In the absence of other causes of the previously listed factors (such as DIC or a thrombotic microangiopathy)

Treatment includes:
- Treatment of any precipitating illness such as infection
- Anticoagulation
- Immunosuppression e.g. high-dose IV methylprednisolone
- Plasma exchange or IVIg for severe cases

Anticoagulation for antiphospholipid syndrome

See Table 8.3.

Table 8.3 Antiplatelet and anticoagulation recommendations according to APS features

Obstetric features of APS	Maternal features of APS (previous thrombosis)	Antiplatelet	Anticoagulation
No	No		None
Yes or no	Yes	Aspirin 75 mg OD from pre-conception	On warfarin before conception: Therapeutic LMWH. Not on warfarin before conception: Prophylactic LMWH
Yes (1st trimester loss)	No	Aspirin 75 mg OD from pre-conception	Prophylactic LMWH after conception if previous loss while on aspirin monotherapy
Yes (intrauterine or neonatal death from placental complications such as pre-eclampsia or abruption)	No	Aspirin 75 mg OD (some start from pre-conception although no benefit proven over starting later)	Prophylactic LMWH after conception

Sjögren's syndrome

Background

- Chronic condition that leads to progressive dryness of mouth and eyes because of inflammation of salivary and lacrimal glands

Primary
- Absence of features of a coexisting connective tissue disease

Secondary
- Features of connective tissue disease also present

Clinical features

- Dry eyes and dry mouth are the hallmark of the condition, along with parotid enlargement
- Extra-glandular features can occur, either as a result of the condition or the associated connective tissue disease (Table 8.4)
- ↑ risk of non-Hodgkin lymphoma in individuals with Sjögren's (as well as those with RA and SLE)

Management of Sjögren's syndrome in pregnancy

- Artificial tears/saliva should be prescribed as required
- Assess anti-Ro/La status (➲ see box 8.2)
- Management of complications

Table 8.4 Extra-glandular features of Sjögren's syndrome

Skin	- Xerosis (dry, scaly skin) - Purpura - Cutaneous vasculitis - Erythema nodosum - Livedo reticularis
Muscles	- Proximal myopathy
Thyroid	- Autoimmune thyroiditis
Lungs	- Interstitial lung disease
Cardiac	- Heart block - Myocardial infarction - Acute pericarditis - Myocarditis
Liver	- PBC
Kidneys	- Interstitial nephritis
Neurological	- Peripheral neuropathy
Haematological	- Anaemia - Leucopenia - Thrombocytopenia

Ankylosing spondylitis

Background
- Progressive, inflammatory condition affecting the spine (also known as an axial spondyloarthropathy)
- More common in HLA B27+ve individuals
- More common in ♂ than ♀

Differential diagnosis of spondyloarthropathy
- Psoriatic arthropathy
- Reactive arthropathy
- IBD-associated spondyloarthropathy

Clinical features
- Inflammatory back pain:
  - Onset <45 yrs
  - Worse at night or when at rest
  - Better with activity
  - Often involves the sacroiliac joints
- Other musculoskeletal features include enthesitis and dactylitis
- Synovitis of other extra-axial joints can also occur
- Extra-articular manifestations (Table 8.5)
- Imaging (mostly MRI) can show inflammation of joints
- Various scoring systems used to assess the degree of sacroiliac involvement

Table 8.5 Extra-articular manifestations of ankylosing spondylitis

Pulmonary	• Interstitial lung disease • Restrictive lung disease due to chest wall limitation
Cardiac	• Aortic regurgitation • Aortic root abnormalities • Acute coronary syndromes
Ophthalmic	• Anterior uveitis
Bone	• Osteoporosis
Renal	• 2° amyloidosis • IgA nephropathy
Gastrointestinal	• Inflammatory bowel disease

Management of ankylosing spondylitis in pregnancy
- Pregnancy does not alter the course of this condition
- Symptoms often worsen because of medication changes
- Postpartum flare of symptoms has been reported in ≥50% of ♀
- NSAIDs are the mainstay of treatment and can be used until 24–28 wks
- Steroids have no therapeutic benefit
- Biologics such as the TNFα inhibitors (➔ see table 8.11) can be continued in pregnancy
- Obstetric anaesthetist referral for spinal assessment and suitability for regional techniques

Psoriatic arthritis

Background

- A deforming, inflammatory polyarthropathy with variety of patterns of joint involvement
- 70% have a history of psoriasis:
  - Signs of psoriasis (hidden plaques, e.g. in hair) or associated nail changes
- Pain is typical inflammatory pain (worse in mornings, worse with inactivity, better with exercise)
- Occurs with equal frequency in ♂ and ♀

Clinical features

- PsA is more likely if there is a family history of psoriasis or PsA
- Variety patterns of arthropathy occur:
  - Arthritis mutilans
  - Symmetrical small joint polyarthropathy
  - Spondyloarthritis
  - Asymmetric large joint oligoarthritis
  - Arthritis of distal interphalangeal joints
- Nail changes (onycholysis, nail pitting) more common with PsA than psoriasis
- Dactylitis ('sausage digits') occurs in PsA more than in other arthropathies
- Enthesitis (inflammation at insertion of tendons/ligaments), e.g. Achilles tendonitis, plantar fasciitis occurs in PsA
- No diagnostic autoantibodies associated with psoriatic arthropathy

▶ ANA, anti-rheumatoid factor, and anti-CCP may be found but do not aid diagnosis or prognostication.

> ### Management of PsA in pregnancy
> - ⟳ See p. 518 for management of psoriasis
> - Analgesia:
>   - NSAIDs can be used up to 24–28 wks
> - DMARDs:
>   - May be continued depending on the agent
> - Biologics are ↑ used in severe disease (see table 8.11):
>   - TNFα inhibitors have ↑ safety data
>   - Newer IL12/23 inhibitors (e.g. ustekinumab) have less safety data available but have been used in pregnancy
>   - Continuation may be appropriate in ♀ where the benefits of controlling their severe disease outweigh theoretical risk
> - VTE prophylaxis may be required if disease active and mobility limited

Systemic sclerosis

Background

- Group of rare, progressive disorders featuring thickening of the skin
- Also known as scleroderma or diffuse cutaneous systemic sclerosis
- Localized scleroderma can also occur (known as linear scleroderma and morphoea)
- Limited cutaneous systemic sclerosis or CREST syndrome is a milder variant
- Occasional cases can occur where there is internal organ involvement and no skin manifestations (systemic sclerosis sine scleroderma)

Clinical features

- Limited cutaneous systemic sclerosis (CREST) consists of:
  - Calcinosis
  - Raynaud's syndrome
  - Oesophageal dysmotility
  - Sclerodactyly
  - Telangiectasia
- Can cause multiorgan dysfunction
- Diagnosis aided by anti-Scl70 and anti-centromere antibodies
- See Table 8.6

Table 8.6 Manifestations of systemic sclerosis

Pulmonary	<ul><li>Interstitial lung disease</li><li>Pulmonary hypertension</li><li>Lung cancer</li></ul>
Cardiac	<ul><li>Pericarditis</li><li>Pericardial effusion</li><li>Myocardial infarction</li><li>Heart failure</li><li>Arrhythmias</li></ul>
Renal	<ul><li>Acute kidney injury 'renal crisis'</li></ul>
Haematological	<ul><li>VTE</li></ul>
Gastrointestinal	<ul><li>Dysphagia</li><li>Gastro-oesophageal reflux</li><li>Angiodysplasia</li></ul>
Musculoskeletal	<ul><li>Arthralgia of small joints</li></ul>
Neurological	<ul><li>Myopathies</li><li>Peripheral neuropathies</li></ul>

Management of systemic sclerosis in pregnancy

- Pre-pregnancy counselling should highlight high-risk nature of pregnancy in ♀ with systemic sclerosis, especially if early (<4 yrs from diagnosis) and/or renal involvement
- Often appropriate to continue ACE-I despite known fetal risks as ↓ risk renal crisis and associated mortality
- Assess for organ complications:
  - Lung function tests
  - Echocardiography (pulmonary hypertension)
  - Bloods including renal function
- Aspirin 75 mg OD from 12 wks
- Caution is required with respect to steroid use as can precipitate a renal crisis
- Refer to obstetric anaesthetist
- Early follow-up should be arranged as postpartum deterioration can occur
- Resume ACE-I postpartum immediately even if BP normal

Takayasu arteritis

Background

- Median age of diagnosis is 26 yrs
- ♀ are affected more than ♂
- More common in Japan and SE Asia
- Inflammatory vasculopathy that mostly affects the aorta and its branches

Clinical features

- Symptoms often develop subacutely, so may only appear when vascular consequences have developed (i.e. stenosis or occlusion of vessels)
- Several phases:
  - Early—generalized systemic symptoms
  - Later—vascular tenderness and pain
  - Final—arteritic changes which → occlusion/aneurysms
- Examination findings include absent pulse/s, unequal BPs, bruits over large arteries

Diagnosis

See Box 8.4.

Management of Takayasu arteritis in pregnancy

- Does not appear that severity of the condition prior to pregnancy correlates with pregnancy outcome
- Continuation of immunosuppression
- Vigilance for the development of symptoms and treatment of any acute exacerbation
- Aspirin 75 mg OD from 12 wks
- Careful BP control **but** a stiff vascular tree may mean that BP measurements remain very elevated. Treatment targets ∴ need to be individualized depending on extent of disease
- Imaging of the vascular tree ideally prior to pregnancy
- Fetal growth assessment (↑ incidence of IUGR)
- Not an indication for caesarean section

Box 8.4 Diagnosis of Takayasu arteritis

American College of Rheumatology classification criteria require three or more features to be present:

- Age >40 yrs
- Claudication of the extremities
- ↓ pulsation of one/both brachial arteries
- Difference in upper limb SBP of ≥10 mmHg
- Bruit over abdominal aorta, or one/both subclavian arteries
- Arteriographic narrowing/occlusion of entire aorta, its branches, or large arteries in the proximal upper and lower limbs (not due to other causes)

Temporal arteritis

Background
- Rare large vessel vasculitis, affecting mainly individuals > 50 yrs of age

💥 Not reported in pregnancy but may be seen in future given ↑ age of pregnant ♀

Clinical features
- Inflammation of the temporal arteries causes bilateral headaches and tenderness over the temporal arteries
- Features of polymyalgia rheumatica may also be present
- Other symptoms include jaw claudication, visual loss, and systemic symptoms such as fever or weight loss
- Diagnostic test of choice used to be temporal artery biopsy but this has been superseded by temporal artery USS
- Treatment is with steroids initially then steroid-sparing agents

Management of temporal arteritis in pregnancy
- Immunosuppression
- Aspirin 75 mg OD
- Any suggestion of ophthalmic involvement is concerning as this is potentially sight-threatening so any ♀ with consistent symptoms and visual changes needs urgent review for consideration of steroid treatment

Polyarteritis nodosa

Background
- Necrotizing inflammation of vessels
- Typically affects middle-aged men so occurrence in pregnancy is very unusual
- 2° polyarteritis nodosa can be seen with hepatitis B or C infection

Clinical features

Symptoms
- Systemic including fever, weight loss, and fatigue
- Organ-specific such as renal failure, abdominal pain, and skin lesions

Imaging
- Imaging of vessels by MRI or angiography show patchy aneurysmal dilatation and occlusion of vessels

Diagnosis
See Box 8.5.

Box 8.5 Diagnosis of polyarteritis nodosa

American College of Rheumatology classification criteria require 3 or more features to be present:
- Livedo reticularis
- Myalgia, weakness, or tenderness of legs
- Mono- or polyneuropathy
- DBP >90 mmHg
- ↑ urea/creatinine
- Hepatitis B
- Arteriographic abnormality (aneurysms/occluded vessels)
- Biopsy showing leucocyte infiltration in vessel wall
- Not associated with ANCA positivity

Management in pregnancy
- ☀ Onset during pregnancy may be associated with poorer outcomes
- Continuation of immunosuppression
- Vigilance for the development of symptoms and treatment of any acute exacerbation
- Aspirin 75 mg OD from 12 wks
- Careful BP control
- Imaging of the vascular tree ideally prior to pregnancy
- Fetal growth assessment
- Not an indication for caesarean section

Kawasaki disease

Background
- Self-limiting vasculitis which occurs mainly in children but is occasionally seen in adults

Clinical features
- Acute phase (fever, conjunctivitis, mucositis) can last several days
- Followed by vasculitis complications such as coronary artery aneurysm

Management of pregnant ♀ with previous Kawasaki disease
- Pregnancy after Kawasaki disease generally has a good outcome
- Echocardiography to assess LV function
- Consider coronary artery imaging if not performed prior to conception
- Manage in MDT with cardiology input

Granulomatosis with polyangiitis

Background

- Previously known as Wegener's granulomatosis
- Small vessel vasculitis that 1° affects the upper and lower respiratory tracts and the kidneys
- Most commonly seen in individuals >50 yrs of age but has been reported in pregnancy
- Untreated disease is associated with significant mortality
- Steroid treatment is insufficient in isolation, so immunosuppression such as cyclophosphamide, rituximab, or azathioprine is required

Clinical features

- Systemic symptoms include fever, fatigue, malaise, and weight loss

Diagnosis

See Box 8.6.

Laboratory findings

- Anaemia
- ↑ inflammatory markers (CRP and white cell count)
- ↑ ESR
- Positive PR3-ANCA

Box 8.6 Diagnosis of GPA

American College of Rheumatology classification criteria require 2 or more features to be present:

- Nasal/oral inflammation:
  - Oral ulcer, purulent, or bloody nasal discharge
- Abnormal CXR:
  - Nodules, infiltrates, or cavities
- Urine:
  - Red cell casts in sediment
- Biopsy:
  - Granulomatous inflammation in artery wall or around artery

Management of GPA in pregnancy

Pre-existing

- Continuation of immunosuppression (may require modification depending on agent used)
- Vigilance for the development of symptoms and treatment of any acute exacerbation
- Aspirin 75 mg OD from 12 wks
- Careful BP control
- Imaging of the vascular tree ideally prior to pregnancy
- Fetal growth assessment
- Not an indication for caesarean section

New diagnosis

- Cyclophosphamide or rituximab can be used depending on gestation

Microscopic polyangiitis

Background
- Necrotizing small vessel vasculitis

Clinical features
- As in GPA except upper respiratory tract symptoms less frequent
- Renal and pulmonary involvement predominant
- Often MPO-ANCA positive
- Less commonly PR3-ANCA positive

Management of MPA in pregnancy
- Rare but onset in pregnancy has been reported
- Manage as for GPA

Eosinophilic granulomatosis with polyangiitis

Background
- Formerly known as Churg–Strauss syndrome
- Small vessel vasculitis
- Has been reported in pregnancy and the postpartum period

Clinical features
- Peripheral eosinophilia ($>1.5 \times 10^9$/L)
- Asthma
- Upper respiratory tract symptoms such as sinusitis
▶ The asthma and allergic symptoms can predate the eosinophilic and vasculitic symptoms by years
- MPO-ANCA antibodies may be present in up to 60% of cases

Diagnosis
See Box 8.7.

Box 8.7 Diagnosis of EGPA
American College of Rheumatology classification criteria require 4 or more features to be present:
- Asthma
- Eosinophil count >10%
- Mono- or polyneuropathy
- Transient pulmonary opacities
- Abnormal paranasal sinuses
- Biopsy showing eosinophil accumulation near blood vessels

Management of EGPA in pregnancy
- Rare but has been reported in pregnancy and the postpartum period
- Disease onset in pregnancy may be associated with poorer outcomes
- Similar principles of management can be inferred from other vasculitides
- Needs consideration in the presence of significant eosinophilia and/or worsening asthma symptoms

Henoch–Schönlein purpura

Background

- IgA-mediated small vessel vasculitis most commonly seen in children but can be seen in adults
- Related to IgA nephropathy

Clinical features

- Diagnostic criteria are listed in Box 8.8
- Other features include:
  - Arthritis
  - Renal involvement (including nephrotic syndrome)

Management of HSP in pregnancy

Previous diagnosis of HSP

- Monitor renal function as renal impairment can occur after the acute episode has resolved
- Baseline urine dipstick/PCR

New diagnosis in pregnancy

- Rare but has been reported
- Immunosuppression with low-dose corticosteroid appears sufficient to → resolution

Box 8.8 Diagnosis of HSP

American College of Rheumatology classification criteria require 2 or more features to be present:

- Palpable purpura (in absence of thrombocytopenia)
- Age ≤20 yrs at onset
- Abdominal pain/bloody diarrhoea (suggestive of bowel ischaemia)
- Histology showing granulocytes in arteriole/venule walls

Inflammatory myopathies

Background

- Characterized by immune-mediated muscle injury
- Includes:
  - Dermatomyositis
  - Polymyositis
  - Inclusion-body myositis
  - Immune-mediated necrotizing myositis
  - Drug-associated myositis (e.g. statins)

Clinical features

- Muscle injury reflected by muscle pain and tenderness
- ↑ plasma CK from muscle damage
- Myositis-specific autoantibodies may be present:
  - Anti-Jo-1
  - Anti-PL-7
  - Anti-PL-12
  - Anti-SRP
- Anti-Ro antibodies also often found (➡ see box 8.2)
- Cutaneous manifestations are seen in dermatomyositis:
  - Gottran's papules (scaly, red patches on the hands)
  - Heliotropic rash over eyelids
- Consider antisynthetase syndrome if features of interstitial lung disease are also present (up to 30% of patients with inflammatory myopathies)

Management of inflammatory myopathies in pregnancy

- Treat as high risk for pre-eclampsia and give aspirin 75 mg OD unless contraindications
- Continue appropriate immunosuppression
- Careful monitoring for the development of complications, particularly respiratory
- Assess anti-Ro/La antibody status

Antisynthetase syndrome

Background
- Autoimmune inflammatory condition characterized by autoantibodies against aminoacyl tRNA synthetases (ASAs)
- Found in ≤30% of individuals with polymyositis or dermatomyositis

Clinical features
- Myositis in conjunction with interstitial lung disease
- Other features include:
  - Fever
  - Small joint arthritis
  - Raynaud's
  - 'Mechanic's hands'
  - Rash
- Common associated antibodies include anti-Jo 1, anti EJ, anti PL-7, and anti PL-12

Management of antisynthetase syndrome in pregnancy
- Very few cases have been reported in pregnancy but the same management principles apply as in other rheumatic conditions
- Review immunosuppressive medication and continue treatment in pregnancy to control disease
- Lung function tests
- Echocardiography (to look for pulmonary hypertension)
- Aspirin 75 mg OD from 12 wks

Osteoporosis

Normal bone changes in pregnancy
- Little information on changes to bone mineral density
- Markers of bone turnover ↑ 2–3×
- No evidence for ↑ fracture risk with ↑ parity
- No association with lactation and post-menopausal fractures

Background
- A condition of low bone mineral density:
  - ↑ risk of fractures, particularly in non-trauma settings
- Post-menopausal ♀ are most at risk
- Conditions such as hyperthyroidism, coeliac disease, and other malabsorptive syndromes ↑ risk of developing osteoporosis
- May be seen with previous steroid use or a diagnosis of osteogenesis imperfecta/juvenile osteoarthritis

Clinical features
- Blood tests including calcium, phosphate, alkaline phosphatase, and 25-hydroxycholecalciferol are usually normal
- Plain radiography shows fractures but the bones may otherwise appear normal

Diagnosis of osteoporosis and assessment of fracture risk
- Based on DXA scan results
- Measures bone mineral density of lumbar spine and neck of femur
- T-scores reflect the difference between the measurement of the patient and that of a young healthy adult
- Traditionally osteoporosis is defined by a T-score ≥2.5 standard deviations below the mean, and osteopenia defined by a T-score 1–2.5 standard deviations below the mean
- However, it is now clear that bone mineral density alone does not correlate well with fracture risk

FRAX score

Scoring tool that gives an estimate of the ♀'s 10 yr fracture risk, based on factors including age, sex, weight, height, presence of other medical conditions that predispose to osteoporosis, smoking status, and bone mineral density of the femoral neck (⅊ http://www.sheffield.ac.uk/FRAX). Treatment can then be targeted at those at highest risk of fracture.

Treatment
- Treatment options in non-pregnant or postpartum ♀ include:
  - Vitamin D ± calcium, depending on dietary intake
  - Bisphosphonates
  - Strontium ranelate
  - Calcitonin or teriparatide
  - Denosumab

Management of pregnancy in a ♀ with pre-existing osteoporosis or osteopenia

- Stop bisphosphonates/strontium/calcitonin/denosumab
- Vitamin D supplementation:
  - At least 1000 IU/day, more if ↓ vitamin D levels
- Assessment of calcium intake:
  - Low threshold for calcium supplementation (2.5 g/day calcium carbonate, or 1 g/day elemental calcium, i.e. 1 pint milk)

Pregnancy and lactation-related osteoporosis

- Usually diagnosed when fractures occur
- ⚠ No appropriate bone density test for pregnancy
- Bilateral neck of femur fractures and vertebral fractures reported
- Often present with vitamin D deficiency, so there may be overlap with osteomalacia and osteoporosis

Management of pregnancy-related osteoporosis

- Surgical fixation of fractures if needed
- Bloods for calcium, phosphate, and vitamin D
- Vitamin D and calcium supplementation
- DXA scan is recommended after cessation of breastfeeding
- Consider bisphosphonates depending on bone status postnatally
- Use of other treatments including teriparatide and denosumab have been described in case reports, but this is usually in association with weaning
- Some physicians advise limiting lactation duration in future pregnancies which may ↓ recurrence

Transient osteoporosis of hip

- First described in pregnant ♀ with hip pain and osteopenia
- Subsequently identified in other patient groups
- MRI shows bone marrow oedema of the femoral head and neck, but the distinction from avascular necrosis of the femoral head (associated with the use of corticosteroids and conditions such as sickle cell disease) and other joint conditions (sacroiliitis, spondyloarthropathies) can be difficult

Management of transient osteoporosis of the hip

- Plain radiography:
  - May identify fractures or osteopenia
- MRI
- If fracture—surgical treatment as needed
- No fracture—conservative management to ↓ fracture risk
- Analgesia

Osteomalacia

Background

- Deficiency of mineralization of newly formed bone
- Often results from vitamin D deficiency (➲ see p. 440) (dietary deficiency or lack of sun exposure)

Clinical features

- Symptoms and signs include bone pain and proximal myopathy, but can be asymptomatic
- Consider in any ♀ at risk of vitamin D deficiency who develops bone pain

Investigations

- Blood test abnormalities:
  - ↓ vitamin D
  - ↓ or normal calcium
  - ↓ or normal phosphate
  - ↑ alkaline phosphatase
  - ↑ parathyroid hormone
- Imaging may show characteristic changes in vertebral bodies on plain radiographs:
  - Looser zones (lines with sclerotic borders) can be seen particularly on the pelvis bones or femurs
  - Usually bilateral and symmetrical
- Bone mineral density assessment (i.e. DXA scan) shows ↓ in bone mineral density but there are no specific features that distinguish osteomalacia from osteoporosis, so the diagnosis is made in combination with the plain radiograph findings ± bone biopsy
- Bone biopsy is only required in rare cases when the diagnosis is not clear from the tests listed
- Treatment is with vitamin D and calcium supplementation (even if bone mineral density is ↓, other treatments such as bisphosphonates are not indicated)

Familial Mediterranean fever

Background

- Inherited inflammatory condition with recurrent episodes of fever and serositis
- Most commonly the 1st episode occurs in childhood, but occasional individuals do not have any episodes until later in life
- Inheritance is usually autosomal recessive and most commonly 2 mutations in the *METV* gene are seen
- Most common in certain populations (Ashkenazi Jews and Mediterranean countries such as Greece, Italy, and Turkey)
- Colchicine is used for long-term prophylaxis (starting or ↑ dose in an acute attack does **not** have any effect on severity or duration)
- If ♀ are resistant to colchicine other treatments including IL-1 blockade, e.g. anakinra, can be tried

Clinical features

- A typical attack features:
  - Fever >38°C (may be absent if patient already on colchicine)
  - Pain due to serositis, e.g. abdominal pain, pleuritic pain, or joint pain (usually 1 joint rather than many)
  - Feels the same as previous attacks
  - Lasts up to 3 days
- Blood tests show ↑ inflammatory markers
- Proteinuria may be present:
  - If persistent between episodes suggests underlying amyloidosis
- Complications include 2° amyloidosis and small bowel obstruction related to adhesions
- Incomplete attacks are painful and recurrent, but do not fulfil the criteria for a typical attack (e.g. involving joints other than those specified, no signs of peritonism, etc.)
- Diagnostic criteria are listed in Box 8.9.

Management of FMF in pregnancy

- 1/3 of patients experience an improvement in symptoms, 1/3 a deterioration, and the remainder stay stable
- Advisable to continue colchicine throughout pregnancy as the benefits to the mother outweigh any theoretical risk to the fetus
- No adverse pregnancy outcomes have been reported in ♀ who start or continue anakinra throughout pregnancy
- Not an indication for induction of labour or caesarean section
- No contraindication to breastfeeding on colchicine, anakinra, or other IL-1 inhibitors

Box 8.9 Diagnosis of FMF

A diagnosis is suggested by 1 or more major criteria, 2 or more minor criteria, or 1 minor and 5 supportive criteria.

Major criteria
- Typical attacks with peritonitis
- Typical attacks with pleuritis or pericarditis
- Typical attacks with monoarthritis of hip, knee, or ankle
- Typical attacks with fever alone

Minor criteria
- Incomplete attacks involving chest pain
- Incomplete attacks involving monoarthritis
- Exertional leg pain
- Favourable response to colchicine

Supportive criteria
- Family history of FMF
- Appropriate ethnic origin
- <20 yrs of age at onset
- Spontaneous remission of attack
- Symptom-free interval between attacks
- Episodic proteinuria and/or haematuria
- Negative laparotomy
- Attacks associated with raised inflammatory markers
- Parental consanguinity

➲ See also https://www.tandfonline.com/doi/abs/10.1080/030097498440949

Haemophagocytic lymphohistiocytosis

Background

⚠ Potentially life-threatening condition of excessive activation of inflammatory cells (lymphocytes and macrophages) resulting in overproduction of inflammatory cytokines (Box 8.10).

- Can occur in the setting of another illness (Table 8.7) and it is appropriate to look for a 2° cause, but the development of HLH is more immediately life-threatening than the underlying diagnosis
- Treatment involves immunosuppression (e.g. steroids, ciclosporin) with other agents such as etoposide added at an early stage
- If central nervous system involvement, intrathecal chemotherapy is required
- Stem cell transplantation may be indicated.

Clinical features

- Multisystem dysfunction can occur including:
  - Cardiovascular: hypotension
  - Respiratory: acute respiratory distress
  - Neurological: seizures, cognitive changes, and PRES
  - Haematological: anaemia, neutropenia, thrombocytopenia, and coagulopathy
  - Biochemical: renal and/or liver dysfunction, hyponatraemia, ↑ LDH, and very high ferritin
- Examination may find lymphadenopathy and organomegaly

Investigations

- Imaging that can aid diagnosis include CXR, abdominal USS, and MRI brain if neurological involvement
- Bone marrow—in all patients with cytopenias
- Immunological tests—including immunoglobulins, but other tests depend on clinical presentation and local availability
- CSF analysis
- Genetic testing

Box 8.10 Diagnosis of HLH

Known genetic mutation or 5 or more of the following:

- Fever >38.5°C
- Splenomegaly
- Cytopenia of 2 or 3 lineages in peripheral blood: Hb <90 g/L, neutrophils <1.0 × 10^9/L, platelets <100 × 10^9/L
- Hypertriglyceridaemia (fasting triglycerides ≥3.0 mmol/L) and/or hypofibrinogenaemia (fibrinogen ≤1.5 g/L)
- Haemophagocytosis in bone marrow or spleen (and no evidence of malignancy)
- ↓ or absent natural killer cell activity
- Ferritin ≥500 mcg/L
- Soluble CD25 ≥2400 units/mL

Table 8.7 Causes of haemophagocytic lymphohistiocytosis (HLH)

1° familial	A number of mutations in genes involves in immunoregulation have been identified, often autosomal recessive	
2° infections	Viral	EBV, CMV, HSV, parvovirus, HIV
	Bacterial	Gram-negative bacteria, Brucella spp., Mycobacterium tuberculosis
	Parasitic	Malaria
Malignancy	• Leukaemia • Lymphoma • Occasionally other solid tumours (often an infective trigger to HLH in this group)	
Inflammatory[a]	• RA • SLE • Mixed connective tissue disease • Systemic sclerosis • Ankylosing spondylitis	
Immune deficiency	• Post transplant • HIV/AIDS • Inherited immune deficiencies	

[a] Macrophage activation syndrome is the term used to describe the occurrence of HLH in association with rheumatological conditions.

Management of HLH in pregnancy

⚠ Significant maternal mortality (cause of 4 maternal deaths in a recent triennium reported by MBRRACE-UK).

- Has been reported in pregnancy with a variety of associated illnesses including EBV, CMV, HSV, and parvovirus infection, and rheumatological conditions such as SLE and Still's disease
- Diagnostic uncertainty is common with HLH:
  - Non-pregnant ♀ are treated for infective and/or inflammatory conditions without success before the diagnosis is made
  - Overlap with features of pregnancy-specific conditions such as HELLP add further challenges to the diagnosis
- Treatment options in pregnancy depend on:
  - Severity of disease
  - Gestation
  - Presence of absence of severe liver dysfunction
  - Central nervous system involvement

⚠ The decision to deliver depends on the individual circumstances, but fetal compromise may occur if the mother is unwell with a cytokine storm, and delivery may aid maternal supportive care.

Adult-onset Still's disease

Background
- Systemic inflammatory condition of unknown aetiology

Clinical features
- Features are often non-specific and can cause diagnostic difficulty, mimicking infection or malignancy such as lymphoma
- Diagnostic criteria are shown in Table 8.8

Investigations
- FBC may reveal anaemia, neutrophilia, and thrombocytosis
- LFTs often abnormal
- Serum ferritin is often greatly ↑
- ↑ ESR and CRP
- Immunological testing to identify other rheumatological conditions with similar features → ANA, rheumatoid factor, and anti-CCP antibodies are recommended

Management of adult-onset Still's disease in pregnancy
- Only a small number of pregnancies reported
- Non-pregnant ♀ are immunosuppressed, with steroids as 1st line, with other biological treatments long term as required:
  - Anakinra (IL-1 receptor blocker)
  - Tocilizumab (humanized anti IL-6 antibody)
- As with all inflammatory conditions, it may improve in pregnancy and worsen postpartum
- Immunosuppression should be reviewed prior to conception, but most agents can be continued during pregnancy as needed
- Flares may require pulsed IV corticosteroids

Table 8.8 Diagnostic criteria for adult-onset Still's disease

5 features, at least 2 of which are 'major', as well as the exclusion of alternative diagnoses such as infection or another rheumatological condition

Major	• Fever of ≥39°C for at least 7 days
	• Arthralgia or arthritis for ≥2 wks
	• Salmon-pink maculopapular rash on trunk or limbs during episodes of fever
	• Neutrophilia (total count >10 × 10⁹/L, with >80% neutrophils)
Minor	• Sore throat
	• Lymphadenopathy
	• Hepatomegaly or splenomegaly
	• Abnormal liver function tests
	• Negative ANA and rheumatoid factor

$\Rightarrow$ The Yamaguchi criteria (*J Rheumat* 1992, 19(3):424–430).

Differential diagnosis of a very high ferritin

High ferritin (>1000 mcg/L)
• Malignancy
• Iron overload syndromes including hereditary haemochromatosis
• Iatrogenic iron overload, e.g. from repeated transfusions
• Inflammation/sepsis

Very high ferritin (>10,000 mcg/L)
• Adult-onset Still's disease
• Systemic juvenile idiopathic arthritis
• HLH/macrophage activation syndrome

Kikuchi disease

Background
- Rare condition that mainly affects ♀ of childbearing age
- Features necrotizing lymphadenitis of unknown aetiology

Clinical features
- Presenting symptoms include:
  - Fevers
  - Painful lymphadenopathy
  - Systemic symptoms such as sweats, chills, and malaise

Management in pregnancy
- Rarely reported in pregnancy, but both maternal and fetal outcomes in the reported cases have been good
- Corticosteroids can be used in pregnancy as they are in non-pregnant ♀, but require vigilance for hyperglycaemia
- Hydroxychloroquine can also be used

Behçet's disease

Background

- An inflammatory condition
- Most commonly seen in people of Mediterranean or Eastern origin, particularly from Turkey, along the old Silk Road
- Associated with HLA-B51

Clinical features

- Can feature a vasculopathy, including:
  - Superficial and deep vein thrombosis
  - Arterial aneurysms
  - Pulmonary vasculitis
- Diagnostic criteria are outlined in Box 8.11

Box 8.11 Diagnostic criteria for Behçet's disease

- Oral ulceration:
  - Minor aphthous, major aphthous, or herpetiform ulceration
  - At least 3 times in a 12 mth period
And two of the following:
- Recurrent genital ulceration:
  - Aphthous ulceration or scarring
- Eye lesions:
  - Anterior or posterior uveitis
  - Cells in vitreous on slit-lamp examination
  - Retinal vasculitis
- Skin lesions:
  - Erythema nodosum, pseudofolliculitis or papulopustular lesions, or acneiform nodules in post-adolescent ♀ not on corticosteroid treatment
  - Positive pathergy test (read by physician at 24–48 hrs)

Management of Behçet's disease in pregnancy

- Symptomatic improvement often seen during pregnancy
- In 25–30% a flare of their symptoms occurs
- Immunosuppressive medication should be reviewed before or at conception and continued
- Prophylactic LMWH if evidence of active vasculitis or previous un-provoked thrombosis
- Genital ulceration is not an indication for caesarean section
- Pathergy (non-infective skin lesions or ulceration) can occur at the site of episiotomy or caesarean section wound, which may benefit from topical corticosteroid treatment
- Rarely, transplacental transfer of antibodies can occur, resulting in transient oral and genital ulceration in the neonate

Ehlers–Danlos syndromes

Background
- A group of connective tissue disorders
- Commonly feature skin and joint abnormalities

Clinical features
See Table 8.9.

Management of EDS in pregnancy
All types of EDS
- Pre-pregnancy assessment for:
  - Characterization of phenotype
  - Identification of genotype (if appropriate)
- If the genotype is known, pre-implantation genetic diagnosis or pre-natal testing can be offered
- May benefit from physiotherapy to help with joint pain and about advice for positions at time of delivery
- Pregnancy can ↑ joint pain and risk of tendon rupture
- ↑ risk of PPH and poor wound healing

Vascular EDS
⚠ **Associated with significant maternal morbidity and mortality, so pregnancy is advised against.**
- Requires referral to a high-risk pregnancy unit and close monitoring in pregnancy because of ↑ risk of vascular aneurysm formation or dissection
- Preterm elective caesarean section may be advised because of the risk of uterine rupture with an increasingly gravid uterus
- Anaesthetic input

Joint hypermobility syndrome
- Features overlap those of EDS hypermobile type
- Often functional overlay with non-inflammatory pain syndromes/fibromyalgia
- ↑ risk of:
  - Very fast labour and delivery
  - Preterm complications such as rupture of membranes

Table 8.9 Clinical features of different Ehlers–Danlos syndromes

Type	Previous label	Features	Genetics
Classic	EDS I and II	Fragile, stretchy skin, flexible joints, herniae	Autosomal dominant mutation in collagen genes COL5A1 and COL5A2
Hypermobile[a]	EDS III	Soft, smooth skin, very flexible joints, frequent joint subluxation/dislocation, joint pain. Postural orthostatic tachycardia syndrome may be seen	Autosomal dominant pattern, gene unknown
Vascular	EDS IV	Easy bruising, normal large joints, some hypermobility of small joints, risk of arterial dissection or aneurysm formation	De novo or autosomal dominant mutations in type III collagen
Kyphoscoliosis	EDS VI	Kyphoscoliosis, joint hypermobility and dislocations, ophthalmological issues such as scleral fragility and risk of globe rupture	Autosomal recessive due to mutations in PLOD1
Arthrochalasia	EDS VII A and B	Hypermobility with joint subluxation, scoliosis and short stature, fragile skin	Autosomal dominant abnormalities in genes involved in type I collagen formation
Dermatosparaxis	EDS VIIC	Severe skin fragility, hernias, blue sclerae	Autosomal recessive mutations in ADAMTS2 gene causing a deficiency

[a] The features of this overlap with joint hypermobility syndrome.

Medications used in rheumatology

See Table 8.10.

Table 8.10 Medications used for the treatment of rheumatological conditions

Drug	Recommendations in pregnancy	Recommendations for breastfeeding
Hydroxychloroquine	• Can be continued throughout pregnancy	• Can be used

Steroids	Fluorinated steroids (betamethasone, dexamethasone)
	  • Cross placenta readily thus preferred for fetal lung maturation
	Non-fluorinated steroids (hydrocortisone, prednisolone)
	  • Do not cross placenta readily so fetal dose much smaller than maternal dose
	• All steroids:
	  • Can predispose to hyperglycaemia so glucose monitoring advised
	  • If on for >3 wks, then requires stress-dose steroids at delivery
		• Can be used

Sulfasalazine	• Can be continued in pregnancy (requires concurrent 5 mg folic acid daily while on treatment)	• Can be used
Azathioprine	• Can be continued throughout pregnancy • A TPMT level is needed if starting this in pregnancy	• Can be used
Methotrexate	• Causes miscarriage and congenital malformations so contraindicated in pregnancy • Should be stopped before conception	• Should be avoided

Drug	Recommendations in pregnancy	Recommendations for breastfeeding
Leflunomide	• Causes miscarriage and congenital malformations so contraindicated in pregnancy • Should be stopped before conception	• Should be avoided
Mycophenolate mofetil	• Associated with miscarriage and congenital malformations so contraindicated in pregnancy • Ideally stop 6–12 wks prior to conception	• Very limited information available so should be avoided
Ciclosporin	• Can be continued throughout pregnancy	• Can be used
NSAIDs (non-selective COX inhibitors, e.g. ibuprofen)	• Can be used in 1st and 2nd trimesters • Use in 3rd trimester associated with closure of the ductus arteriosus so should be avoided	• Can be used
COX II inhibitors (e.g. celecoxib, etoricoxib)	• Insufficient information available so use should be avoided	• Celecoxib—can be used • Others—use advised against
Cyclophosphamide	• Causes an embryopathy if used in 1st trimester, but can be used later in pregnancy if required	• Very limited information so alternative agent preferred if possible • Neutropenia reported in 2 infants whose mothers received cyclophosphamide postnatally

Biologics in pregnancy

See Table 8.11.

Table 8.11 Summary from EULAR and BSR guidelines

Agent	Compatible for use in early pregnancy		Gestation to discontinue		Breastfeeding	
	EULAR	BSR	EULAR	BSR	EULAR	BSR
Infliximab	Yes	Yes	Up to 20 wks[a]	Stop at 16 wks	Yes	Yes
Etanercept	Yes	Yes	Up to 32 wks[a]	Not compatible with 3rd trimester	Yes	Yes
Adalimumab	Yes	Yes	Up to 20 wks[a]	Not compatible with 3rd trimester	Yes	Yes
Certolizumab	Yes	Yes	Use throughout pregnancy	Compatible with 3rd trimester	Yes	No data
Golimumab	No ↑ in malformations[b]	No	Use another agent[b]	No data	Yes	No data
Anakinra	Yes	No[c]	Only if no other options	No	No data	No data
Tocilizumab	[b]	Stop 3 mths prior[c]	Avoid[b]	No	No data	No data
Ustekinumab	No ↑ malformations[b]	–	Use another agent[b]	–	No data	–
Abatacept	[b]	No	No[b]	No data	No data	No data

	In exceptional circumstances	Stop 6 mths prior[c]	Not specified[d]	No	No data	No data
Rituximab	No ↑ in malformations[b]	No[c]		No		
Belimumab	No[b]		No	No data	No data	

[a] Can be used throughout pregnancy if indicated; [b] insufficient evidence; [c] insufficient data to recommend drug, but unintentional exposure in the 1st trimester is unlikely to be harmful; [d] neonatal B cell depletion if used in late pregnancy. BSR, British Society for Rheumatology; EULAR, European League Against Rheumatism;, – not covered by publication.
Source: Soh and Moretto 2019, Obstetric Medicine.

Haematology

Physiological changes

Normal pregnancy results in changes in many haematological factors:
- ↓ Hb due to iron deficiency and haemodilution
- MCV ↑ later in pregnancy
- ↑ WBC count up to 20×10^9/L due to ↑ neutrophils (which may also demonstrate a left shift)
- Platelet count ↓
- ↑ ESR (up to 70 mm/hr), due to ↑ fibrinogen and globulin (whereas CRP remains normal)
- ↑ factors V, VWF, VIII, and X and fibrinogen
- ↓ levels of protein S
- Impaired fibrinolysis (placental PAI-2, ↑ PAI-1)
- ↓ Th1-mediated immunity (cellular)
- ↑ Th2-mediated immunity (humoral)

⚠ The resulting hypercoagulability has the evolutionary advantage of ↓ the risk of blood loss at delivery but results in a 6-fold ↑ risk of VTE during pregnancy.

Biochemical markers in pregnancy

Ferritin
- Iron binds to ferritin and is stored in the liver
- An excellent marker of body iron stores
- ⚠ An acute phase protein so unreliable in acute inflammation
- ➲ See page 297 for causes of very high ferritin

Serum iron
- Measurement of Fe^{3+} ions bound to serum transferrin
- Not a reliable marker of iron status in isolation as the level is very variable throughout the day, and influenced by inflammation, infection, and eating

Transferrin
- Main protein that transports iron
- ↑ in iron deficiency to maximize the circulation of available iron

Total iron binding capacity
- Laboratory calculation that measures the total amount of iron the body can carry (an indirect measurement of transferrin)

Transferrin saturation
- Measurement calculated from serum iron and transferrin
- A healthy ♀ has a transferrin saturation of ~30%
- Useful test for the diagnosis of iron deficiency as <16% consistent with iron deficiency anaemia
- Also useful as ↑ in hereditary haemochromatosis

Vitamin B₁₂
- Levels ↓ in pregnancy, so routine testing is not recommended

Folate
- Serum folate and red cell folate ↓ in pregnancy but should be tested in anaemia with normal iron indices
- Dietary deficiency is not uncommon in pregnancy and has been associated with profound anaemia

Anaemia
See Table 9.1.

Anaemia in pregnancy

1st trimester:	Hb <110 g/L
2nd and 3rd trimesters:	Hb <105 g/L
Postpartum:	Hb <100 g/L

➲ British Society of Haematology (2012). Management of iron deficiency anaemia in pregnancy guideline: ⌖ https://b-s-h.org.uk/guidelines/guidelines/management-of-iron-deficiency-in-pregnancy/

Table 9.1 Causes of anaemia by MCV

Microcytic	Normocytic	Macrocytic

• Iron deficiency anaemia
• Thalassaemia
• Sideroblastic anaemia:
  • Congenital
  • Lead poisoning
  • Alcohol
  • Drugs (e.g. isoniazid)
• Vitamin B_6 deficiency
	• Acute blood loss
	• Early iron deficiency anaemia
	• Anaemia of chronic disease
	• Bone marrow suppression
	• Chronic renal failure
	• Hypopituitarism
		• Megaloblastic:
		  • Folate deficiency
		  • Vitamin B_{12} deficiency
		• Alcohol
		• Some bone marrow disorders including:
		  • Myelodysplasia
		  • Multiple myeloma
		  • Aplastic anaemia
		• Liver disease
		• Reticulocytosis
		• Severe hypothyroidism
		• Drug that affect DNA synthesis (e.g. azathioprine)

Iron deficiency anaemia

Definition
In an anaemic individual, ferritin <15 mcg/L is diagnostic.

Overview
- Iron deficiency (with or without anaemia) is common worldwide
- Prevalence of 40–70% in low- and middle-income countries, where hookworm infection is often a contributory factor
- Microcytic RBCs but MCV may be normal
- Only around 15% of dietary iron is absorbed
- Pregnancy has ↑ iron requirement (~3-fold compared to menstruating ♀)
- Absorption of iron ↑ 3-fold by 3rd trimester
- Many factors affect gut absorption of iron:
  - ↑ absorption with ascorbic acid in orange juice
  - ↓ absorption with tannins in tea or calcium in dairy products
- In 1st trimester is associated with adverse fetal outcomes such as low birthweight babies:
  - Iron replacement in 2nd and 3rd trimesters does not ↓ this risk

---

Iron replacement in pregnancy
- Oral iron is beneficial for maternal health
- ↓ need for blood products in the event of PPH
- Oral iron is associated with side effects, which are mostly GI and related to dose of elemental iron
- No significant variation in side effect profile with different iron preparations
- 100–200 mg elemental iron/day is required to replenish stores (e.g. ferrous sulfate 200 mg dose contains 65 mg elemental iron, Pregaday® contains 100 mg, Pregnacare® 17 mg)
- Need to continue for 3 mths following correction of Hb

☛ IV iron preparations have historically been associated with adverse events including anaphylaxis
- Newer preparations such as Ferinject® are associated with far fewer adverse events and there have been no reported cases of anaphylaxis to date
- Doses of IV iron can be calculated in a similar way to that of a non-pregnant individual, but it is prudent to use a lower Hb target for pregnant ♀

⮕ RCOG (2015). Blood transfusion in obstetrics (green-top guideline no. 47): ℜ https://www.rcog.org.uk/en/guidelines-research-services/guidelines/gtg47/

Management of iron deficiency anaemia in pregnancy

- Trial of oral iron for normocytic or microcytic anaemia (ferritin not required prior to this in uncomplicated ♀)
- Further investigations if no rise in Hb after 2–4 wks (and compliant with oral iron) including:
  - Ferritin
  - Folate
- Parenteral iron if:
  - Oral iron not tolerated
  - Approaching term and not enough time for oral supplementation to be effective
  - Malabsorptive condition present that means oral iron unlikely to be sufficient

Ferritin measurement

- Unselected screening with ferritin is not recommended
- Ferritin measurement advisable in ♀ with:
  - Known anaemia (iron, folate, or vitamin B$_{12}$ deficiency)
  - Haemoglobinopathy
  - Conditions that may impair iron absorption (IBD, gastric surgery, coeliac disease)
  - Conditions that may → ↑ iron requirement (multiple pregnancy, age <20 yrs, previous pregnancy <1 yr before)
  - High bleeding risk (previous PPH, placenta praevia)
  - Beliefs that lead them to decline blood products (therefore iron repletion is crucial)

➲ British Society of Haematology (2012). Management of iron deficiency anaemia in pregnancy guideline: ⅋ https://b-s-h.org.uk/guidelines/guidelines/management-of-iron-deficiency-in-pregnancy/

Sickle cell disease

Introduction
- Autosomal recessive condition which results in production of abnormal globin chains
- Abnormal chains distort RBCs, resulting in a sickled shape → microvascular injury which can affect any organ

Types of sickling disorder
- Homozygous for haemoglobin S:
  - Sickle cell anaemia
- Compound heterozygotes:
  - Hb SC disease
  - Hb S β-thalassaemia
  - Others including Hb SD Punjab

Specific mutations

Haemoglobin S
- Mutation in the β-globin gene
- The 6th amino acid (glutamic acid) is replaced by valine

Haemoglobin C
- Mutation in the β-globin chain
- The sixth amino acid (glutamic acid) is replaced by lysine
- This abnormal haemoglobin **does not** result in the same deformity of red cells that is seen in HbS → vaso-occlusive crises do not occur in homozygous individuals, but HbSC does result in sickling

---

Diagnosis
- Diagnosis suggested by high reticulocyte count and/or findings on blood film (e.g. target cells, Howell–Jolly bodies, sickle poikilocytes)
- FBC
- Sickle solubility test
- High-performance liquid chromatography can confirm the diagnosis and has largely replaced the use of Hb electrophoresis
- Manifestations of the haemoglobinopathies are outlined in Table 9.2

Complications of sickle cell disease
- Vaso-occlusive crises (bone, kidney, cerebral, retina, lung)
- Acute chest crisis (fever, chest pain, tachypnoea, pulmonary infiltrates)
- Thromboembolic disease
- ↑ risk of infection, e.g. UTI and pneumonia
- Splenic infarction resulting in hyposplenism
- Cholelithiasis
- PH (described in up to 30%)
- Retinal disease
- Pulmonary disease
- Avascular necrosis
- Complications of iron overload
- Red cell alloimmunization

Table 9.2 Manifestations of haemoglobinopathies

Name	Manifestations	Haematological abnormalities
HbAC Haemoglobin C trait	• Asymptomatic	• Normal Hb • ↓ MCV • Target cells
HbCC Haemoglobin C disease	• Mild haemolytic anaemia	• Mild ↓ Hb • ↓ MCV • Target cells
HbS Sickle carrier	• Symptoms only if hypoxic or very dehydrated	• Normal Hb • Normal MCV • Normal blood film
HbSC Haemoglobin SC disease	• Mild haemolytic anaemia • Sickle crises, often less frequent than in HbSS • Thrombosis • Vaso-occlusive osteonecrosis and retinal disease occur	• Mild ↓ Hb • Mild reticulocytosis • Blood film: • Target cells, Poikilocytes, boat cells, etc.

HbSS
Sickle cell disease
	• Highly variable
	• Can have severe and frequent vaso-occlusive crises
	• Haemolytic anaemia
	• Chronic organ damage
	• Complications are common
		• Hb 60–90 gL
		• Normal MCV
		• Blood film:
		  • Sickle cells
		  • Target cells
		  • Howell–Jolly bodies

Management of sickle cell disease

Maternal complications

- ↑ incidence pre-eclampsia
- More frequent vaso-occlusive crises
- Anaemia requiring top-up or exchange transfusion
- Sepsis especially pneumonia and puerperal sepsis
- VTE
- Sequestration
- Atypical thromboses (cerebral venous sinus, mesenteric, splenic)
- Cardiomyopathy

Fetal risks

- Miscarriage and stillbirth (perinatal mortality ↑ 4–6-fold)
- IUGR
- Prematurity

Sickle cell crises

- Associated with pain, ischaemia, and end-organ damage
- 'Acute chest syndrome' is associated with significant mortality
- Precipitant may be evident from history or examination:
  - Infection
  - Hypoxia
  - Dehydration
  - Acidosis
- Often no precipitant is identified

⚠ Management of a sickle cell crisis in pregnancy

- ↑ risk of crises in 3rd trimester

Management is the same as in non-pregnant ♀

- If >20 wks admit to bed on HDU
- May need opioid analgesia
- Oxygen
- Aggressive rehydration
- Antibiotics if infective precipitant suspected
- Transfusion as guided by haematologist
- Exchange transfusion may be required in severe crises
- Needs anaesthetic review ± patient-controlled analgesia
- Fetal monitoring appropriate to gestation

Management of sickle cell disease in pregnancy

- MDT involvement
- Discuss inheritance and partner screening ± prenatal diagnosis
- FBC and ferritin:
  - Regular Hb and % of sickled Hb
  - Only give iron if ↓ ferritin
  - Stop iron-chelating agents before conception
  - Regular top-up or exchange transfusion may be required depending on type of SCD, Hb, % sickled Hb (extended phenotype matching for antigens other than rhesus is required in those receiving long-term transfusion therapy)
- Assess for and manage complications:
  - Echocardiogram for evidence of PH and/or if history of iron overload
  - Retinal assessment
  - Renal function
  - Screen for bacteriuria

Medications
- Folic acid 5 mg OD prior to conception and throughout pregnancy
- Stop medications such as hydroxycarbamide and ACE-I
- Thromboprophylaxis
- Aspirin 75 mg OD from 12 wks
- Phenoxymethylpenicillin V 250 mg BD in all ♀ (functional hyposplenism)
- Review vaccination history (especially meningitis C, *Haemophilus influenzae* type B, hepatitis B, and influenza)

Fetal monitoring
- Monthly growth scans in 3rd trimester

Delivery plans
- Aim for vaginal delivery avoiding hypoxia and dehydration
- Caesarean section for fetal indications

Postpartum management of sickle cell disease

- Thromboprophylaxis
- Prevention of crises:
  - Exchange transfusion
  - Physiotherapy
  - Continuous positive airway pressure ventilation sometimes used
- Contraception

Thalassaemia

- Group of conditions involving defective production of globin chains
- Usually autosomal recessive conditions involving a variety of deletions or mutations
- Carriership is often referred to as 'trait'
- Symptoms and treatment depends on the type and severity

Types of haemoglobin

See Table 9.3.

α thalassaemia

- 4 α globin genes
- 2 inherited from each parent
- The severity depends on the combination of absent genes (Table 9.4)
- High prevalence of α plus carriers: African, Caribbean, Indian, Pakistani, Bangladeshi populations
- High prevalence of α zero carriers: Taiwan, Laos, Vietnam, Malaysia, Hong Kong, China, Cyprus, Burma, Turkey, Greece, Singapore
- Complete absence of α chain production is incompatible with life and is a common cause of stillbirth in countries where the prevalence of α zero is high

β thalassaemia

- β chains are not a component of fetal Hb, so the fetus is unaffected *in utero*:
  - Results in ↓ β-globin synthesis
  - This alone in heterozygous individuals does not cause any significant clinical consequences
- Types and complications (Table 9.4)
- There is a risk of iron overload in ♀ receiving regular transfusions
- Compound heterozygosity can → severe thalassaemia

Table 9.3 Types of haemoglobin

HbA	2 α chains 2 β chains	• Main Hb in adults
HbA$_2$	2 α chains 2 γ chains	• 2–3% of adult Hb
HbF	2 α chains 2 γ chains	• 50–98% of fetal Hb at birth • 1–2% in adults • Can ↑ in pregnancy to 5–10% total Hb

Table 9.4 Genetic phenotypes in the thalassaemias

	Genetic abnormality	Complication outside pregnancy	Complications in pregnancy
Alpha (α) thalassaemia			
α plus thalassaemia carrier	1 or 2 gene deletions (α–/αα or α–/α–)	• Often silent • Slight ↓ in MCV may be seen	
α zero thalassaemia carrier	2 gene deletions (– –/αα)	• Usually asymptomatic • MCH <25 pg	• May become symptomatic of anaemia • Risk to offspring of α thalassaemia major if both parents are carriers
α thalassaemia intermedia (haemoglobin H disease)	3 gene deletions (– –/–α)	• Hb 70–100 g/L; MCH 15–25 pg • Microcytic, hypochromic indices • Splenomegaly	• Anaemia may worsen
α thalassaemia major	4 gene deletions (– –/– –)	• Usually fatal to fetus • Massive hepatosplenomegaly and hydropic	• Mother of an affected fetus may develop early pre-eclampsia ('mirror syndrome')
Beta (β) thalassaemia			
β thalassaemia trait	1 gene abnormal	• Asymptomatic • Hb rarely <100 g/L • Microcytic hypochromic appearances • ↑ HbA$_2$	• May become anaemic

| β thalassaemia intermedia | 2 genes abnormal → mild to moderate ↓ in synthesis of β globin | • Varying severity of phenotype:
 • Some asymptomatic, some require regular transfusion
 • Hb usually 100–120 g/L, can be as low as 50 g/L
 • Hepatosplenomegaly | • Variable, depends on phenotype
 • May become anaemic |
| β thalassaemia major | 2 genes abnormal → severe ↓ in synthesis of β globin | • Untreated → skeletal deformities and hepatosplenomegaly
 • Often transfusion dependent, so may need iron chelation therapy
 • Iron overload can → hepatic and endocrine dysfunction | • Very few pregnancies reported (iron overload can → endocrine dysfunction and subfertility) |

Management of thalassaemia

Treatment of anaemia

- Folic acid 5 mg OD prior to conception and throughout pregnancy
- Regular FBC
- Ferritin at booking
- Only give iron if ferritin/iron markers confirm iron deficiency
- Blood transfusion requirements ↑ and those not normally transfused may require it during pregnancy or after delivery:
  - Target 100 g/L in β-thalassaemia major
  - A lower target may be appropriate in other types

Iron overload
- Occurs in β-thalassaemia major
- Multiple causes:
  - Multiple blood transfusions
  - ↑ GI iron absorption
  - Ineffective erythropoiesis
- Can cause serious complications:
  - Endocrine (hypogonadotropic hypogonadism, hypothyroidism)
  - Cardiac failure
  - Liver
  - Pancreatic insufficiency and 2° DM

History of iron overload

- Iron chelation therapy:
  - Chelating agents should be optimized prior to pregnancy and stopped during pregnancy
  - ♀ with unintentional exposure to chelators in pregnancy have not exhibited adverse fetal outcomes
  - Can be considered during pregnancy if the risks of cardiac complications are high, but this requires specialist input
  - Deferiprone and deferasirox should be withheld while breastfeeding, but desferrioxamine can be used
- Regular MDT involvement
- Assessment for complications:
  - Oral GTT at 24–28 wks (earlier if diagnosis suspected or history of GDM)
  - Thyroid function
  - Cardiac assessment (may need MRI if not done prior to pregnancy)

History of splenectomy

- Prophylactic phenoxymethylpenicillin
- ↑ risk of thrombosis

Other complications

- Thromboprophylaxis after delivery and if other risk factors present
- Calcium and vitamin D supplements, especially if there is a history of osteoporosis/osteopenia (bisphosphonates should be stopped)

Screening for haemoglobinopathies

Introduction

- SCT (NHS Sickle Cell and Thalassaemia) screening programme provides guidance in the UK for screening in pregnancy
- All ♀ should have an FBC at booking:
  - If low MCV or mean corpuscular Hb, suspect thalassaemia
  - If microcytic and hypochromic, ferritin should be checked
- Prevalence of haemoglobinopathies determines next screening steps:
  - The Family Origin Questionnaire (FOQ) indicates risk of haemoglobinopathies (Fig. 9.1)
  - In low-prevalence areas, offer Hb variant screening to ♀ if they or the baby's father have high-risk family origins
  - In high-prevalence areas, offer Hb variant screening to all ♀, irrespective of FOQ answers
  - HPLC to identify Hb variant and quantify HbA_2

Positive screening

- If the ♀ is identified as a carrier, the partner should be tested
- If both parents are carriers, confirm by DNA analysis
- Provide genetic counselling
- Offer prenatal genetic testing for the fetus (CVS or amniocentesis)
- Use to determine presence and severity of haemoglobinopathies

➔ NHS SCT guidance: ℘ https://www.gov.uk/topic/population-screening-programmes/sickle-cell-thalassaemia

➔ NICE guidance on antenatal care for uncomplicated pregnancies (CG62): ℘ https://www.nice.org.uk/Guidance/cg62

Public Health England

NHS Sickle Cell and Thalassaemia Screening Programme

Family Origin Questionnaire

NHS

If using a pre-printed label please attach one to each copy

Hospital number ....
NHS number ....
Estimated delivery date ....
Surname ....
Forename ....
Date of birth ....
Address 1 ....
Address 2 ....
Post code ....

Gestation at ime of sample (weeks and days) ☐

Screening test declined ☐

Report destination (such as community midwife, GP, antenatal clinic, obstetrician)
....

Is pregnancy the result of IVF? If yes, complete the form including SECTION H.

What are your and your family's origins?

Please tick all boxes in ALL sections that apply to the woman and the baby's biological father.

	Woman	Biological father
A. AFRICAN OR AFRICAN-CARIBBEAN (BLACK)		
Caribbean Islands	☐	☐
Africa (excluding North Africa)	☐	☐
Any other African family origins	☐	☐
B. SOUTH ASIAN (ASIAN)		
India or African-Indian	☐	☐
Pakistan, Bangladesh, Sri Lanka	☐	☐
C. SOUTH EAST ASIAN (ASIAN)		
China including Hong Kong. Taiwan	☐ #	☐ #
Singapore, Thailand, Indonesia	☐ #	☐ #
Malaysia, Vietnam, Philippines	☐ #	☐ #
Cambodia, Laos, Myanmar	☐ #	☐ #
Any other Asian family origins	☐ #	☐ #
D. OTHER NON-EUROPEAN (OTHER)		
North Africa, South America	☐	☐
Middle East, Saudi Arabia, Iran	☐	☐
Any other non-European family origins	☐	☐
E. SOUTHERN AND OTHER EUROPEAN (WHITE)		
Sardinia	☐ #	☐ #
Greece, Turkey, Cyprus	☐ #	☐ #
Italy, Portugal, Spain	☐	☐
Albania, Czech Republic	☐	☐
Poland, Romania, Russia	☐	☐
Any other Mediterranean country	☐	☐
F.* UNITED KINGDOM (WHITE) refer to the list on the back		
England, Scotland, Northern Ireland, Wales	☐	☐
G.* NORTHERN EUROPEAN (WHITE) refer to the list on the back		
Austria, Belgium, Switzerland, Scandinavia	☐	☐
Eire, France, Germany, Netherlands	☐	☐
Australia, North America, South Africa	☐	☐
Any other European family origins	☐	☐
* Hb Variant Screening Requested by (F) and/or (G)		
# Higher risk for alpha zero thalassaemia		
H. DON'T KNOW		
Adoption/unknown ancestry	☐	☐
Donor egg/sperm (of pregnancy results from donor egg, order test for mother and offer biological father test immediately)	☐	☐
Bone marrow transplant (if mother has had a bone marrow transplant, order test for mother and offer biological father test immediately)	☐	☐
I. DECLINED TO ANSWER	☐	☐

All women need to be informed that routine analysis of blood may identify them as a thalassaemia carrier. In low prevalence areas OFFER haemoglobin variant screening to all women if they or the baby's father have answers in any yellow box. In high prevalence areas OFFER haemoglobin variant screening to all women irrespective of answers.

Signed _____ Print name _____ Hospital _____ Date _____
(By health care professional completing the form)

Fig. 9.1 The Family Origin Questionnaire (FOQ). Reprinted under the Open Government License V3 ♒ https://www.nationalarchives.gov.uk/doc/open-government-licence/version/3/

Major obstetric haemorrhage

RCOG definition

>1000 mL blood loss and continuing to bleed **or** in shock (Table 9.5).

⚠ Pregnant ♀ generally tolerate blood loss even better than non-pregnant individuals (as a result of ↑ circulating volume).

⚠ Cardiovascular parameters are maintained until about 30–40% of blood volume is lost therefore estimated blood loss can be underestimated.

Causes of MOH

Antepartum
- Placental abruption
- Placenta praevia
- Severe chorioamnionitis or sepsis
- Severe pre-eclampsia (including hepatic rupture)
- Retained dead fetus

Intrapartum
- Intrapartum abruption
- Uterine rupture
- Amniotic fluid embolism
- Complications of caesarean section: angular or broad ligament tears
- Abnormally invasive placenta (accreta/increta/percreta)

Postpartum
- 1° PPH is usually due to:
  - Atonic uterus ('tone')
  - Genital tract trauma ('trauma')
  - Coagulopathy ('thrombin')
  - Retained products of conception ('tissue')
- 2° PPH is due to:
  - Infection (associated with retained products of conception)
  - Rarely gestational trophoblastic disease or uterine arteriovenous malformation including a pseudo-aneurysm

---

Table 9.5 Blood loss and cardiovascular parameters in a pregnant ♀

Blood loss	Heart rate	Systolic BP	Tissue perfusion
10–15%	Normal	Normal	Postural hypotension
15–30%	↑ +	Normal	Peripheral vasoconstriction
30–40%	↑ ++	70–80 mmHg	Pallor, oliguria, confusion, restlessness
>40%	↑ +++	<60 mmHg	Collapse, anuria, dyspnoea

Initial measures for resuscitation in MOH

Seek assistance
- Call for help; include alerting senior obstetrician, anaesthetist, haematologist, hospital porter, blood bank, theatres

Initial resuscitation
- Left lateral tilt if antepartum (relieve venocaval compression and improve venous return)
- High-flow facial O_2 (regardless of O_2 saturation)
- Assess airway and respiratory effort (intubation may be indicated if there is ↓ level of consciousness due to ↓ BP)
- Two large-bore IV cannulae (14 gauge):
  - Take blood while cannulating for FBC, cross-match, U&Es, LFTs, coagulation screen, fibrinogen
  - Start warm IV crystalloid to correct hypovolaemia
- Catheterize and measure hourly urine output

Blood transfusion
- O rhesus –ve blood until cross-matched blood is available

Replace clotting factors (as per RCOG guidelines)
- FFP alongside packed red cells
- Cryoprecipitate to maintain fibrinogen >2 g/L
- Platelet transfusion if platelet count <75 × 10⁹/L
- Ongoing replacement determined by haemostasis markers (PT, APTT, fibrinogen, and thromboelastography if available)

Tranexamic acid
- WHO recommend 1 g of tranexamic acid for all cases of PPH irrespective of the source of blood loss:
  - As soon as possible after onset of bleeding
  - Can be repeated after 30 mins if ongoing bleeding

Further considerations
- As soon as appropriate, transfer the ♀ to a place where there is adequate space, lighting, and equipment (usually theatre)
- Assess need for a central venous line
- Interventional radiological procedures

▶ 1 team member should be assigned to record the vital signs, urinary output, fluid replacement, drugs, and timeline of events.

⮌ RCOG (2016). Prevention and management of postpartum haemorrhage (green-top guidance no. 52): ℗ https://obgyn.onlinelibrary.wiley.com/doi/epdf/10.1111/1471-0528.14178

Principles for stopping obstetric bleeding
- Empty uterus (fetus or tissue)
- Treat uterine atony (physically, medically, surgically)
- Repair genital tract trauma

Folate deficiency

- Folic acid cannot be synthesized by humans:
  - Humans dependent on external sources
  - Found in a wide variety of meat and plant-based sources
- Most common cause of folate deficiency is dietary insufficiency:
  - ↑ prevalence in low- and middle-income countries
  - ↓ prevalence in countries with food fortification programmes
- Deficiency can also result from:
  - Malabsorptive syndromes
  - Haemolysis
  - Myeloproliferative conditions
  - Anticonvulsants
- Can be measured either in a serum sample or a red cell folate assay but the British Society of Haematology advocates performing serum folate

Folate deficiency in pregnancy

- Red cell folate assays are not a reliable marker in pregnancy
- Folate deficiency (even mild) is associated with neural tube defects

Folate supplementation

- 3/12 prior to conception
- Throughout 1st trimester
- Ongoing supplementation for ♀ with low dietary intake of folate
- ↑ dose (5 mg rather than 400 mcg daily) advised in ♀ who:
  - Are on anticonvulsant medications
  - Have conditions associated with greater red cell turnover
  - Have had a previous pregnancy with a neural tube defect
- Confirmed folate deficiency should be treated with 5 mg TDS, after investigation for vitamin B_{12} deficiency

Vitamin B$_{12}$ deficiency

Background

- Cobalamins, including cyanocobalamin (vitamin B$_{12}$), are required for methionine synthesis
- Important for DNA and protein synthesis
- Mostly derived from meat, fish, and dairy products

Causes

- Dietary deficiency can result from vegan diet preferences
- ↓ GI absorption can also cause insufficiency, as vitamin B$_{12}$ absorbed particularly in the terminal ileum
- ↓ GI absorption can result from:
  - Pernicious anaemia: autoimmune lack of intrinsic factor, antibodies may or may not be present
  - Achlorhydria from proton pump inhibitor use
  - Resection of upper parts of the GI tract
- Body stores take 3 or more years to deplete

Clinical features

Megaloblastic anaemia

- Characteristic changes on blood film include:
  - Oval macrocytes
  - Hypersegmented neutrophils
  - Thrombocytopenia and leucopenia are also often present
- Clinical indicators of deficiency include:
  - Gradually worsening anaemia
  - Neurological, e.g. subacute combined degeneration of the cord
  - Neuropsychiatric symptoms
  - Angular stomatitis

Management of vitamin B$_{12}$ deficiency in pregnancy

- True vitamin B$_{12}$ deficiency is rare but ↓ vitamin B$_{12}$ levels are not uncommon
- ↓ vitamin B$_{12}$ levels in pregnancy compared to non-pregnant (↓ ≤50% in 3rd trimester) and return to normal rapidly after delivery
- Testing only recommended in pregnancy therefore if:
  - Macrocytic anaemia
  - Symptoms of deficiency
  - Known malabsorptive condition
- Parenteral supplementation should be considered if deficiency identified **and** felt to be clinically significant
- Oral supplementation can be offered in the small number of ♀ where deficiency is due to diet alone

Lactation

- Cobalamins are important for the developing infant, so adequate dietary vitamin B$_{12}$ should be ensured, particularly in ♀ on strict vegan diets, or ♀ with a history of gastric bypass surgery

Haemolysis in pregnancy

See Tables 9.6 and 9.7.

Table 9.6 Tests for haemolysis

Test	Findings in haemolysis
FBC	• Anaemia
Blood film	• Polychromasia • Red cell fragmentation (schistocytes) (MAHA/thrombotic microangiopathy) • Spherocytes (immune) • Red cell agglutination (cold AIHA) • All sorts of other poikilocytes, e.g. blister/ghost cells (G6PD, sickle cell, etc.)
Reticulocyte count	↑
Haptoglobins	↓ (if intravascular)
Direct antiglobulin test	Positive in immune-mediated haemolysis
LDH	↑
Bilirubin	↑

Table 9.7 Causes of haemolysis

Type	Examples
Haemoglobinopathies	• Sickle cell disease
Red cell membrane defects	• Spherocytosis
Autoimmune	• Haemolytic anaemia • 'Warm'—usually IgG mediated • 'Cold'—usually IgM mediated
MAHA	• TTP/HUS • HELLP
Enzyme deficiency	• G6PD deficiency • PK deficiency
Heart valve pathology	• Severe aortic stenosis • Prosthetic valve
Infections	• Severe malaria • *Clostridium perfringens*
Other	• Liver disease • Hypersplenism • Oxidative drugs, e.g. dapsone • Wilson's disease • Paroxysmal nocturnal haemoglobinuria • Transfusion of incompatible blood

Haemolytic anaemia

Autoimmune haemolytic anaemia

- Commonest acquired cause of haemolysis but remains rare in pregnancy
- RBC destruction by red cell antibodies:
  - 'Warm' AIHA: IgG-mediated
  - 'Cold' AIHA: IgM- and complement-mediated (cold agglutinins)
- Neonatal haemolysis is rarely severe even with transplacental passage of IgG antibodies
- The main features are:
  - RBC fragmentation on a blood film
  - Positive direct antiglobulin test (previously known as 'Coombs test')
  - ↑ LDH
  - ↑ bilirubin
  - ↓ haptoglobins

⚠ Non-immune haemolytic anaemia can occur in many conditions (particularly conditions associated with pregnancy) ∴ important to assess a pregnant ♀ with possible haemolytic anaemia thoroughly.

Microangiopathic haemolytic anaemia

- Non-immune haemolytic anaemia, with intravascular haemolysis
- The main features are:
  - RBC fragmentation on a blood film
  - Negative direct antiglobulin test
  - ↑ LDH
  - ↑ bilirubin
  - ↓ haptoglobins
- Can result from:
  - Mechanical intravascular devices (e.g. prosthetic heart valve)
  - Thrombotic microangiopathy associated with thrombocytopenia

---

Disorders associated with MAHA and thrombocytopenia

- HELLP syndrome
- Severe hypertension
- Systemic infection such as bacterial endocarditis and HIV
- Systemic malignancies
- Rheumatic conditions such as SLE, APS, and systemic sclerosis
- Drug regimens used in stem cell transplantation
- TTP and HUS

Management of haemolytic anaemia in pregnancy
- Look for underlying cause
- The specific management depends on the cause
- Specialist haematology input
- Blood transfusion can be given but may be complicated by the presence of antibodies, and may require blood warmer if 'cold' AIHA identified
- Steroids and IVIg can be used in pregnancy if indicated
- Folic acid 5 mg OD given ↑ RBC turnover
- Thromboprophylaxis
- Inform neonatologists prior to delivery

Thrombotic thrombocytopenic purpura

- Deficiency of the ADAMTS13 enzyme (levels <10%)
- ADAMTS13 is a metalloproteinase responsible for cleaving multimers of von Willebrand factor
- Large multimers accumulate → platelet aggregation and thrombi

Clinical features

- The 5 cardinal features of this condition are:
  - MAHA
  - Thrombocytopenia
  - Fever
  - Neurological involvement
  - Renal involvement

▶ The diagnosis can be made and treatment instituted without all 5 features being present.

▶ Renal function may be relatively preserved, in contrast to other thrombotic microangiopathies, despite microvascular involvement of the kidney.

Causes of TTP

Congenital
- Upshaw–Schulman syndrome

Autoimmune
- Antibodies to ADAMTS13

2° *(40%)*
- Cancer
- Bone marrow transplantation
- Pregnancy
- Medications (quinine, clopidogrel, ciclosporin)
- HIV-1 infection

Management of TTP in pregnancy

Investigate cause
- Can be:
  - 1st presentation
  - Recurrent presentation of known congenital TTP
  - Acquired TTP arising *de novo*

▶ Diagnosis should be confirmed by an ADAMTS13 activity level.

⚠ Plasma exchange must be initiated urgently in an acute presentation and specialist haematology input is required.

Pregnancy-specific considerations
- A decision about pregnancy continuation depends on:
  - Gestation
  - Any coexistent placental insufficiency
  - Likelihood that delivery will improve the clinical condition
- Regular plasma therapy (either infusion or exchange) can be undertaken throughout pregnancy, usually every 1–2 wks, to provide adequate ADAMTS13 levels
- Prophylactic LMWH should be given to all ♀ with a history of VTE, as long as platelet count >50 × 10^9/L
- RBC transfusions can be given as clinically indicated
- Platelet transfusions usually avoided due to the potential ↑ in thrombotic events that can result, but can be given if severe haemorrhage occurs

Haemolytic uraemic syndrome

- Previously divided into:
  - Typical: diarrhoea-positive HUS
  - Atypical: diarrhoea-negative HUS
- Classification has now been altered to 1° and 2° HUS

1° HUS (with no underlying disease)

- Complement gene mutations
- Antibodies to complement factor H

2° HUS

- Infections:
  - Shiga toxin-producing enterohaemorrhagic *Escherichia coli* or *Shigella*
  - *Streptococcus pneumoniae*
  - HIV
- Drug toxicity (e.g. solid organ transplant recipients)
- Pregnancy (also known as pregnancy-associated atypical HUS, or p-aHUS)
- Underlying autoimmune disorders

Features of HUS

- MAHA
- Thrombocytopenia
- AKI
- Other organ involvement:
  - Central nervous system—seizures, coma, stroke, cortical blindness
  - Cardiovascular—severe hypertension, cardiac dysfunction
  - GI tract—severe haemorrhagic colitis, bowel necrosis, perforation
  - Pancreas—glucose intolerance, transient DM
  - Liver—hepatomegaly, ↑ serum transaminases
  - Haematological—leucocytosis

Management of HUS in pregnancy

- High index of suspicion is required as the features overlap with pre-eclampsia/HELLP
- Close monitoring of renal function
- Send stool sample for culture
- Low threshold for plasma exchange and/or eculizumab if renal impairment
- Cautious transfusion of RBCs given haemolysis
- Screening for mutations in genes that encode components of the complement pathway identified in non-Shiga toxin-related HUS should be offered for:
  - ♀ developing HUS in pregnancy without identifiable precipitant
  - Individuals with a personal or family history of HUS
- Risk of recurrence of HUS in future pregnancies is not clear

Eculizumab

- Eculizumab is a monoclonal antibody to C5 that blocks the terminal complement cascade
- Can be used in pregnancy, options include:
  - Continuing eculizumab throughout pregnancy
  - Using it from before delivery and the early postpartum period
  - Waiting to institute treatment if complications develop
- The exact approach can be individualized to the ♀ based on their history and severity of the condition

⚠ Associated with ↑ risk of meningococcal infection so advise meningococcal vaccination alongside *H. influenza* type B and *S. pneumoniae* vaccination.

Paroxysmal nocturnal haemoglobinuria

- Rare condition characterized by haemolytic anaemia, bone marrow failure, and thromboembolism
- Caused by a clonal expansion of haematopoietic stem cells that → a ↓ of complement inhibitory proteins CD55 and CD59

PNH in pregnancy

- Presenting features of PNH overlap with HELLP ∴ sometimes difficult to distinguish the aetiology
- Diagnosis should be suspected in anyone presenting with:
  - Anaemia and/or thrombocytopenia
  - Intravascular haemolysis
  - Thrombosis in unusual locations

Maternal risks

- Haemolysis can ↑ even in ♀ well controlled when not pregnant
- Pregnancy is associated with maternal morbidity and mortality, commonly due to thromboembolic events often in atypical sites (e.g. hepatic veins)

Fetal risks

- Adverse fetal outcomes include miscarriage and premature delivery

Management of PNH in pregnancy

- Multidisciplinary input required
- RBC and platelet transfusion as clinically indicated
- 5 mg folic acid OD prior to conception and throughout pregnancy
- Iron supplementation throughout pregnancy
- Thromboembolic risk associated with PNH means that therapeutic anticoagulation throughout pregnancy is advisable
- Regular blood tests:
  - FBC
  - Reticulocyte count
  - U&E
  - LFTs
  - LDH
- Fresh frozen plasma should be used with caution due to the high complement concentration (↑ risk of haemolysis and thrombosis)
- Eculizumab

Neutropenia

- A normal neutrophil count is $1.5-4.0 \times 10^9/L$
- Neutropenia is an abnormally low level of neutrophils, i.e. $<1.5 \times 10^9/L$
- However, in definitions of febrile neutropenia the threshold for treatment is normally ↓, i.e. 0.5 or $1.0 \times 10^9/L$ depending on protocol

---

Causes of neutropenia

- Benign ethnic neutropenia (common in people of African descent or some Middle East populations)
- Autoimmune
- Drug related:
  - Chemotherapy agents
  - Antithyroid drugs, e.g. carbimazole, propylthiouracil
  - Antibiotics, e.g. penicillins, co-trimoxazole
- Infections:
  - Viral, e.g. EBV, CMV
- ↓ production from bone marrow (often not isolated):
  - Malignancy
- Vitamin deficiency, e.g. vitamin B_{12}

Management of neutropenia in pregnancy

⚠ Warn ♀ on medication that it may cause agranulocytosis to ensure that if they develop infective symptoms such as a sore throat they seek medical attention (for review and FBC)

- Regular urine screening → treat if bacteriuria identified
- Active management when membranes rupture
- If sepsis develops, ensure local guidelines for antibiotics in neutropenic sepsis are followed
- Consider the use of G-CSF if unwell and neutrophils remain low
- Ensure paediatricians aware as occasional cases of neonatal neutropenia have been reported due to transplacental transfer of anti-neutrophil antibodies

➔ See 'Neutropenic sepsis' p. 507.

Thrombocytopenia

- The normal range of platelets is 150–400 × 10⁹/L
- Thrombocytopenia is therefore a platelet count of <150 × 10⁹/L
- This is common in pregnancy (seen in ~13% pregnant ♀ at term)

Causes of thrombocytopenia in pregnancy

Pregnancy related
- Gestational
- Hypertensive syndromes (pre-eclampsia/HELLP/AFLP)
- DIC
- Folate deficiency

Other
- ITP
- Viral infection: HIV
- HUS/TTP
- Hereditary
- Marrow infiltration
- Hypersplenism
- Drugs
- Platelet clumping *in vitro*

Gestational thrombocytopenia

- Platelet count ↓ during normal pregnancy
- Tends to be mild, but sometimes it ↓ as low as 70 × 10⁹/L
- 75% of thrombocytopenia at term is gestational thrombocytopenia
- No impact on the fetus as it is not antibody mediated, but may affect plans for regional analgesia
- The platelet count rapidly recovers in the weeks after delivery

Differentiating gestational thrombocytopenia from other causes
- Can be challenging
- The lower the platelet count, the more likely it is to be due to a cause other than gestational thrombocytopenia
- ITP is a diagnosis of exclusion and other causes should be considered before ITP is diagnosed
- A previous history of thrombocytopenia is present in 2/3 of cases of ♀ with ITP presenting in pregnancy

---

Newly identified thrombocytopenia in pregnancy

- Repeat sample
- Blood film (clumping or large platelets seen in ITP and some hereditary causes such as Bernard–Soulier disease)
- Maternal bleeding history and previous results if available
- Review medications
- Examination for hepatomegaly and splenomegaly
- Any suggestion of autoimmune condition

Immune thrombocytopenia

Monitoring
- At least monthly in the 1st and 2nd trimesters
- Fortnightly in 3rd trimester
- Weekly from 36 wks

Treatment in the antenatal period
- Should be restricted to those who:
  - Have very low platelet counts (<20 × 10^9/L)
  - Have bleeding complications
  - Are near term and require higher count at delivery
- A trial of steroids can be helpful in the early 3rd trimester to assess response to enable planning treatment for nearer delivery

Treatment options
- Steroids, e.g. prednisolone 20 mg OD for 1 wk, ↑ to 60 mg OD for 1 wk if no response (start at 60 mg if significant bleeding)
- IVIg where rapid response needed
- Anti-D in non-splenectomized rhesus D-positive ♀
- Platelet transfusion only if significant bleeding
- IV methylprednisolone is only used in life-threatening bleeding or in refractory cases
- In refractory cases, splenectomy, tranexamic acid, azathioprine, or rituximab may have a role

Fetal considerations
- Anti-platelet antibodies can cause fetal thrombocytopenia
- Severity of fetal manifestations does not correlate with maternal platelet count
- Main concern is fetal intracranial haemorrhage, but this is rare:
  - Thrombocytopenia can occur in the neonate, ~10% have platelet count <50 × 10^9/L, <5% have platelet count <20 × 10^9/L, but the incidence of intracranial haemorrhage is <1%

Delivery considerations for ♀ with low platelets

- Use of regional anaesthesia is determined by platelet count
- Thresholds for inserting epidural catheters differ between guidelines so seek local advice but in general at $<80 \times 10^9$/L most anaesthetists would not advise it
- No evidence that caesarean section ↓ incidence of intracranial haemorrhage in babies at risk
- Induction of labour may be warranted if the ↑ in platelet count is very transient after treatment
- Advisable to avoid in ♀ with ITP (or where the platelet count is low and the diagnosis is unclear):
  - Fetal scalp electrode (FSE)
  - Fetal blood sampling (FBS)
  - Ventouse delivery
  - Rotational forceps

Neonatal considerations with ITP

- Neonatal thrombocytopenia is more likely if:
  - Previous sibling affected by thrombocytopenia
  - Mother had a splenectomy prior to pregnancy
  - Severe maternal disease
- Inform neonatal team prior to delivery
- Cord platelet count at birth:
  - If normal, no further tests required
  - If low, venous sample required
- Avoid IM injections
- Regular FBC as platelets often fall after birth, reaching a nadir at day 4 or 5
- Treatment if platelets $<20 \times 10^9$/L (with IVIg) and cranial USS
- Testing for paternal platelet incompatibility is advised if severe thrombocytopenia is identified in the neonate

Fetal/neonatal alloimmune thrombocytopenia

- Rare condition that occurs when antibodies develop to paternal platelet antigens
- Antibodies cross the placenta and react against the fetal platelets
- Results in thrombocytopenia in the neonate
- Consequences are mostly mild, e.g. petechiae
- Can occasionally be severe, e.g. intracranial haemorrhage

Diagnosis

- May only be apparent:
  - After neonate develops a bleeding complication
  - After detection of an antenatal fetal intracranial haemorrhage, in a mother who has no history of a bleeding disorder and a normal platelet count during pregnancy
- In contrast to rhesus disease of the newborn, this disorder can occur in a 1st pregnancy
- FNAIT tends to worsen in subsequent pregnancies
- Platelet antibodies can develop after (multiple) platelet transfusions, so this phenomenon can also occur in ♀ with platelet disorders and a history of (multiple) platelet transfusions

Management of subsequent pregnancies after FNAIT

- No evidence for routine screening
- Fetal blood sampling and platelet transfusion is no longer recommended due to the risks associated with in utero transfusion
- Weekly IVIg (1 mg/kg/wk) is commonly used in pregnancies viewed as high-risk
  - Advised to start at 16–18 weeks of gestation
  - No evidence for steroids in addition

Delivery advice

- Elective caesarean delivery at 37 weeks is the preferred option but generally evidence is weak
- Vaginal delivery in a multiparous woman can be considered, with avoidance of:
  - Fetal scalp blood sampling
  - FSE placement
  - Instrumental delivery especially ventouse or rotational forceps
- Inform neonatologist and ensure prompt investigation and treatment of the potentially affected neonate

RCOG Scientific Impact Paper on Prenatal Management of Pregnancies at Risk of Fetal Neonatal Alloimmune Thrombocytopenia (FNAIT) ℘ https://www.rcog.org.uk/en/guidelines-research-services/guidelines/sip61/

Recurrence

See Table 9.8.

Table 9.8 Risk of recurrence of FNAIT and intracranial haemorrhage

	Recurrence risk (%)
Father homozygous for the responsible anti-platelet antibody	100
Father heterozygous for the responsible anti-platelet antibody	50
Intracranial haemorrhage (ICH)	
Affected sibling had an ICH and survived	72
Affected sibling had an ICH and did not survive	79
Affected sibling had FNAIT without an ICH	7

Platelet function disorders

Glanzmann thrombasthenia (GT)

- Rare autosomal recessive disorder with normal platelet count but ↓ platelet aggregation
- Results from abnormalities of the platelet receptor GPIIb/IIIa
- Higher prevalence in areas where consanguinity is common
- Usually diagnosed in childhood in the presence of mucocutaneous bleeding symptoms:
  - Easy bruising
  - Epistaxis
  - Gingival bleeding
  - Menorrhagia

▶ Haemarthrosis, haematuria, and GI bleeding can also occur

Bernard–Soulier syndrome (BSS)

- Rare inherited platelet disorder, usually with thrombocytopenia and large platelets
- Usually autosomal recessive
- Higher prevalence in areas where consanguinity is common
- Results from a variety of defects in membrane glycoprotein IIb–IX–V complex:
  - This complex mediates platelet adhesion to vessel walls by binding von Willebrand factor
  - It enhances the capacity of thrombin at low concentrations to activate platelets
- Bleeding severity is variable, usually less severe than GT
- Severe bleeding complications can occur, including epistaxis, gingival bleeding, and menorrhagia.

Treatment of GT and BSS

- Tranexamic acid or local compression in the event of a minor bleed
- Platelet transfusions (from HLA-matched single donor) can be considered:
  - Some ♀ become refractory to these
  - Can produce HLA or GPIIb/IIIa antibodies
- Activated recombinant factor VII (rVIIa)—can be used to treat bleeding episodes in patients who are refractory to transfusion or have developed antibodies (but only licensed for use in GT)
- Desmopressin
- Menorrhagia may improve with oral contraceptive use

Management of GT and BSS in pregnancy

MDT management
- In a tertiary centre where possible

PPH risk
- Planned use of haemostatic agents at delivery
- Recombinant factor VIIa and tranexamic acid recommended for un-complicated vaginal deliveries
- HLA-matched platelets with tranexamic acid recommended for cae-sarean section, or if bleeding at time of vaginal delivery
- Avoidance of platelet transfusion if possible because of the risk of antibody formation
- Aggressive use of uterotonics
- Avoidance of traumatic delivery
- Tranexamic acid can ↓ the risk of 2° PPH for up to 6 wks postnatally

Antibodies
- Monitor for anti-HLA and anti-GPIb antibodies
- Transplacental transfer of maternal antiplatelet antibodies → FNAIT → ↑ risk of bleeding complications including intracranial haemorrhage
- Management as for FNAIT
- Steroids and plasmapheresis have been used to ↓ antibody levels and ↑ response to platelets

Analgesia/anaesthesia
⚠ Regional procedures are not recommended because of the risk of haematoma formation.

Inherited thrombophilias

- Associated with ↑ risk of VTE compared to the normal population
- Controversy over testing for these mutations in pregnancy → no universal agreement as to which ♀ should be screened
- For management see RCOG Green-top Guideline 37a

Antithrombin deficiency

- Most severe thrombophilia with a 50% lifetime risk of VTE
- Antithrombin is a potent anticoagulant
- Acts by binding the active serine of thrombin and activated factor X
- LMWH potentially acts in 2 ways:
  - On antithrombin, inhibiting the action of factor Xa converting prothrombin to thrombin
  - Longer LMWH chains also inhibit factor IIa (thrombin)
- RCOG guidelines recommend 50–100% of therapeutic LMWH dose antenatally, and for 6 wks postpartum
- Doses can be guided by anti-Xa levels but this depends on the source of antithrombin utilized by the assay
- Antithrombin concentrate is short acting but can be useful, e.g. at delivery when anticoagulants are not given
- Types are given in Table 9.9

Table 9.9 Types of antithrombin deficiency

Type 1	Quantitative ↓ in antithrombin
Type 2	Qualitatively abnormal antithrombin protein
	• Type 2 reactive site (RS)
	• Type 2 heparin-binding site (HBS)
	• Type 2 pleiotropic (PE)

Protein C deficiency

- Protein C is a vitamin K-dependent anticoagulant made in the liver
- Activated by thrombin on the endothelial surface
- APC ↓ generation of thrombin by inactivating factors VIIIa and Va

▶ Protein C measured levels are not affected by pregnancy in some studies, but are ↑ in others, ∴ results obtained in pregnancy should be interpreted cautiously and the tests repeated postpartum if in doubt

Protein S deficiency

- Protein S is a vitamin K-dependent anticoagulant made in the liver
- Co-factor for the APC-mediated inactivation of the factors
- About 60% is bound to a binding protein and therefore inactive

▶ Protein S levels ↓ as pregnancy progresses so it is not possible to accurately diagnose protein S deficiency in pregnancy

RCOG GTG 37a 'Reducing the Risk of Venous Thromboembolism during Pregnancy and the Puerperium' ℘ https://www.rcog.org.uk/globalassets/documents/guidelines/gtg-37a.pdf

G20210A mutation
- Polymorphism in the prothrombin gene is associated with:
  - 30% ↑ in prothrombin levels
  - Small ↑ in VTE

Factor V Leiden
- Factor V is a co-factor that is required for thrombin generation
  - Has no co-factor activity until cleaved by thrombin or factor Xa
- Once activated it is inactivated by APC
- Factor V Leiden is a polymorphism in which APC binding and inactivation is ↓, → APC resistance
- It is found in at least 4% of the Caucasian population and 15% of those with a 1st thromboembolic event
- Previously diagnosed by demonstrating ↑ APC resistance; largely superseded by genetic analysis
- As APC resistance can occur in pregnancy, this cannot be used to screen for factor V Leiden in pregnant ♀

Thrombophilia screening

☙ Thrombophilia testing in pregnancy is controversial:
- The physiological changes mean that many of the tests are not reliable if performed in pregnancy (Table 9.10)
- Many results will not alter management even if positive
- The exception is antithrombin testing or antiphospholipid antibodies in ♀ with a personal or family history of VTE, where a positive result would change management in pregnancy

☙ The evidence does not support screening for inherited thrombophilias in placental-mediated pregnancy complications.

Table 9.10 Pregnancy-specific considerations for thrombophilia screening

Heritable	
Antithrombin deficiency	Levels ↓ by 20% in pregnancy
Protein S deficiency	Levels ↓ with advancing gestation
Protein C deficiency	Studies vary; some suggest protein C is unchanged, others suggest levels ↑ Should be interpreted cautiously and the tests repeated postpartum if in doubt
Factor V Leiden	Genetic test so results not altered by pregnancy APC ratio cannot be used in pregnancy
Prothrombin G20210A	Genetic test so results not altered by pregnancy
Acquired	
Antiphospholipid syndrome	Antibodies can be present in up to 5% of population with no maternal or fetal complications

Haemophilia

- Inheritance is shown in Table 9.11
- X-linked condition with a deficiency in:
  - Factor VIII → haemophilia A
  - Factor IX → haemophilia B
- Haemophilia A is 4× more common than haemophilia B
- Clotting factor levels determine the severity of bleeding:
  - Mild (0.05–0.40 IU/mL)
  - Moderate (0.01–0.05 IU/mL)
  - Severe (<0.01 IU/mL)
- ♀ carriers have 1 abnormal gene:
  - Wide variation in level of clotting factor
  - ↑ risk of PPH and bleeding with invasive procedures
- Up to 1/3 of neonatal ♂ with severe haemophilia have no family history:
  - In these cases, there is a 90% chance that the mother is a carrier

Changes in factors VIII and IX in pregnancy
- Levels of factor VIII ↑ in unaffected ♀ and haemophilia carriers:
  - Desmopressin can be used to ↑ factor VIII levels (➔ see 'Von Willebrand disease', p. 348)
  - Recombinant factor VIII can be given to non-responders
- Levels of factor IX do **not** ↑ in pregnancy:
  - Haemophilia B carriers are at ↑ risk when pregnant
  - Recombinant factor IX can be used to ↑ levels
- Aim for factor VIII/IX levels of at least 0.5 IU/mL to cover surgical or invasive procedures:
  - If treatment required, treat until levels are 1.0 IU/mL

Table 9.11 Inheritance in haemophilia

	Sons		Daughters	
Carrier ♀	50% unaffected	50% affected	50% unaffected	50% carriers
Affected ♂	All unaffected		All carriers[a]	

[a] This is not synonymous with asymptomatic or unaffected.

Management of haemophilia in pregnancy

Pre-pregnancy counselling
- Genetic counselling should be provided to ♀ at risk
- ♀ at risk should be tested for the genetic mutation (if known)
- Measure baseline clotting factor level
- Carriers of severe haemophilia should be offered pre-implantation genetic diagnosis

Antenatal care
- MDT management including haematologist with expertise in the field
- Carriers of severe haemophilia should be offered sex determination using cell-free fetal DNA from 9 wks
- If ♂ fetus, offer prenatal diagnosis with CVS at 11–14 wks or amniocentesis
- If no early invasive testing performed, amniocentesis in 3rd trimester is offered to guide delivery options
- Measure maternal clotting factors at booking and 34 wks, and any other time if clinically indicated
- Hepatitis serology if previous exposure to blood products

Intrapartum care
- This is not an absolute contraindication to vaginal delivery
- Check maternal clotting factor level (target is >0.5 IU/mL):
  - If <0.5 IU/mL treat with desmopressin or recombinant clotting factor concentrates
- Group and save (consider cross-match if factor level very low)
- If fetus is affected, or the status of a ♂ fetus is unknown, avoid FSE, FBS, ventouse and rotational forceps deliveries
- Epidural anaesthesia can be used if factor level >0.5 IU/mL

⚠ Levels should be checked and normalized prior to epidural catheter removal

Postpartum care
- Active 3rd stage of labour
- Send cord blood of ♂ infants for clotting factor levels
- Maintain factor levels at least >0.5 IU/mL for:
  - 3 days after uncomplicated vaginal delivery
  - 5 days after instrumental or caesarean delivery
- Tranexamic acid for at least 5 days
- Avoid IM injections in infants with possible haemophilia
- Caution with use of non-steroidal analgesia and IM injections in mothers with low factor levels
- Decisions about LMWH should be individualized as these depend on factor levels and other risk factors for VTE

⮑ RCOG (2017). Management of inherited bleeding disorders in pregnancy (green-top guideline no. 71): ⌇ https://obgyn.onlinelibrary.wiley.com/doi/epdf/10.1111/1471-0528.14592

Von Willebrand disease

- VWF is a large multimeric protein released from Weibel–Palade bodies in endothelial cells in response to many stimuli
- 2 important roles in haemostasis:
  - Mediates adhesion of platelets to sites of vascular injury
  - Binds factor VIII
- Deficiency or abnormal function → impaired haemostasis and bleeding
- See Table 9.12.

Pregnancy and VWD

- Levels of VWF and factor VIII ↑ in pregnancy and ↓ rapidly after
- The main maternal risk is PPH
- If the fetus has inherited the condition, they are at risk of intracranial bleeding at the time of delivery

Medications for VWD and low factor VIII levels

Desmopressin
- Synthetic analogue of antidiuretic hormone
- Acts on type 2 vasopressin receptors found in various locations, including endothelial cells, where it triggers release of VWF from Weibel–Palade bodies
- Given IV or SC which causes an ↑ in both VWF and factor VIII that may last for several hours
- Response significantly varies between individuals: most type 1s respond unless severe, few type 2s, no type 3
- Test dose recommended with measurement of factor VIII and VWF levels and activity at 1 and 4 hrs post dose
- 1 litre fluid restriction for 24 hrs following a dose

Alternatives
- Cryoprecipitate was previously used but this cannot be treated to inactivate viruses
- Plasma-derived concentrates are available:
  - Contain both VWF and factor VIII (Voncento®, Wilate®)
  - Higher purity VWF-containing concentrates (Willfact®)
- Recombinant VWF is being developed

Pre-pregnancy counselling

- Genetic counselling should discuss type of inheritance according to maternal VWD type as well as variable penetrance and expression

Neonate

- Tests for VWD should be repeated at 6–12 mths of age, as cord blood levels can be unreliable and of limited diagnostic use
- Avoid IM injections if factor VIII levels ↓
- Prolonged pressure required after blood tests including heel prick

Table 9.12 Von Willebrand disease subtypes

Type 1 (75–80%)	Quantitative deficiency: • Mild/moderate reduction in VWF level • Normal multimer structure	Autosomal dominant	Desmopressin can be used in some cases (stimulates VWF release from endothelial cells)
Type 2 (15–20%)	**2A** • Loss of high and intermediate weight multimers		
	2B • Loss of high-molecular-weight multimers • Gain of function to avidly bind platelets, resulting in thrombocytopenia		Anecdotally, may be associated with higher rate of fetal morbidity due to the thrombocytopenia
	2M • Normal VWF multimers • Poor platelet binding	Autosomal dominant	
	2N • Mutation in VWF protein → reduced factor VIII binding		
Type 3 (<5%)	Complete absence	Autosomal recessive (more common in consanguineous marriage)	Severe
Platelet type	Hyper-reactive platelets		

Management of VWD in pregnancy

Antenatal care

- MDT management including haematologist with expertise in the field
- Measure at booking, 34 wks, and prior to invasive procedures:
  - VWF antigen (VWF:Ag)
  - Activity (usually VWF:RCo)
  - Factor VIII levels
- For ♀ with type 2B, also measure platelet count
- If factor VIII and VWF:RCo levels are ≤0.5 IU/mL and an invasive procedure or delivery is anticipated, treat with desmopressin (should not be used in ♀ with pre-eclampsia)

Intrapartum care

- Consider tranexamic acid in all ♀
- Repeat tests if factor VIII or VWF:RCo <0.5 IU/mL
- Type 1: levels often normalize
- Type 2/3: most need VWF-containing concentrates rather than desmopressin
- Type 2B: may require platelets
- Vaginal delivery can be undertaken if no additional obstetric issues
- Avoiding a prolonged 2nd stage is advisable:
  - ↓ risk of trauma and uterine atony, which can ↑ risk PPH
- Epidural anaesthesia is usually avoided in ♀ with type 2 or 3 VWD, but may be possible in type 1 depending on level
- If a fetus is suspected to have type 2 or 3 VWD or severe type 1, then the same management applies, as in suspected haemophilia:
  - Avoid FBS and FSE
  - Avoid ventouse or rotational forceps delivery
  - Cord blood for VWD testing

Postpartum care

⚠ ↑ risk of 1° and 2° PPH in ♀ with VWD

- Active management of the 3rd stage
- Avoid aspirin and NSAIDs if possible
- Tranexamic acid for at least 5 days
- Regular Hb and VWF:RCo
- In ♀ with type 2 or 3 disease, or severe type 1, VWF:RCo should be maintained >0.5 IU/mL for:
  - 3 days after uncomplicated vaginal delivery
  - 5 days after instrumental or caesarean delivery
- Decisions about LMWH should be individualized as these depend on factor levels and other risk factors for VTE

Factor XI deficiency

- Associated with a very variable bleeding phenotype, even within families
- Severe deficiency is defined as <0.15–0.2 IU/mL
- Risk of significant bleeding does not correspond with factor level
- Low factor XI can cause a prolonged APTT
- Normal APTT does not exclude mild deficiency especially in pregnancy
  (↑ factor VIII can → a normal APTT even with ↓ factor XI)
- FFP contains factor XI:
  - May be useful for milder cases (dose of 15–20 mL/kg)
  - Rarely sufficient to treat severe deficiency
- Factor XI concentrate:
  - Has a long half-life (>50 hrs) so a single dose will suffice
  - Risks include thrombosis and theoretical risk of infections such as
    prion disease
  - Target post administration should be 0.3–0.7 IU/mL

Management of factor XI deficiency in pregnancy

- Levels should be checked at the booking visit, 28 wks, and 34 wks
- Main risks are of bleeding at the time of procedures or delivery
- In ♀ with severe factor XI deficiency or a bleeding history the risk of
  bleeding can be ↓ by:
  - Active management of the 3rd stage
  - Prophylactic factor XI concentrate or FFP
- In ♀ with no history of bleeding or partial deficiency:
  - Tranexamic acid 1 g TDS can be given while in labour and for at
    least 1 wk postpartum
- Epidural can be sited depending on the maternal factor level and
  bleeding tendency

Myeloproliferative conditions

- Series of rare conditions
- Include:
  - Polycythaemia vera
  - 1° thrombocythaemia (essential thrombocythaemia)
  - Myelofibrosis
  - Chronic myeloid leukaemia
- ↑ risk of both thrombosis and haemorrhage
- Also a risk of transformation to acute myeloid leukaemia
- Pregnancy does not alter the risk of transformation

Chronic myeloid leukaemia

- Can occur in ♀ of childbearing age
- 95% have a balanced translocation of the *BCR* and *ABL* genes:
  - Resulting combination is known as the Philadelphia chromosome
- Treatment has been transformed by the introduction of tyrosine kinase inhibitors, including imatinib and nilotinib:
  - Tyrosine kinase inhibitors not recommended in pregnancy as associated with congenital abnormalities
  - If pregnancy is being considered, change to interferon-α
  - Use also associated with ↓ fertility in both ♂ and ♀, but currently insufficient evidence to prove this

Primary myelofibrosis

- Very rare in ♀ of childbearing age
- Diagnostic features are:
  - Splenomegaly
  - ↑ bone marrow fibrosis
  - Leucoerythroblastic blood film (including tear-shaped red cells)
  - Exclusion of other causes of marrow fibrosis, e.g. metastatic malignancy, lymphoma, TB, and leishmaniasis

Risk factors for pregnancy complications in myeloproliferative conditions

- Marked sustained ↑ in platelet count to >1500 × 10⁹/L
- Previous maternal venous or arterial thrombosis
- Previous haemorrhage attributed to myeloproliferative disease
- Previous pregnancy complication that may be attributable to 1° thrombocythaemia:
  - Significant antepartum or postpartum haemorrhage
  - Severe pre-eclampsia
  - IUGR
  - Stillbirth with no other cause evident
  - 3 previous early pregnancy losses (<10 wks)
  - ≥1 later pregnancy losses (>24 wks)

Primary thrombocythaemia

- 1° (essential) thrombocythaemia is a diagnosis of exclusion
- Associated with mutations including Janus kinase 2 (*JAK2*, positive in ~50%), *CALR*, and *MBL*
- Placental thrombosis can occur, increasing the risk of:
  - Fetal loss
  - Preterm delivery
  - IUGR
  - Placental abruption

Causes

See Table 9.13.

Table 9.13 Causes of thrombocythaemia

Spurious	• Mixed cryoglobulinaemia
Reactive	
Haematological causes	• Acute blood loss
	• Acute haemolytic anaemia
	• Iron deficiency anaemia
	• Rebound after treatment of ITP
Post procedure	• Post splenectomy
Infections	• TB
	• Chronic infection
Inflammatory conditions	• Inflammatory bowel disease
	• Vasculitides
	• Rheumatological disorders
Malignancies	• Metastatic malignancy
	• Lymphoma
Autonomous	• Polycythaemia vera
	• Chronic myeloid leukaemia
Primary	• 1° thrombocythaemia

Management of 1° thrombocythaemia in pregnancy

Preconception
⚠ Cytoreductive therapy including hydroxycarbamide has been associated with teratogenicity in animal studies
- Stop hydroxycarbamide or anagrelide before conception

In pregnancy
- Aspirin 75 mg OD (unless platelet count very high, where there is a risk of bleeding from acquired VWD)
- Thromboprophylaxis antenatally and postnatally if:
  - Previous VTE
  - Platelet count very high >1500 × 10⁹/L
  - Cytoreductive therapy at diagnosis
  - Thromboprophylaxis postnatally only otherwise
- Regular fetal growth scans
- Breastfeeding contraindicated if taking hydroxycarbamide or anagrelide

Polycythaemia vera

- Results from a clonal expansion of erythrocyte progenitor cells (most often mutation in *JAK2*)
- Majority of ♀ have ↑ haematocrit and/or ↑ Hb concentration
- Many also have a leucocytosis and a thrombocytosis
- Causes are described in Table 9.14

Investigations

- Assessment for other causes
- Screening for *JAK2* mutation
- See Table 9.15

Table 9.14 Causes of polycythaemia

Genetic mutations	Appropriately ↑ erythropoietin	Inappropriately ↑ erythropoietin	Other causes
Polycythaemia vera	High altitude	Renal cell carcinoma	Androgen or anabolic steroid use
Congenital methaemoglobinaemia	Pulmonary disease	Cerebellar haemangioblastoma	Exogenous erythropoietin
	Intracardiac shunting	Hepatocellular carcinoma	

Management of polycythemia vera in pregnancy

Preconception

⚠ Cytoreductive therapy including hydroxycarbamide has been associated with teratogenicity in animal studies

- Stop hydroxycarbamide or anagrelide before conception

In pregnancy

- Aspirin 75 mg OD
- Venesection:
  - Physiological haemodilution can ↓ need for venesection
- Interferon-α is the drug of choice if necessary
- VTE assessment and plan for at least postpartum LMWH
- Regular fetal growth scans
- Breastfeeding contraindicated if taking hydroxycarbamide and anagrelide
- Breastfeeding on interferon-α is an individualized decision:
  - It enters breastmilk but there is no evidence of resulting neonatal harm, however the number of cases is small

Fetal consequences

- Placental thrombosis can occur, increasing the risk of:
  - Fetal loss
  - Preterm delivery
  - IUGR

Rhesus isoimmunization

- This is caused by maternal IgG antibodies crossing the placenta and destroying fetal RBCs
- Resulting anaemia can be severe and cause fetal hydrops

Rhesus blood groups

- 3 linked gene pairs:
  - C/c, D/d, and E/e
- Only 5 antigens:
  - d is not an antigen, it implies absence of the D antigen

Pathophysiology of rhesus disease

- Fetal RBCs cross into the maternal circulation in pregnancy:
  - This is ↑ during sensitizing events
- Fetus may have a gene for an antigen the mother does not have:
  - Most commonly rhesus D
  - Can also be c, E, and sometimes Kell or Duffy
- Maternal immune system mounts a response to this 'foreign' antigen:
  - Initially IgM which does not cross the placenta so the 1st pregnancy is not at risk
  - Later IgG (which can cross the placenta)
- Subsequent pregnancies which have same antigen (e.g. D +ve) cause the primed B cells to produce ↑ IgG antibodies
- IgG binds to the fetal red cells which are then destroyed in the reticuloendothelial system
- Causes haemolytic anaemia in the fetus:
  - Severe anaemia causes high-output cardiac failure (fetal hydrops)
  - In milder cases it causes neonatal anaemia or jaundice

Anti-D IgG

- If anti-D IgG is given to the mother it will bind any fetal cells in her circulation carrying the D antigen and prevent her being sensitized
- The dose of anti-D usually used is 1500 IU
- A Kleihauer should be performed after sensitizing events which will indicate if more anti-D IgG is required

▶ Anti-D IgG administration now means sensitization is rare with other antibodies (particularly anti-Kell and anti-c) accounting for >50% of fetal haemolysis 2° to isoimmunization

---

Prevention and management of rhesus isoimmunization

Maternal screening
- All ♀ should be checked for atypical antibodies at booking, 28 wks, and 34 wks
- If Rh D-negative (d/d), then ♀ should be offered fetal blood typing using cell-free fetal DNA testing at 15–16 wks:

Fetus is Rh D negative
- Anti-D is not needed
- Kleihauer is not required at delivery or other potential sensitizing events
- Blood should be sent at 28 and 34 wks for FBC and antibodies

Fetus is Rh D positive
- Anti-D (1500 IU) is given to the mother:
  - At 28 wks after sending bloods for FBC and antibodies
  - After any sensitizing event
  - At delivery

▶ Further doses of anti-D should be guided by the Kleihauer results

---

Potential sensitizing events for rhesus disease
- Termination of pregnancy, surgical management of miscarriage, and ectopic pregnancy
- Vaginal bleeding >12 wks
- Blunt abdominal trauma
- Invasive procedure, e.g. CVS or amniocentesis
- Intrauterine death
- External cephalic version
- Delivery

Antithrombotic drugs

See Table 9.15.

Table 9.15 Anti-thrombotic drugs in pregnancy and breast feeding

Type	Generic name	Use in pregnancy	Use in lactation
Aspirin	Aspirin	• Used at low doses (75–150 mg daily) to ↓ risk of pre-eclampsia • High dose ↑ risk of premature closure of ductus arteriosus and oligohydramnios	• Can be used at low doses ⚠ long periods of high doses advised against
Unfractionated heparin (binds antithrombin, increasing inactivation of IIa and Xa inhibition)	Heparin	• Can be used in pregnancy (SC or IV) • IV infusion requires either APTT or anti-Xa monitoring (latter may be preferable in later pregnancy due to the effects of increased factor VIII on APTT results)	• Can be used
Low molecular weight heparin (potentiates action of anti-thrombin to inactivate factor Xa)	Enoxaparin Tinzaparin Dalteparin	• Anti-Xa monitoring advised in some groups (extremes of weight, renal impairment, recurrent VTE) if therapeutic doses used • Do not cross placenta, so can be used throughout pregnancy • ↑ GFR means higher doses are required, so use pregnancy specific dosing	• Can be used • Non-pregnant doses
Vitamin K antagonists (inhibits factors II, VII, IX and X)	Warfarin	• Teratogenic so generally avoided in pregnancy (change to LMWH); only used in highest risk ♀ e.g. with metallic heart valves • Crosses placenta and antagonizes fetal vitamin K (present in lower doses than in adults) so risk of fetal bleeding	• Can be used
Fondaparinux (potentiates antithrombin in factor Xa inhibition)	Fondaparinux	• Can be used • Long half life means 36–42 hours advised before regional anaesthesia	• Can be used
Factor Xa inhibitor	Rivaroxaban Apixaban Edoxaban	• Evidence of teratogenicity in animal models (rivaroxaban, edoxaban) so advised to avoid in pregnancy	• Not advised
Thrombin inhibitor	Dabigatran	• Associated with fetal growth restriction, not advised in pregnancy	• Not advised

Blood products

See Table 9.16.

Table 9.16 Blood products and their indications

	Constituents	Indications	Dosing

Red blood cells	RBCs in additive solution	• Acute blood loss >1.5 L
		• Sickle cell crisis
		• Symptomatic anaemia with Hb <70 g/L if no cardiovascular disease
			• 1 unit should be expected to ↑ Hb by 10 g/L
			• Irradiated cells required for:
			  • ♀ at risk of transfusion-associated graft vs host disease
			• Washed cells required for:
			  • ♀ with recurrent/ severe allergic or febrile reactions to red cells
			  • Severe IgA deficiency when RBCs from an IgA deficient donor are not available
			⚠ CMV-negative blood required for all pregnant ♀

Fresh frozen plasma	All coagulation factors	• Bleeding due to multiple clotting factor deficiencies, e.g. DIC • Inheritable factor deficiencies where a factor concentrate is not yet available	

Platelets	Platelets from either pooled donors or from a single donor (from apheresis)	Platelets <50 × 10⁹/L:
		• Major surgery with active bleeding
		Platelets <10 × 10⁹/L
		• Stable, non-bleeding
			• Irradiated platelets (as for RBCs)
			• Additive solution (washed as for RBCs)
			• HLA-selected platelets:
			  • Indicated for ♀ refractory to random platelets because of the development of antibodies after previous transfusions
			• HPA-selected platelets:
			  • Indicated for babies with FNAIT (HPA–1a/5b negative platelets)

Cryoprecipitate	High concentration of factor VIII, VWF, and fibrinogen	• Massive haemorrhage or transfusion	• Average adult dose is 2 pools of 5 units (or 1 unit per 5–10 kg body weight)
Prothrombin complex concentrate	Factors II, VII, IX, and X	• Rapid reversal of warfarin overdose • Coagulopathy associated with liver disease	• 25–50 IU/kg
Recombinant factor VIIa	Recombinant factor VIIa	• Severe platelet disorders: either bleeding or immediately prior to an invasive procedure • Factor VII deficiency • Acquired haemophilia	• Initial dose 90 mg/kg; repeated every 90–120 mins until haemostasis achieved • Has been associated with VTE and arterial thrombosis when used for severe PPH in ♀ without platelet disorders
Recombinant factor VIII	Recombinant factor VIII	Haemophilia A	• Dose depends on indication and severity of haemorrhage • Seek specialist haematology advice
Recombinant factor IX	Recombinant factor IX	Haemophilia B	• Dose depends on indication and severity of haemorrhage • Seek specialist haematology advice

HPA, human platelet antigen.

Venous thromboembolism

Thromboprophylaxis

- VTE is a major cause of maternal mortality and morbidity
- LMWH is 1st-line agent (Table 10.1)
- Every pregnant ♀ should have a risk assessment for VTE at their 1st antenatal visit and whenever the clinical situation changes (e.g. inpatient admission, at delivery) (Table 10.2)
- Many risk assessment tools are available
- If the threshold is reached, pharmacological thromboprophylaxis is recommended
- Anti-embolism stockings are recommended in some ♀, e.g. those who are hospitalized or where pharmacological prophylaxis is contraindicated

History of previous VTE

- ♀ with a history of VTE require anticoagulation in pregnancy (unless related to a transient precipitant, e.g. a surgical procedure)
- If not on daily anticoagulation when not pregnant → require prophylaxis in pregnancy and until 6 wks postpartum
- Long-term anticoagulation, e.g. warfarin or direct oral anticoagulant → change to therapeutic LMWH as soon as a pregnancy test positive and continue for the entire pregnancy and for 6 wks postpartum

Thromboprophylaxis and early pregnancy events

- No clear guidance exists for duration of thromboprophylaxis for ♀ at risk of VTE after a miscarriage or termination of pregnancy

💣 The risks of thrombosis after these events compared to a term delivery are not clear

💣 The decision has to be individualised depending on thrombotic risk, gestation and details of pregnancy/event: some women may require 7–10 days, some may need the equivalent of 6 weeks postnatal prophylaxis.

Table 10.1 Prophylactic doses of LMWH

Bodyweight (kg)	Dalteparin	Enoxaparin	Tinzaparin
<50	2500 units OD	20 mg OD	3500 units OD
50–90	5000 units OD	40 mg OD	4500 units OD
91–130	7500 units OD	60 mg OD	7000 units OD
131–170	10,000 units OD	80 mg OD or 40 mg BD	9000 units OD
>170	75 units/kg/day	0.6 mg/kg/day	75 units/kg/day

Source: data from RCOG GTG 37a 'Reducing the Risk of Venous Thromboembolism during Pregnancy and the Puerperium' ჷ https://www.rcog.org.uk/globalassets/documents/guidelines/gtg-37a.pdf

Table 10.2 Risk factors for VTE

Pre-existing	• Previous VTE
	• Thrombophilia:
	• **Inherited**, e.g. antithrombin deficiency, protein C/S deficiency, factor V Leiden
	• **Acquired**, e.g. antiphospholipid antibodies
	• Age >35 years
	• BMI ≥30 kg/m²
	• Parity ≥3
	• Smoking
	• Gross varicose veins (i.e. symptomatic, above knee or if associated with phlebitis or oedema)
	• Immobility, e.g. paraplegia
	• Medical comorbidities, e.g. cancer, active IBD or joint disease, active SLE, nephrotic syndrome
	• Current IV drug user
Obstetric	• Multiple pregnancy
	• Pre-eclampsia
	• Caesarean section
	• Prolonged labour (>24 hrs)
	• Mid-cavity or rotational operative delivery
	• Stillbirth
	• Preterm birth
	• PPH (>1 l or requiring blood transfusion)
Transient	• Any surgical procedure in pregnancy (except perineal repair)
	• Hyperemesis gravidarum, dehydration
	• Ovarian hyperstimulation syndrome
	• Admission or immobility (>3 days of bed rest)
	• Current systemic infection (requiring IV antibiotics or hospital admission)
	• Long-distance travel

Source: data from RCOG GTG 37a 'Reducing the Risk of Venous Thromboembolism during Pregnancy and the Puerperium' https://www.rcog.org.uk/globalassets/documents/guide-lines/gtg-37a.pdf

Deep vein thrombosis

Background
- In pregnancy they occur more in the left leg than the right
- Higher incidence of ilio-femoral DVT

Clinical features

Symptoms
- Pain
- Swelling
- Erythema and ↑ temperature

Signs
- Mild fever
- ↑ leg circumference compared to the non-affected side

⚠ A large, proximal DVT can cause 'phlegmasia alba dolens' (painful white leg) or 'phlegmasia caerulea dolens' (painful blue leg).

⚠ These presentations require urgent treatment and often vascular intervention (catheter-directed thrombolysis).

Investigations
- Blood tests may show a mild leucocytosis and ↑ CRP
- Doppler USS
- MR venography

⚠ D-dimer should not be used for VTE risk stratification of pregnant ♀.

⚠ A negative D-dimer does not exclude VTE in pregnancy.

> ### Management of DVT in pregnancy
> ⚠ No role for pre-test probability scores (e.g. Well's score) in pregnant ♀ with suspected VTE
> - Doppler USS will usually confirm the diagnosis
> - If initial USS is negative then:
>   - Low clinical suspicion or another diagnosis more likely
>   → no further investigation required
>   - High clinical suspicion, signs suggestive of proximal DVT
>   → consider MRI abdomen for possible ilio-femoral DVT
>   - High clinical suspicion, signs suggestive of distal DVT
>   → discontinue anticoagulation, repeat USS on day 3 and/or 7
>
> ⚠ In the absence of contraindications, treatment should be started at presentation rather than waiting for confirmatory imaging
> - Pregnancy-specific doses of LMWH are required
> - If there are concerns regarding empirical anticoagulation, urgent imaging is required irrespective of the time of day
> - No urgency for delivery purely for the DVT, in fact allowing some time for clot stabilization is probably preferable (this could be ≥14 days)

Upper limb venous thrombosis

⚠ Upper limb DVT accounts for ~4–10% of all DVTs.

Additional risk factors include:

- Indwelling intravascular devices such as central venous catheters
- Some repetitive physical activities ('effort thrombosis' or Paget–Schroetter syndrome), e.g. baseball, wrestling, and martial arts
- Thoracic outlet abnormalities

Management of upper limb VTE in pregnancy

- Doppler USS is usually sufficient to make the diagnosis
- 1st-line treatment, i.e. anticoagulation with LMWH, is the same as in lower limb DVT

✦ Early thrombolysis and thoracic outlet decompression are performed in upper limb DVT and give better clinical results compared to conservative management (anticoagulation, analgesia, and elevation) but not all guidelines support this more aggressive approach.

➲ RCOG (2015). VTE during pregnancy (green-top guideline no. 37a): ℘ https://www.rcog.org.uk/globalassets/documents/guidelines/gtg-37a.pdf

Pulmonary embolism

Background

- Potentially life-threatening and is a cause of death in most reports of the Confidential Enquiry into Maternal Deaths in the UK (now known as MBRRACE-UK)
- Incidence in pregnancy is ↓ due to ↑ use of thromboprophylaxis

Clinical features

Symptoms

- Pleuritic chest pain
- Breathlessness (may be just on exertion)
- Palpitations
- Haemoptysis

Signs

- Hypoxia (at rest but may only occur on exertion)
- Tachypnoea
- Tachycardia
- Hypotension
- Mild fever

Basic investigations

- Bloods including troponin should be sent
- CXR often normal, but may show areas of relative oligaemia or wedge infarcts
- Confirmatory investigations for PE ➔ see p. 369

⚠ D-dimer should not be used to risk-stratify pregnant ♀ with possible PE.

Massive PE

- Haemodynamic compromise (hypotension not responsive to fluids ± inotropes and not explained by another cause)

Submassive PE

- Myocardial necrosis but no haemodynamic compromise
  Or
- Evidence of RV dysfunction defined as the presence of at least one of the following:
  - Systolic dysfunction on echocardiogram
  - RV dilation on echocardiogram or CT
  - Elevation of brain natriuretic peptide (BNP) or N-terminal pro-BNP
  - ECG changes (new or incomplete right bundle branch block, anteroseptal ST elevation/depression, or TWI)

Investigations for PE

Bilateral Doppler USS

- Performed if symptoms/signs of DVT are present
- If positive for VTE, further chest imaging is not required

CXR

- To ensure no other pathology is causing the symptoms
▶ Radiation dose is equivalent to eating 140 g of brazil nuts

V/Q scan

- Ventilation (V):
  - Nebulized radioisotope, e.g. Tc-99m DTPA is inhaled
- Perfusion (Q or quotient):
  - Injection of Tc-99 microaggregated albumin (MAA)
- Gamma camera then creates images of the emission pattern from each isotope
- Radiation exposure is low, but can be further ↓ by:
  - Omitting the V component (if CXR is normal)
  - Using a half dose for the Q scan
▶ The fetal dose of ionizing radiation used in this scan is very low, lower than the dose associated with an ↑ in childhood malignancy.

> **Practical considerations for a V/Q scan**
> - Low doses of radioactivity present for a few hours afterwards
> - It is ∴ recommended that the ♀:
>   - Avoids prolonged close contact with their baby (e.g. >30 mins cuddling) in the 12 hrs after the scan
>   - Avoids breastfeeding for 12 hrs (express and discard)
>   - Is not cared for by pregnant staff (bodily fluids can show low levels of radioactivity)

CTPA

- First line investigation if CXR abnormal
- Fetal dose of ionizing radiation is lower than that of a V/Q scan
- Dose to maternal breast tissue is higher vs V/Q:
  - Previously thought to be associated with ↑ lifetime risk of breast cancer, but newer scanning techniques mean that this increase is likely to be negligible

> **Practical considerations for a CTPA**
> - More likely to achieve suboptimal opacification of the pulmonary arteries due to the ↑ cardiac output in pregnancy (the timing of the contrast administration does not make allowances for this)
> - No need to stop breastfeeding after the scan

2019 ESC Guidelines on Acute Pulmonary Embolism. https://www.escardio.org/Guidelines/Clinical-Practice-Guidelines/Acute-Pulmonary-Embolism-Diagnosis-and-Management-of

Management of PE

Management of PE in pregnancy
⚠ No role for pre-test probability scores in pregnant ♀
- CXR to ensure no other causes of symptoms are identified
- Imaging using a V/Q scan or CTPA (➔ see p. 369)
- Pregnancy-specific doses of LMWH should be started empirically while awaiting imaging (unless contraindications to anticoagulation are present)
- If concerns about empirical anticoagulation, then urgent imaging is required irrespective of the time of day
- If haemodynamically unstable (i.e. hypotensive and tachycardic) for IV fluid resuscitation, early senior input and urgent imaging (consider echocardiogram if too unwell to go to Radiology department)
- If imaging positive for PE: ensure ♀ is in a suitable location where appropriate levels of medical monitoring can be performed

Submassive PE
- Current guidelines do not advocate the use of systemic or catheter-directed thrombolysis

Massive PE
- Thrombolysis should be considered

⚠ Scoring systems for PE severity (e.g. PE severity index 'PESI' score) are not validated for pregnancy

Anticoagulation
For choice of agents, see Table 9.15.

Systemic thrombolysis
- Indicated for massive PE
- Tissue plasminogen activator (tPA) is the agent of choice in pregnancy:
  - No ↑ in bleeding events or adverse pregnancy outcomes reported
  - Some cases describe the use of half-dose tPA

Catheter-directed thrombolysis
- Catheter inserted into the pulmonary artery, followed by disruption of the thrombus and local administration of thrombolytic agent
- Continuous infusion of thrombolytic agent for 24 hrs
- In non-pregnant individuals, has been shown to improve clinical parameters and right heart function
☛ Long-term benefits are not clear and it is not yet part of any guidelines for management of VTE in pregnancy

IVC filters
- Used infrequently as often associated with problems with removal postpartum
- RCOG guidelines advocate their use in ♀ with iliac vein VTE or ♀ with recurrent PE despite appropriate anticoagulation

Bleeding while anticoagulated

Initial resuscitation

ABCDE approach to assessment and immediate resuscitation
- Large-bore IV access
- Urgent bloods for FBC, coagulation
- Cross-match blood
- Fluid resuscitation with fluid or blood
- Haematology input with advice on possible agents for reversing the anticoagulant

Therapies
See Table 10.3.

Table 10.3 Specific therapies for bleeding on anticoagulants

Prothrombin complex concentrate	• Reverses the effects of warfarin within 15 mins
	• Vitamin K needs to be prescribed alongside this
	• If an individual is on warfarin and comes in with potentially life-threatening bleeding, this should be given immediately, i.e. before an INR result is available
Protamine	• Binds unfractionated heparin effectively and LMWH less effectively

➔ See Table 9.16, p. 360, for blood products.

Superficial vein thrombosis

Background
- Most commonly occurs in the 1st month postpartum
- Can be associated with DVT so anticoagulation may be indicated

💮 No clear consensus is available regarding who to treat or duration

Superficial phlebitis
- Inflammation of a superficial vein not associated with thrombosis

Superficial thrombophlebitis
- Inflammation of a superficial tributary vein, associated with thrombosis

Superficial venous thrombosis
- Inflammation and thrombosis of the short or long saphenous veins

Clinical features
- Usually presents as a painful lump or erythema, which may be linear and follow the course of a superficial vein
- Features that are associated with a greater risk of DVT:
  - >5 cm affected vein
  - Affected segment <5 cm from the saphenofemoral or saphenopopliteal junction
  - The presence of other risk factors for VTE

Management of superficial venous thrombosis in pregnancy

Low-risk lesions
- Analgesia
- Elevation of limb
- Avoid bed rest
- Compression stockings may be of benefit

Higher-risk lesions
- Anticoagulant decision depends on the background and the features of the thrombosis

💮 Appropriate duration of anticoagulation is unclear (evidence in non-pregnant ♀ suggests at least 45 days)

Associated DVT/PE already present
- Treatment as per VTE guidelines

Diabetes mellitus

For the purposes of this chapter 'diabetes' is used to cover 'diabetes mellitus'

Type 1 and type 2 diabetes

Type 1 diabetes
- Usually develops in childhood or young adult life but can occur at any age
- Autoimmune destruction of insulin-producing pancreatic β cells
- The diagnosis can be helped by:
  - Anti-islet cell antibodies (present in 70–80%)
  - Anti-GAD antibodies (present in 70–80%)
  - C-peptide (biochemical marker of endogenous insulin; ↓/absent level indicates insulin deficiency and supports diagnosis)
- Other autoimmune diseases are more common, e.g. Addison's disease, vitiligo

Type 2 diabetes
- Often develops later in life but ↑ seen in young adults and even children
- More common with obesity
- Combination of insulin resistance and insufficient insulin production:
  - Oral hypoglycaemic agents are often sufficient to treat hyperglycaemia
- Also seen with some medications e.g. steroids, atypical 2nd-generation antipsychotics (olanzapine)
- In the setting of other medical conditions:
  - Cystic fibrosis
  - Hereditary haemochromatosis
  - Chronic pancreatitis
  - Cushing's syndrome
  - Acromegaly
  - Other rare hormone-secreting tumours e.g. glucagonomas, somatostatinomas

General complications of diabetes

- Ketoacidosis:
  - Due to inadequate insulin levels to suppress ketogenesis; common causes include poor compliance with insulin therapy or illness
  - Ketone production ↑ resulting in a metabolic acidosis which can be life-threatening
  - More common in T1DM; rare in T2DM
- Hypoglycaemia:
  - Insulin or oral hypoglycaemic agent administration with inadequate food intake
- Microvascular complications:
  - Nephropathy
  - Retinopathy
  - Neuropathy
- Macrovascular complications:
  - Ischaemic heart disease
  - Peripheral vascular disease
  - Cerebrovascular disease

Gestational diabetes

Who to test for GDM
- If any risk factors for GDM, offer GTT at 24–28 wks
- Risk factors include:
  - Family history of diabetes (1st-degree relative with diabetes)
  - Previous macrosomic baby weighing ≥4.5 kg
  - Obesity (BMI >30 kg/m²)
  - Minority ethnic family origin with high prevalence for diabetes, e.g. South Asian, Black Caribbean, Middle Eastern
- With a history of GDM in a previous pregnancy offer:
  - Early self-monitoring of blood glucose
    Or
  - 2 hr oral GTT as soon as possible after booking, if normal repeat at 24–28 wks
- Diagnostic criteria are shown in Table 11.1

Oral glucose tolerance test

Preparation
- Overnight fast (≥8 hrs)
- Water only during this time
- No smoking

Method
- Baseline fasting plasma glucose
- 75 g glucose load*
- 1 hr plasma glucose (advised in IADPSG but not NICE guidelines)
- 2 hr plasma glucose

* The sugar content of Lucozade® was ↓ in the UK in 2017 so if this is used, a larger volume is required than was previously the case, but alternatives are likely to be preferable, e.g. Polycal®.

Table 11.1 Diagnosis of GDM

	WHO/IADPSG criteria	NICE guidelines
Fasting	≥5.1 mmol/L	≥5.6 mmol/L
1 hr	≥10.0 mmol/L	N/A
2 hrs	≥8.5 mmol/L	≥7.8 mmol/L

IADPSG, International Association of the Diabetes and Pregnancy Study Groups.

GDM and driving (in the UK)

The DVLA regards GDM as a temporary indication for insulin, so an individual on insulin for GDM does not have to routinely inform the DVLA that they have started insulin, unless it is anticipated that they will be taking this for ≥3 months postpartum.

Women should be advised to discuss the commencement of insulin with their motor insurance provider.

Management of GDM

All ♀
- Refer to dietician to educate about appropriate diet including:
  - Low glycaemic index foods
  - Carbohydrate and protein content of meals
- Teach self-monitoring of blood glucose levels; targets as per NICE guidelines:
  - Fasting <5.3 mmol/L
  - 1 hr post meal <7.8 mmol/L
  - 2 hr post meal <6.4 mmol/L
- Regular exercise

Fasting plasma glucose <7 mmol/L
- Trial of dietary modification and exercise
- Offer metformin if targets are not met within 1–2 wks
- Offer insulin if:
  - Metformin not tolerated
  - Previously listed measures do not result in glucose targets being met

⚠ Immediate insulin treatment if complications such as macrosomia or polyhydramnios are present.

💊 Glibenclamide is occasionally used if metformin is insufficient, and if insulin is not an option.

Fasting plasma glucose >7 mmol/L
- Immediate treatment with insulin
- Changes in diet and exercise
- Metformin should be started alongside insulin

🠖 NICE (2015). Diabetes in pregnancy guidelines: 🕭 https://www.nice.org.uk/guidance/ng3

Monogenic diabetes

- Previously categorized as 'maturity-onset diabetes in the young' or 'MODY'
- Responsible for up to 2% of all diabetes diagnosed in people <45 yrs
- Often misdiagnosed

Clues to the diagnosis of monogenic diabetes

- Lack of characteristics of T1DM:
  - Negative antibodies
  - Low or no requirement for insulin after 5 years
  - Persistently detectable C-peptide levels
  - No episodes of DKA
- Lack of characteristics of T2DM:
  - Normal BMI
  - No lipid abnormalities
- Strong family history

Glucokinase mutations

- Autosomal dominant inheritance of a mutation in the *GCK* gene
- GCK is an enzyme acting as the glucose sensor of pancreatic β cells
- Heterozygous inactivating mutation:
  - Lifelong, mild fasting hyperglycaemia with a mildly elevated HbA1c
- Homozygous inactivating mutations (very rare):
  - Severe neonatal diabetes

Pregnancy

- Often misdiagnosed as GDM, but glucose measurements remain stable and abnormal after delivery
- BMI <25 kg/m^2
- Fasting glucose 5.5–8 mmol/L and HbA1c <64 mmol/mol (8%)
- Heterozygous: no glucose-lowering treatment or self-monitoring required
- Micro- and macrovascular complications are very rare

Effects on the fetus

- Fetus **without** the inherited mutation:
  - Produces ↑ insulin in response to maternal hyperglycaemia ∴ is at risk of macrosomia
- Fetus **with** the inherited mutation:
  - Recognizes the maternal hyperglycaemia as a normal level
  - ∴ does not produce ↑ insulin
  - ∴ growth is normal

⚠ There is a risk of ↓ fetal growth if maternal glucose is ↓.

Management

- Regular measurement of fetal growth
- Start treatment if this is over the 75% percentile

Monogenic diabetes: HNF-1A

- Progressive insulin secretion defect; initially post-prandial hyperglycaemia, then fasting hyperglycaemia is also seen
- Low renal glucose threshold; glycosuria occurs before frank diabetes
- Microvascular and macrovascular complications do occur
- Most present young and are misdiagnosed as T1DM
- Differ from T1DM:
  - Absent antibodies
  - No DKA when insulin omitted
  - Low insulin requirement
- Aids to diagnosis include:
  - ↑ high-density lipoprotein
  - Low highly sensitive CRP

Treatment
- Low-dose sulfonylureas, e.g. glibenclamide rather than insulin
- Some will progress to needing insulin therapy

Effects on the fetus
- None seen

Monogenic diabetes: HNF-4A

- Similar phenotype to HNF-1A (except normal renal glucose threshold)

Treatment
- As for HNF1A-MODY

Effects on the fetus
- 50% of babies with HNF-4A mutations are macrosomic
- Can cause neonatal hyperinsulinaemic hypoglycaemia in infants

⚠ A macrosomic baby with neonatal hypoglycaemia in a mother **without diabetes** should raise suspicion about a paternal HNF-4A mutation.

Monogenic diabetes: HNF-1B

- Inheritance autosomal dominant, less commonly a *de novo* mutation
- Typical phenotype is coexistent diabetes and renal developmental disorders (horseshoe or single kidney, renal dysplasia, or cysts)
- Genital tract malformations can also occur with renal abnormalities
- Other features include gout, hyperparathyroidism, and abnormal liver transaminases
- Unlikely to cause diabetes in the absence of renal disease

Treatment
- Usually requires insulin therapy

Effects on the fetus
- Fetal and neonatal assessment for renal and urogenital abnormalities is indicated

⚠ Women with renal and genital tract abnormalities should be assessed for HNF-1B mutations, and if found should prompt monitoring for complications and genetic counselling.

Pregnancy and diabetes

Effect of pregnancy on diabetes
- General anaesthesia → a ↑ risk of hypoglycaemia and higher rate of aspiration (higher resting gastric volume)
- ↑ tendency to ketosis particularly in the 3rd trimester
- Insulin requirements may ↑ to ≥2× the pre-pregnancy dose
- ↑ hypoglycaemia unawareness, particularly in the 1st trimester

Effects of diabetes on pregnancy
- Poor glycaemic control in the 1st trimester is associated with ↑ risk of congenital malformations
- Fetal hyperglycaemia → hyperinsulinaemia which can cause:
  - Macrosomia
  - Organomegaly
  - Erythropoiesis
  - Fetal polyuria (polyhydramnios)
  - Neonatal hypoglycaemia
  - Respiratory distress syndrome
- Fetal hyperinsulinaemia does not resolve immediately, so there is a risk of neonatal hypoglycaemia after delivery:
  - This may resolve with feeding
  - Some neonates require parenteral glucose supplementation on a special care baby unit
- Complications are shown in Table 11.2

Factors associated with poor pregnancy outcome
- Maternal social deprivation
- Lack of contraceptive use in previous year
- No folic acid intake
- Suboptimal:
  - Self-management
  - Preconceptual care
  - Glycaemic control before pregnancy
  - Maternity care
- Suboptimal surveillance of macrosomic fetuses
- Pre-existing complications

Table 11.2 Complications of diabetes in pregnancy

Maternal	Fetal	Neonatal
UTI	Miscarriage	Polycythaemia
Vulvovaginal candidiasis	Congenital abnormalities[a]	Jaundice
Gestational hypertension Pre-eclampsia	Neural tube defects	Hypoglycaemia
Obstructed labour	Microcephaly	Hypocalcaemia
Operative deliveries	Cardiac abnormalities	Hypomagnesaemia
Retinopathy	Sacral agenesis	Hypothermia
Nephropathy	Renal abnormalities	Cardiomegaly
Cardiac disease	Preterm labour	Birth trauma: • Shoulder dystocia[b] • Fractures • Erb's palsy • Asphyxia
	Polyhydramnios (25%)	Respiratory distress syndrome
	Macrosomia (25–40%)	
	Intrauterine growth restriction	
	Unexplained stillbirth	

[a] In ♀ with poorly controlled diabetes in the 1st trimester.

[b] More common at all birthweights than in babies of ♀ without diabetes.

Preconceptual advice

Glycaemic control

- Needs to be optimized as the rate of congenital malformations correlates with HbA1c; target HbA1c is 48 mmol/mol (6.5%)
- Advise postponing pregnancy if HbA1c is >86 mmol/mol (10%)
- Daily capillary blood glucose monitoring, ideally at least 6 times a day
- Ensure effective contraception until glycaemic control optimized and pregnancy desired

Medications when planning pregnancy

- 5 mg folic acid OD (3 months preconception to >12 wks)
- Continue metformin (can be used as an adjunct to insulin therapy)
- Discontinue all other oral hypoglycaemic agents (with the exception of glibenclamide in some ♀ with monogenic diabetes), replace with insulin
- Start insulin if required for optimal glycaemic control
- Review other medications and substitute for pregnancy-appropriate medications, e.g. antihypertensives and statins
- Advise aspirin required from 12 wks

Complications

See Table 11.3.

Table 11.3 Complications to consider preconceptually or at booking

Risk	Action
Risk of DKA	• Discuss and offer ketone meter to all ♀ with T1DM
Risk of hypoglycaemia and unawareness especially 1st trimester	• Counsel regarding risk and potential atypical symptoms
Hypoglycaemia	• Discuss symptoms and management • Ensure has emergency glucagon injection (1 mg IM) if on insulin • Consider continuous glucose monitoring or insulin pump if recurrent and severe
Retinopathy	• Fundoscopy • Formal retinal imaging • Arrange assessment and treatment of proliferative retinopathy or maculopathy if present
Nephropathy	• Baseline creatinine and microalbuminuria (when not taking ACE-I if appropriate) • Consider renal referral before contraception cessation if: • Serum creatinine >120 micromol/L • Urinary PCR >30 mg/mmol • eGFR <45 mL/min/1.73 m^2 • If nephrotic (protein >3 g/24 hrs, or PCR >300 mg/mmol), prescribe antenatal LMWH prophylaxis
Coronary artery disease	• Ideally treat before conception

Antenatal care

Glycaemic control
- Needs to be optimized
- Glucose monitoring
- HbA1c in 1st trimester
- Dietician review

Fetal complications
- Offer Down's syndrome screening:
  - Consider nuchal translucency, cell-free fetal DNA or invasive testing
  - Serum screening is affected by diabetes (↑ αFP) so less accurate unless appropriate nomograms used
- Offer fetal echocardiography
- Offer assessment of fetal growth and amniotic fluid volume by USS every 4 wks between 28 and 36 wks
- Diabetes is not a contraindication to tocolysis if required but β agonists should be avoided due to risk of triggering ketoacidosis
- Diabetes is not a contraindication to antenatal steroids for fetal lung maturation but glucose monitoring is required ± additional insulin

---

Falling insulin requirements in pregnancy
⚠ This is concerning and should always be taken seriously.

- Any symptoms or signs of adrenal insufficiency:
  - Especially in ♀ with T1DM
- Assess renal function:
  - Impaired renal function can → ↓ insulin excretion
- Consider placental insufficiency:
  - Growth scans
- Discuss timing of delivery (Table 11.4)

Table 11.4 Suggested birth timings in diabetes

Diabetes type	Complications?	Birth timing
T1DM and T2DM	No	• 37^{+0} to 38^{+6} wks
	Yes	• Consider before 37^{+0} wks
GDM	No	• No later than 40^{+6}
	Yes	• Consider earlier than 40^{+6}

Intrapartum management with diabetes

Delivery options
- Vaginal delivery usually preferred
- Caesarean section for obstetric reasons

Gestational diabetes
- Regular capillary blood glucose monitoring:
  - Start variable rate IV insulin infusion (previously known as a 'sliding scale') if capillary blood glucose >8 mmol/L

T1DM/T2DM
- Insulin pump:
  - Continue as normal unless unable to self-manage pump
- Continue SC insulin until in established labour then change to variable rate IV insulin infusion
- If elective delivery planned, start variable rate IV insulin infusion on the morning of the procedure
- Continue long-acting SC insulin while on any IV insulin infusion

Postnatal care

Maternal considerations

GDM

- Discontinue all medications and monitor glucose closely
- Lifestyle advice
- Fasting glucose at, or after 6 wks postpartum (Table 11.5)
- If a fasting glucose not done, HbA1c can be performed after 13 wks postpartum
- Do not routinely offer an oral GTT postpartum
- Offer annual HbA1c testing to those with normal fasting glucose:
  - Up to 50% of ♀ with GDM develop T2DM within 5 yrs

Pre-existing diabetes

- Half the infusion rate of the IV insulin at delivery and ensure supplementary IV glucose is running
- If a general anaesthetic is used, monitor blood glucose every 30 mins until fully conscious
- Resume SC insulin when eating and drinking:
  - At the pre-pregnancy dose if not breastfeeding
  - At 2/3 of the pre-pregnancy dose if breastfeeding
  - If pre-pregnancy dose unknown, half the last dose
- Stop insulin infusion 1 hr after SC insulin dose

All ♀

- Antibiotics and thromboprophylaxis as per local guidelines according to mode of birth
- Breastfeeding should be encouraged in all ♀ with diabetes as it ↓ the risk of:
  - T2DM in ♀ with GDM
  - Cardiovascular disease in later life
  - Childhood obesity in the offspring
- If breastfeeding:
  - Metformin or glibenclamide can be resumed but other oral hypoglycaemics should be avoided
  - Insulin doses may need to be ↓ further (significantly ↑ risk of hypoglycaemia)
- Discuss contraception

Neonatal considerations

- Monitor the infant for hypoglycaemia
- Assess for other complications including:
  - Jaundice
  - Respiratory distress
  - Unidentified malformations.

Table 11.5 GDM: postpartum testing (at 6 wks)

Fasting blood glucose levels	Fasting plasma glucose <6 mmol/L Or HbA1c <39 mmol/mol (5.7%)	Fasting plasma glucose 6.0–6.9 mmol/L Or HbA1c 39–47 mmol/mol (5.7–6.4%)	Fasting plasma glucose ≥7 mmol/L Or HbA1c ≥48 mmol/mol (6.5%)
Risk of diabetes	Low probability of pre-existing diabetes	High risk of developing T2DM	Likely to have T2DM
Management	Lifestyle advice and dietary modification	Lifestyle advice and dietary modification	If FBG used, then confirm with HbA1c If HbA1c used, diagnose and treat as per guidelines for T2DM
Further tests	Annual HbA1c	Annual HbA1c	

NICE (2015). Diabetes in pregnancy guidelines: ⌕ https://www.nice.org.uk/guidance/ng3

Target capillary glucose levels

▶ Advise pregnant ♀ with any form of diabetes to maintain their capillary plasma glucose below target levels if achievable without causing problematic hypoglycaemia (Tables 11.6 and 11.7).

⚠ If on insulin or glibenclamide, the capillary glucose level should be maintained at >4 mmol/L

Table 11.6 Target capillary plasma glucose levels

Timing	Maximum plasma glucose level (mmol/L)
Fasting	5.3
1 hr after meal	7.8
2 hrs after meal	6.4

➔ See also NICE (2015). Diabetes in pregnancy guidelines: ⟳ https://www.nice.org.uk/guidance/ng3

Table 11.7 Suggested capillary glucose monitoring regime

Type of diabetes	Selection	Regime
T1DM	• All ♀	• Fasting • Pre-meals • 1 hr post meals • Bedtime
T2DM	• Multiple daily doses of insulin	• Fasting • Pre-meals • 1 hr post meals • Bedtime
	• Diet controlled • Oral therapy • Single dose of intermediate or long-acting insulin	• Fasting • 1 hr post meal
GDM	• Multiple daily doses of insulin	• Fasting • Pre-meals • 1 hr post meals • Bedtime
	• Diet controlled • Oral therapy • Single dose intermediate or long-acting insulin	• Fasting • 1 hr post meal

Continuous glucose monitoring

- Monitors interstitial glucose concentration very frequently
- Improves rates of normoglycaemia
- Use during pregnancy:
  - ↓ incidence of macrosomia
  - ↓ birthweight
  - ↓ HbA1c
- Unrecognized postprandial hyperglycaemia and nocturnal variability can be identified
- These devices are not advised for use in inpatient settings, e.g. alongside IV insulin infusion
- Now available to all ♀ with T1DM in pregnancy (in the UK) due to improvement in neonatal outcomes seen in CONCEPTT study

Consider its use for pregnant ♀ on insulin if:

- Problematic severe hypoglycaemia ± hypoglycaemia unawareness
- Unstable blood glucose
- To gain information about blood glucose level variability

Insulin pumps in pregnancy

- Insulin pumps are small battery-powered pumps which administer subcutaneous rapid/short-acting insulin e.g. Novorapid® or Humalog® as a continuous infusion, with the option to bolus when required
- They have been shown to result in better control throughout the preconception period, antenatally and postnatally, with ↓ complications such as maternal or neonatal hypoglycaemia, and ↓ maternal weight gain
- Potential problems associated with pump use include inadvertent cannula removal, air bubbles in the tubing, or running out of insulin
- These can be continued during labour and delivery, but can be changed to a variable rate IV insulin infusion if problems arise or the ♀ is unable to manage her pump independently

⚠ Offer ♀ with insulin-treated diabetes continuous SC insulin infusion if adequate blood glucose control is not achieved with multiple daily doses of insulin without significant hypoglycaemia occurring

⮕ NICE (2015). Diabetes in pregnancy guidelines: ℘ https://www.nice.org.uk/guidance/ng3

HbA1c

- Measurement of glycosylated haemoglobin reflects the glucose level over the previous 3 months
- Normal range changes in pregnancy (↑ turnover of red blood cells, see Table 11.8)
- Does not correlate with complications such as macrosomia
- Should not be used to assess glycaemic control in the 2nd and 3rd trimester routinely

☛ IFCC (International Federation of Clinical Chemistry) expressed HbA1c in mmol/mol (preferred use in NICE guidelines)

☛ DCCT (Diabetes Control and Complications Trial) expressed HbA1c as a percentage (see Table 11.9 for conversion)

▶ mmol/mol is now the more widely used measurement and enables easier comparison across international studies

- Normal HbA1c in an individual without diabetes is <42 mmol/mol (4–5.9%)
- Target HbA1c in a non-pregnant individual with diabetes is <48 mmol/mol (6.5%), but this may be higher if the person is prone to problematic hypoglycaemia

Table 11.8 Measurement of HbA1c

Timing	Notes
At booking	• Pre-existing T1DM or T2DM
On diagnosis of GDM	• High level makes underlying T2DM more likely
2nd and 3rd trimester	• Consider in pregnant ♀ with pre-existing diabetes to assess level or risk

➔ See also NICE (2015). Diabetes in pregnancy guidelines: ⌾ https://www.nice.org.uk/guidance/ng3

Table 11.9 Comparison of values for HbA1c

DCCT (%)	IFCC (mmol/mol)
5	31
6	42
7	53
8	64
9	75
10	86
11	97
12	108

➔ For an example of a converter, see: ⌾ https://www.diabetes.co.uk/hba1c-units-converter.html

Types of insulin

See Table 11.10.

Table 11.10 Types of insulin and uses in pregnancy

Speed of action	Type	Benefits	Notes on usage
Rapid	Insulin analogues e.g. insulin aspart, insulin lispro	• Faster onset and shorter duration of action than soluble insulin	• Not associated with adverse pregnancy outcomes • Can be taken before, during, or after a meal
Short-acting	Soluble human insulin	• Can be given SC, IM, or IV • SC: onset of action 30–60 mins, peak action 2–4 hrs, duration up to 8 hrs • IV: very short half-life (5 mins)	• Most appropriate for use in diabetic emergencies • Needs to be given 30–45 mins before meal
Intermediate	Isophane insulin (suspension of insulin with protamine)		• Isophane insulin historically preferred in pregnancy
Long-acting	Human insulin analogues e.g. insulin detemir, glargine, degludec	• Long duration of action so should protect against ketosis	• Should be continued if taking prior to pregnancy and achieving good glycaemic control

Diabetic retinopathy

See Table 11.11.
- Pregnancy can → ↑ progression of diabetic retinopathy
- More common with:
  - Severe retinopathy
  - Poor glucose control
  - ↑ BP
- **Not** a contraindication to vaginal delivery
- ♀ with pre-proliferative diabetic retinopathy should have follow up for at least 6 months after delivery

⚠ Rapid optimization of glucose control is advised against in non-pregnant ♀ with diabetes until their retinopathy has been treated.

⚠ Not a contraindication to rapid optimization of glucose control in pregnant ♀ who were previously poorly controlled.

Table 11.11 Diabetic retinopathy

Condition	Assessment

Pre-existing diabetes *without* retinopathy	**Preconception**
	 • Offer retinal assessment (unless has been done in last 6 mths)
	 • Perform yearly if normal
	 When pregnancy confirmed
	 • Offer retinal assessment:
	  • At booking
	  • At 28 wks

Pre-existing diabetes *with* known retinopathy	• Offer retinal assessment:
	  • At booking
	  • At 16–20 wks
	  • At 28 wks

Hypoglycaemia

Definition
- A blood glucose <4.0 mmol/L in a ♀ with diabetes.
- Can become more frequent during pregnancy, especially at night
- Hypoglycaemia unawareness is also common, particularly in the 1st trimester
- If persistent despite appropriate changes to insulin regimen, then a continuous subcutaneous insulin infusion or 'insulin pump' should be considered
- Any ♀ on insulin therapy should always carry a fast-acting glucose-containing food or drink
- Glucagon injections should be provided to ♀ with T1DM, and their close contacts educated on its use if appropriate

Fasting glucose in ♀ without diabetes:
⚠ A fasting glucose of ~3.5 mmol/L is normal in a non-pregnant individual who does not have diabetes.

⚠ In pregnancy, fasting glucose can be 10–15% lower than this, therefore caution is required before diagnosing true hypoglycaemia in ♀ without diabetes, particularly in pregnancy.

Treatment
See Table 11.12.

Hypoglycaemia after glucose load
- Occasionally an oral GTT will show significant hypoglycaemia following a glucose load
- If fasting glucose normal and ♀ is not unwell or on any glucose-lowering medications:
  - Diagnosis is likely postprandial hypoglycaemia
  - No further tests are routinely required
  - Advise patient about regular meals and snacks
- If fasting glucose also abnormally low:
  - Investigations required for an underlying cause (e.g. insulinoma)

Table 11.12 Treatment for hypoglycaemia

Oral administration (1st line)	Non-oral administration
• Tablets containing glucose • Buccal glucose gel • Drinks containing glucose	• IV glucose: • Bolus of 10% or 20% glucose • Can be repeated • IM glucagon: • 1 mg (one-off dose)

Causes

See Table 11.13.

Table 11.13 Causes of hypoglycaemia

Drugs	• Insulin
	• Oral hypoglycaemic agents, e.g. gliclazide, glibenclamide
	• Other drugs, e.g. quinine, pentamidine
Hormonal	• Cortisol deficiency
	• Hormone-secreting tumours, e.g. insulinoma
Renal	• Renal impairment → accumulation of insulin/oral hypoglycaemics
Liver	• Liver impairment
Infections	• Sepsis
	• Malaria
Post-prandial	• Reactive hypoglycaemia
	• After gastric bypass (post-prandial hyperinsulinaemic hypoglycaemia; previously known as 'late dumping' syndrome)
Alcohol	

Diabetic ketoacidosis

Background
- In pregnancy, ketosis occurs more readily
- DKA should be considered even at lower blood glucose levels
- DKA is associated with significant fetal mortality (historically reported with the use of sympathomimetics as tocolytics)
- ↑ risk of DKA if education and/or compliance with treatment are poor

⚠ Steroids for fetal lung maturation should be given with caution in ♀ with diabetes as this could precipitate ketosis, and close blood glucose monitoring should be performed

Management of DKA in pregnancy

Consider the appropriate location
- May be ITU/HDU

Look for the cause
- Compliance or missed doses
- Intercurrent illness, e.g. infection, pancreatitis
- New diagnosis

IV insulin
- A fixed rate IV insulin infusion is preferred in DKA
- Starting rate is 0.1 units/kg/hr
- ↑ rate each hour if the glucose and ketones do not ↓ sufficiently rapidly (e.g. a ↓ in glucose <3 mmol/L per hour, or a ↓ in ketones <0.5 mmol/L per hour)

Fluid resuscitation
- Rapid replacement as these individuals are often very fluid depleted

Potassium replacement
- Insulin drives K^+ into cells
- Significant ↓ K^+ can develop if replacement is not aggressive enough

Other considerations
- Avoidance of IV sodium bicarbonate or phosphate replacement is advised
- Fetal monitoring as determined by gestational age

Endocrinology

Hormones and pregnancy

See Table 12.1.

Table 12.1 Hormones and pregnancy

Hormone	Effect of pregnancy	Explanation
Luteinizing hormone	Undetectable during pregnancy	Suppressed by ↑ levels of oestrogen and progesterone
Follicle-stimulating hormone	Undetectable during pregnancy	Suppressed by ↑ levels of oestrogen and progesterone
Growth hormone	Total GH level ↑	Placenta produces GH Most assays cannot distinguish placental from pituitary GH
Adrenocorticotropic hormone	Level doubles after 1st trimester	Placenta produces cortisol-releasing factor and ACTH Pituitary ACTH secretion is unchanged
Insulin-like growth factor 1	↑ in normal pregnancy	Production is stimulated by human placental lactogen
Antidiuretic hormone	↓ ADH	Placenta produces vasopressinase
Prolactin	Progressive ↑ throughout pregnancy	↑ oestrogen stimulates pituitary prolactin release Prolactin is synthesized by decidual tissue but little enters the fetal and maternal circulations
Renin	↑ up to 4× by 20 wks then plateaus	↓ total peripheral resistance and resulting afterload ↓ therefore allowing plasma volume expansion
Aldosterone	↑ up to 3× in 1st trimester and 10× in 3rd trimester	Response to ↑ renin and ↑ angiotensin II
Angiotensin II	↑ 3×	↑ renin ↑ angiotensinogen
Catecholamines	No known change in reference range	

Table 12.1 Continued

Hormone	Effect of pregnancy	Explanation
Parathyroid hormone	No known change in reference range	
Cortisol	Serum cortisol (reflecting total cortisol) ↑ up to 3×	↑ cortisol-binding globulin
		↑ cortisol-releasing hormone
		↑ progesterone
	Urinary cortisol (reflecting free cortisol only) ↑	
	Suppression by exogenous corticosteroid is blunted	
Thyroid hormones: T_3, T_4, and thyroid-stimulating hormone	50% ↑ thyroid hormone requirement	↑ thyroid-binding globulin
	↑ iodine requirement	De-iodination in placenta
	↑ T_4 production suppresses TSH (particularly in 1st trimester)	↑ renal iodine clearance
		Fetal iodine uptake
	↓ Upper end of normal range for free T_3 and T_4 in late pregnancy	Structural similarity of TSH and HCG → HCG-mediated stimulation of TSH receptors
	↑ levels of total T_3 and T_4	Haemodilution

Prolactinoma

Background
- Most common pituitary tumour in ♀ of childbearing age
- Diagnosis in non-pregnant individuals is made by ↑ serum prolactin (usually >2000 mU/L, lower values suggest non-functioning lesion and hyperprolactinaemia) and pituitary lesion on CT or MRI (Table 12.2):
  - Microadenoma <1 cm diameter
  - Macroadenoma >1 cm diameter
- Treatment may result in rapid return of fertility

⚠ Serum prolactin ↑ up to 10× in normal pregnancy, so prolactin levels are not useful for diagnosis or monitoring.

Clinical features
- Amenorrhoea/infertility
- Galactorrhoea
- Visual field defects (bitemporal hemianopia)
- Headache

Causes of hyperprolactinaemia
- Normal pregnancy and breastfeeding
- Hypothalamus or stalk lesions
- Empty sella syndrome
- Hypothyroidism
- Chronic renal failure
- Drugs, e.g. phenothiazines, metoclopramide, methyldopa

Management of prolactinoma in pregnancy
- Regular review
- Imaging (MRI) if any change in visual fields or symptoms

Treatment
- Dopamine agonists (Table 12.3):
  - If tumour does not respond, surgical resection is an option

Table 12.2 Macro- and microprolactinomas in pregnancy

	Macroadenoma	Microadenoma
Expansion risk during pregnancy	Likely; highest in 3rd trimester	Low
Treatment	May be appropriate to continue dopamine agonist	Stop dopamine agonist at conception
Formal visual field assessment	Each trimester	If symptoms develop

Table 12.3 Drug treatments for prolactinoma

	Side effects	Pregnancy considerations
Bromocriptine (short-acting ergot derivative)	• Nausea • Nasal stuffiness • Orthostatic ↓ BP • Raynaud-like symptoms in hands • Unmasking of depression and/or psychosis	• Good safety record • May suppress milk production
Cabergoline (long-acting ergot derivative)	• Headache • Nausea • Postural ↓ BP • Fatigue	• No association with fetal or maternal complications • Concerns regarding valvular heart disease
Quinagolide (not ergot related)		Not recommended if pregnant or planning to be: • ↑ miscarriage rate • ↑ congenital malformations

Ergot derivatives and valvular heart disease

- Cabergoline has been associated with valvular heart disease when used in high doses in patients with Parkinson's disease (?2° to potent 5-HT 2B receptor activation)
- No ↑ incidence of valvular disease seen with doses used in prolactinomas (much lower than that used in Parkinson's)

📌 Theoretical risk of maternal and fetal cardiac valve fibrosis but no studies to support this

📌 UK Medicines and Healthcare products Regulatory Authority (MHRA) advice (October 2008) is to:
- Exclude pregnancy before administration of cabergoline
- Advise ♀ planning pregnancy to stop taking cabergoline 1 mth before trying to conceive

📌 Bromocriptine has been shown to have mild 5-HT 2B receptor activation therefore could have a similar effect but data is sparse

➔ MHRA: ⌖ https://www.gov.uk/drug-safety-update/ergot-derived-dopamine-agonists-risk-of-fibrotic-reactions

Acromegaly

Background

- Caused by excess production of GH and subsequent ↑ IGF-1
- Changes can be subtle and insidious, often leading to a delay of several years between the onset of symptoms and diagnosis
- Majority are caused by GH-secreting pituitary adenomas (more likely to be macroadenomas than microadenomas)
- Few are caused by GHRH-secreting lesions such as carcinoid tumours, or ectopic GH secretion
- If untreated, sequelae include cardiovascular disease and T2DM

Clinical features

See Box 12.1.

Pregnancy

- Uncommon in ♀ with acromegaly because:
  - Majority undergo curative surgery
  - Stalk compression can cause ↑ prolactin and infertility
- Diagnosis is difficult to make in pregnancy because:
  - Most assays cannot distinguish pituitary from placental GH
  - IGF-1 ↑ in pregnancy

Risks in pregnancy

- ↑ risk of GDM
- ↑ risk of ↑ BP
- Cardiac complications can arise for the 1st time (coronary artery disease, cardiomyopathy)

 Potential for tumour growth and pituitary apoplexy so macroadenomas should be monitored in the same way as macroprolactinomas (see Table 12.2, p. 400).

Management of suspected acromegaly in pregnancy

Diagnosis

- Biochemical tests confirm by:
  - ↑ IGF-1 level
  - Failure of GH levels to suppress in response to 75 g oral glucose load
- If excess GH confirmed, imaging is indicated (MRI pituitary ± other sites if other sources suspected)

Treatment

- 1° surgical, i.e. resection of adenoma
- 1st-line medical treatment is somatostatin analogues (octreotide or lanreotide) is used in those not cured by surgery

---

Box 12.1 Clinical features of acromegaly
- Headaches
- Fatigue, lethargy
- Sweating
- ↑ shoe size
- Sleep apnoea
- Changes in facial appearance such as supra-orbital bossing, coarse features, interdental separation
- Deepening of voice
- Enlargement of hands, feet, jaw (macrognathia)
- Peripheral neuropathies such as carpal tunnel syndrome
- Symptoms and signs of ↑ prolactin (from stalk compression)

Somatostatin analogues and examples of dosing regimens
- Octreotide: 50–200 mcg SC TDS
- Lanreotide sustained release (SR): 30 mg IM every 7–14 days or 60 mg deep SC every 28 days depending on preparation used
- Octreotide long-acting release (LAR): 10–30 mg IM every 4–6 wks

Side effects
- Gallstones (1%/yr develop symptomatic gallstones)
- Nausea
- Abdominal cramps
- Steatorrhoea

🔅 *Considerations for use of somatostatin analogues in pregnancy*
- Cross the placenta ∴ have the potential to affect fetal development (somatostatin receptors are widespread in fetal tissues)
- Very limited safety data in pregnancy
- Stopping treatment for 9 mths is unlikely to affect the overall course of the condition

🔅 Despite the issues, if symptomatic tumour enlargement occurs, medication may be preferable to surgery in pregnancy.

Other tumours

TSHomas
- Rarely reported in pregnancy
- Octreotide may be required if tumour growth occurs or if hyperthyroidism develops (as thionamides may be ineffective)

Non-functioning adenomas
- Tumour growth is rare
- Symptoms may result from growth of surrounding lactotroph cells causing displacement of the tumour and compression of the optic chiasm

Hypopituitarism

Background

- Underactivity of the pituitary gland, can arise from several pathologies (Box 12.2) and cause various manifestations
- Onset of symptoms can be insidious, and there can be a significant delay between symptom development and diagnosis
- Can be life-threatening if untreated
- Production of hormones can be affected to varying degrees
- Diagnosis is made by measuring oestradiol/testosterone, LH, FSH, TSH, T_4, ACTH, cortisol, and GH

Clinical features

- Depends on the hormone deficiency
- Symptoms and signs of hypocortisolaemia (from ACTH deficiency) including ↓ weight, ↓ appetite, fatigue, postural ↓ BP, hypoglycaemia
- Symptoms and signs of hypothyroidism (from TSH deficiency)
- Symptoms and signs of ↓ FSH and ↓ LH: hypogonadotropic hypogonadism, i.e. anovulatory infertility, oligo- or amenorrhea
- Symptoms and signs of GH deficiency—including changes in body fat mass, abnormal lipid profile
- ↓ prolactin resulting in lactation failure

Fertility

- Ovulation induction with gonadotropins may be required
- If pregnancy achieved, oestrogen and progesterone production from the feto-placental unit can sustain the pregnancy

Pregnancy

- If adequate hormonal replacement has been achieved before pregnancy, no effect on maternal or fetal outcome
- If inadequately treated, or not diagnosed, can be associated with:
  - Maternal hypoglycaemia
  - Maternal hypotension
  - Miscarriage
  - Stillbirth
- Lactation may be impaired due to inadequate prolactin production

---

Box 12.2 Causes of hypopituitarism

- Pituitary surgery
- Radiotherapy
- Pituitary tumours
- Infarction (e.g. Sheehan's syndrome)
- Lymphocytic hypophysitis

Diagnosis of suspected hypopituitarism in pregnancy
- Diagnosis cannot be confirmed until after pregnancy (altered hormone levels in pregnancy prevent certainty)
- ACTH stimulation test (Synacthen® test) not helpful in acute pituitary insufficiency, as the adrenal response remains normal; cortisol levels are also altered in pregnancy leading to difficulty in interpretation of the results
- Insulin tolerance tests should **not** be performed in pregnancy
- Prolactin measurement may be of use if the level is abnormally low

Management
See Table 12.4.

Management of suspected hypopituitarism in pregnancy
- Identification and treatment of the cause if possible
- Replacement of the deficient hormones
- TFTs may initially be normal due to the long half-life of thyroxine, so repeated measurements are important
- Empirical steroid treatment is reasonable until diagnosis can be confirmed after delivery

Table 12.4 Management of pre-existing hypopituitarism in pregnancy

Drug	Pregnancy considerations
Levothyroxine	• May require ↑ dose as pregnancy progresses
Glucocorticoids	• Continue normal dose • Parenteral steroid replacement during labour
Growth hormone	• Lack of confirmatory safety data in pregnancy • Therapy usually discontinued
Desmopressin	• Symptoms of DI may worsen • May need to ↑ dose

Lymphocytic hypophysitis

Background
- An inflammatory disorder, characterized by lymphocyte infiltration and enlargement of the pituitary gland
- Cause is often unknown
- More common in ♀ (~5♀:1♂)
- 20% have coexisting autoimmune disease, particularly Hashimoto's thyroiditis

Clinical features
- 60% present with symptoms of mass effect, e.g. headache, visual symptoms
- 85% have features of hypopituitarism ± ↑ prolactin
- Isolated ↓ ACTH can occur
- Imaging often shows an enlarged anterior pituitary, which can appear similar to an adenoma

Common hormonal changes in lymphocytic hypophysitis
- ↓ ACTH
- ↓ ADH
- ↓ TSH
- Normal LH
- Normal FSH
- Normal GH
- Prolactin may be normal, mildly ↑ or mildly ↓

Pregnancy
- ↑ frequency in pregnancy and the postpartum period
- Can be difficult to diagnose as a result of the changes in LH, FSH, and cortisol that occur in normal pregnancy

Management of lymphocytic hypophysitis in pregnancy
- Treatment is often not required as spontaneous resolution may occur
- Hormone deficiencies should be treated
- Surgery—if significant visual symptoms

❥ Steroid treatment is controversial, may → an improvement but recurrence of symptoms can occur as dose is ↓.

Sheehan's syndrome

Background

- In a normal pregnancy, the pituitary gland enlarges to 2–3× normal size
- Hypotension resulting from PPH can cause avascular necrosis of the enlarged pituitary → partial or complete pituitary failure
- Pregnancy can occur after this diagnosis

Clinical features of Sheehan's syndrome

Acute
- ↓ BP and ↑ HR despite blood product administration
- Hypoglycaemia
- Failure of lactation

Chronic
- Persistent amenorrhoea
- Loss of pubic and axillary hair
- Breast atrophy
- Fatigue
- Hypothyroidism
- Symptoms of adrenal insufficiency including:
  - Nausea
  - Abdominal pain
  - Postural ↓ BP
- Polydipsia and polyuria are rare

Management of Sheehan's syndrome in pregnancy

- Is the same as for ♀ with hypopituitarism from other aetiologies

Treatment
- Treatment of the identified hormone deficiencies

Diabetes insipidus

Background
See Table 12.5.
- Failure in ADH axis resulting in inappropriately dilute urine
- Can be either:
  - Cranial/central (defect in production of ADH)
  - Nephrogenic (resistance to ADH action in the kidney)

Clinical features
- Symptoms include polydipsia and polyuria
- Associated biochemical abnormalities result from ↑ water loss (Box 12.3)

Pregnancy
- Pregnancy ↓ the plasma osmolality at which ADH is released:
  - 5 mOsmol/kg less than in the non-pregnant ♀
- 50% of ♀ deteriorate:
  - ↑ placental vasopressinase production → ↓ ADH levels
- Desmopressin may need to be ↑ during pregnancy, but then rapidly ↓ after delivery
- Thiazide diuretics can be used if required

⚠ Water deprivation tests should be avoided as may result in alterations of placental perfusion and uterine irritability

⚠ DI can occur 2° to acute fatty liver of pregnancy (see p. 162)

Management of DI in pregnancy

Central DI

Desmopressin
- Stereoisomer of ADH (also known as vasopressin or arginine vasopressin)
- Acts on V2 receptors predominantly
- Longer half-life than native hormone
- Intranasal spray (10–20 mcg), SC or IV routes preferred
- Oral (only 5% absorbed, ↓ by further 50% if taken with meals)

Nephrogenic DI

Thiazide diuretics
- Can ↓ urine output when desmopressin does not work

NSAIDs
- ↓ prostaglandin production (which antagonize ADH)

Considerations for labour
- Cranial DI is associated with ↓ oxytocin production (the other posterior pituitary hormone) l:
  - ↑ risk of failure of progression of labour
  - ↑ risk of uterine atony and PPH

Box 12.3 Common biochemical abnormalities in DI
- Hypernatraemia
- Renal impairment
- Evidence of haemoconcentration:
  - ↑ haematocrit
  - ↑ albumin

Table 12.5 Types of DI

Type	Characteristics

Central (defect in ADH production by posterior pituitary)	• Hereditary causes:
	  • Defect in *AVP-Np2* gene
	  • DIDMOAD syndrome (DI, DM, optic atrophy, blindness)
	• Acquired causes:
	  • Trauma
	  • Sarcoid
	  • TB
	  • LCH
	  • Lymphocytic hypophysitis
	  • Meningitis
	  • Encephalitis
	  • Sheehan's syndrome

Nephrogenic (abnormal response to ADH in kidney)	• Hereditary causes:
	  • X-linked defect of V2 receptor
	  • Autosomal recessive defect in *AQP2* gene which encodes for aquaporin 2
	• Acquired causes:
	  • Drugs (orlistat, demeclocycline, amphotericin)
	  • Metabolic (hypercalcaemia, hypokalaemia, chronic renal disease, post-obstructive uropathy)

Gestational	• Production of placental vasopressinase (↑ 1000× between 4 and 38 wks) • Can recur in subsequent pregnancies • Resolves after delivery • May be seen in ♀ heterozygous for X-linked defect in V2 receptor despite being asymptomatic outside pregnancy

Thyroid antibodies

See Table 12.6.

TSH receptor antibodies

- TSH-R **stimulating** antibodies:
  - Cause Grave's disease
  - Can cross the placenta and cause neonatal hyperthyroidism (see p. 420)
- TSH-R **blocking** antibodies are rare:
  - Cause hypothyroidism
  - Can cross the placenta and cause neonatal hypothyroidism

Thyroid peroxidase antibodies

- Testing is not routinely advocated with 1° hypothyroidism as they are commonly positive in this setting and their presence does not alter management
- Testing is advocated in individuals with a goitre and normal TFTs, or with subclinical hypothyroidism, as presence makes later development of overt hypothyroidism more likely

In pregnancy

↑ TPO antibodies are common and have been associated with risks for both the mother and fetus, even with normal thyroid function.
- Maternal:
  - ↑ risk of overt hypothyroidism
  - ↑ risk of postpartum thyroiditis
- Fetal:
  - ↑ risk of miscarriage
  - ↑ risk of preterm delivery

Anti-thyroglobulin antibodies

- Autoimmune antibody associated with thyroid disease
- Present in ~10% of normal individuals, so presence not sensitive or specific for Grave's disease or autoimmune hypothyroidism

In pregnancy

No association of the presence of these antibodies with adverse pregnancy outcomes, so routine testing of this antibody is not recommended.

When to test for TSH-R stimulating antibodies in pregnancy

- Current treatment for Grave's disease
- Previous treatment for Grave's disease
- History of previous pregnancy complicated by fetal or neonatal hyperthyroidism
- New diagnosis of hyperthyroidism
- Significant biochemical hyperthyroidism in 1st trimester (even if asymptomatic)

If positive
- Consider USS looking for fetal goitre (but practice varies between centres as the presence of a goitre is very rare)
- Neonate needs TFTs at 10 days of age

When to test for TPO antibodies in pregnancy

- If autoimmune condition including T1DM
- Subclinical hypothyroidism

If positive
- Treatment is not indicated for positive TPO antibodies alone if thyroid function normal, even if assisted reproductive technology being considered
- TFTs if any symptoms of thyroid disease develop
- Postpartum TFTs advised, e.g. at 3 and 6 mths postnatally, as postpartum thyroid dysfunction is more likely
- TFTs prior to future conception to ensure optimal thyroid function in 1st trimester

Table 12.6 Antibodies present in autoimmune thyroid disease

Antibody	Frequency
Grave's disease	
TSH-R (stimulating)	• 70–100%
Anti-TPO	• 70–80%
Anti-thyroglobulin	• 30–50%
Autoimmune hypothyroidism	
TSH-R (blocking)	• 10–20%
Anti-TPO	• Majority
Anti-thyroglobulin	• Majority

Hypothyroidism

- Multiple causes, most common is autoimmune (Table 12.7)
- Diagnosis is made by ↑ TSH and ↓ free T_4 or free T_3 levels using pregnancy-specific reference ranges
- Untreated can → ovulation inhibition (amenorrhea ± infertility)

Clinical features of hypothyroidism

Normal for pregnancy
- Lethargy
- Weight gain
- Constipation

Specific to hypothyroidism
- Cold intolerance
- Bradycardia
- Delayed relaxation of tendon reflexes

Treatment

- Mainstay of treatment is levothyroxine (T_4) (PO, OD)
- A minority may be taking liothyronine (T_3)

🖱 ↑ use of alternative thyroid supplements, including those available online. These are not recommended in pregnancy.

Pregnancy

- Present in up to 1% of pregnant ♀
- Aim for optimal control prior to conception
- Avoid overtreatment
- Well-controlled disease has good maternal and fetal outcomes
- Untreated hypothyroidism is associated with:
  - Miscarriage
  - Anaemia
  - Pre-eclampsia
  - Low birthweight babies
- Maternal ↓ iodine can result in neonatal hypothyroidism with abnormal cognitive and physical development
- Maternal hypothyroxinaemia early in pregnancy can cause delayed mental and motor function in the child

---

Poorly controlled hypothyroidism in pregnancy

- Assess for other reasons for ↓ absorption such as nausea/vomiting
- Check maternal compliance
- Check timing of medication administration:
  - Taken when fasting? (this ↑ absorption)
  - Taken at the same time as medication or food such as antacids, iron supplementation, colestyramine or milk? (↓ absorption)

Table 12.7 Causes of hypothyroidism

Type	Cause
Not associated with goitre	• Post treatment to thyroid • Surgery • Radiation or radioiodine • Atrophic thyroiditis • Congenital developmental defect
Associated with goitre	• Autoimmune (Hashimoto's thyroiditis) • Iodine deficiency
Drugs	• Amiodarone • Lithium • Iodine • Anti-thyroid drugs
Pituitary causes	• Hypopituitarism • Isolated TSH deficiency
Hypothalamic causes	• Neoplasm • Sarcoidosis • Infection, e.g. encephalitis
Self-limiting	• Postpartum thyroiditis • Withdrawal of suppressive anti-thyroid therapy

Management of hypothyroidism in pregnancy

- Aim to optimize control preconception and throughout
- Continue pre-pregnancy levothyroxine dose with any ↑ in treatment guided by pregnancy-specific TFTs
  - ↑ levothyroxine is often but not always required
  - May reflect inadequate treatment prior to pregnancy
  - Empirical dose ↑ is not recommended in UK practice
- Recheck TFTs every trimester or 4–6 wks after any dose change
- Endocrine Society guidelines recommend:
  - Target TSH <2.5 mIU/L
  - A high TSH in 1st trimester in the absence of a low T_4 should **not** automatically prompt a change in levothyroxine dose
- ♀ on T_3 (liothyronine) should change to levothyroxine as:
  - Liothyronine does not cross the placenta
  - Fetus depends on maternal thyroid hormones until 2nd trimester
- Levothyroxine is safe when breastfeeding
- Starting dose for newly diagnosed hypothyroidism would be 50 mcg OD (in the absence of cardiac disease)

→ Endocrine Society guidelines: ℛ https://www.endocrine org/guidelines-and-clinical-practice/clinical-practice-guidelines

Subclinical hypothyroidism

Overt hypothyroidism
- TSH >10 mIU/L even if T_4 normal

Subclinical hypothyroidism
- TSH of between 4.0 and 10 mIU/L in pregnancy, in combination with a normal T_4

Normal for pregnancy
- TSH <4.0 mIU/L

Background
- SCH is seen in 3–4% of pregnant ♀
- Older definitions of SCH used a threshold of TSH >2.5 mIU/L which is now outdated and probably led to overtreatment
- Larger studies have shown that a TSH of <4 mIU/L is normal in pregnancy after 7 wks

Treatment
- Advised for overt hypothyroidism
- No evidence that treatment with thyroxine improves outcomes in SCH
- If treatment is started, TFTs should be repeated after 4–6 wks to check for iatrogenic hyperthyroidism
- Antibody positivity does not mandate a different treatment threshold
- In ♀ with SCH undergoing assisted reproductive technology, treatment with thyroxine is advised, with a target TSH of <2.5 mIU/L

Isolated maternal hypothyroxinaemia
- Defined as a low free T_4 in the setting of a normal TSH
- No clear evidence of adverse fetal or neonatal outcomes in this setting, although the exact cut-off for T_4 varies between studies
- Possible causes:
  - Iodine deficiency
  - Antibody interference with assay results
  - 2° hypothyroidism (rare)
- No blood test can be performed to confirm iodine deficiency, it requires repeated urine samples

△ There is a lack of evidence of harm in pregnancy so thyroxine treatment is not routinely recommended

▶ Optimization of iodine intake is recommended in all pregnant and breastfeeding ♀.

🔗 Endocrine Society guidelines for the management of thyroid dysfunction in pregnancy: ℛ https://www.endocrine org/guidelines-and-clinical-practice/clinical-practice-guidelines

Thyroid function tests

Background

- Ideally, pregnancy-specific reference ranges should be used for TFTs in pregnancy, and performed locally to ensure they reflect the population in question, as well as utilizing the same assays
- If local data is not obtainable, then the use of data from a similar population is suggested
- If this is not available, then an upper limit of 4 mIU/L for TSH can be used for 7 wks onwards
- An example of UK-based reference ranges for thyroid function is shown in Table 12.8

Table 12.8 Thyroid function tests

	Normal range (non-pregnant)	1st trimester	2nd trimester	3rd trimester
TSH (mIU/L)	0.3–4.2	0–5.5	0.5–3.5	0.5–4
T_4 (pmol/L)	9–26	10–16	9–15.5	8–14.5
T_3 (pmol/L)	2.6–5.7	3–7	3–5.5	2.5–5.5

Source: data from Cotzias et al (2008) 'A study to establish gestation-specific reference intervals for thyroid function tests in normal singleton pregnancy' *Gynecology and Reproductive Biology* 123(1):61–66 (UK population studied)

➲ 2017 Guidelines of the American Thyroid Association for the Diagnosis and Management of Thyroid Disease During Pregnancy and the Postpartum: ℰ https://www.liebertpub.com/doi/pdf/10.1089/thy.2016.0457

Hyperthyroidism

Background

- Diagnose by ↓ TSH and ↑ free T_4 or free T_3 levels using pregnancy-specific reference ranges
- 95% caused by Grave's disease (TSH-R stimulating antibodies)
- If inadequately treated can be associated with infertility
- See Box 12.4

Treatment

- Anti-thyroid medication (Table 12.9):
  - Thionamides such as carbimazole are usually the 1st-line treatment
  - PTU is associated with idiosyncratic hepatic disturbance so is usually reserved for when carbimazole is not appropriate
  △ Both can → agranulocytosis
- Thyroidectomy
- Radioiodine treatment:
  △ ♀ receiving radioiodine treatment should be counselled to avoid pregnancy for 6 to 12 mths, due to risk of requiring 2nd treatment as well as the risk of hypothyroidism

Pregnancy

- Complicates 1 in 500 pregnancies
- Most ♀ diagnosed before pregnancy will be on medical treatment or had definitive treatment (thyroidectomy or radioiodine)
- Subclinical hyperthyroidism (↓ TSH and normal T_3/T_4) is not associated with adverse pregnancy outcome
- Uncontrolled hyperthyroidism is associated with:
  - Miscarriage
  - Preterm labour
  - Fetal growth restriction
- TSH-R antibodies cross the placenta:
  - Untreated fetal hyperthyroidism has a 15% mortality rate
  - Titre may ↓ from pregnancy-related immunosuppression, but then ↑ postpartum

---

Box 12.4 Signs and symptoms of hyperthyroidism

Normal for pregnancy
- Fatigue
- ↑ HR and palpitations
- Shortness of breath
- Palmar erythema

Specific to hyperthyroidism
- ↓ weight
- Eye signs (proptosis, lid lag, and lid retraction)
- Pretibial myxoedema
- Tremor

Table 12.9 Drugs to treat hyperthyroidism in pregnancy

	Side effects	Pregnancy-specific risks	Breastfeeding
PTU (50–400 mg daily)	1 in 1000 risk of acute liver failure (idiosyncratic reaction) Agranulocytosis	Crosses placenta One study shows an increase in congenital malformations	Considered safe
Carbimazole (5–40 mg daily)	Agranulocytosis	Crosses placenta Suspicion of ↑ risk of aplasia cutis and choanal atresia One study shows an ↑ in malformations, that appears to be dose related	Considered safe If high dose, monitor neonatal thyroid function

Management of hyperthyroidism in pregnancy

▶ TSH-R antibodies should be checked in all ♀ with a history of Grave's disease, irrespective of previous treatment

- In the 1st trimester, treatment should not be started unless there are clinical signs or symptoms of overt hyperthyroidism (Box 12.4) in which case PTU is used
- If hyperthyroidism develops later in pregnancy then carbimazole or PTU can be used
- If a ♀ is taking carbimazole before pregnancy, then European and USA guidelines advocate changing to PTU. Recent data shows thionamides and PTU are associated with an ↑ in congenital malformation rate, and this appeared to be associated with ↑ doses of thionamide. However, this risk is only ↓ if carbimazole is changed to PTU ≥3 mths before conception (i.e. risk not ↓ if changed after pregnancy confirmed)
- If thyroid function is well controlled on a low dose of carbimazole prior to conception, some centres continue this throughout pregnancy
- β blockers (propranolol) can be used for symptom control
- Surgery can be performed if required

⚠ Radioiodine should be avoided in pregnancy and breastfeeding

Causes of hyperthyroidism

Thyroid
- Graves' disease
- Toxic multinodular goitre
- Toxic adenoma
- Subacute thyroiditis
- Drugs, e.g. amiodarone, lithium

Exogenous thyroid hormone
- Over-replacement
- Thyroxine abuse

Pregnancy related
- Hydatidiform mole
- Hyperemesis gravidarum

Indications for surgical thyroidectomy in pregnancy

- Dysphagia
- Stridor
- Suspected carcinoma
- Allergies to both anti-thyroid drugs

β-HCG and TSH

- β-HCG is structurally similar to TSH, so can stimulate TSH-R
- In 1st trimester, TFTs may appear consistent with hyperthyroidism but symptoms and signs related to hyperthyroidism are absent
- This phenomenon is ↑ in conditions with ↑ β-HCG such as:
  - Molar pregnancy
  - Multiple pregnancy
  - Hyperemesis gravidarum

▶ This is **biochemical hyperthyroidism** and does not mandate treatment in the absence of symptoms and signs of thyroid disease.

▶ Close monitoring of thyroid function (i.e. every 4 wks initially) is recommended to ensure TFTs normalize.

Fetal and neonatal hyperthyroidism

Fetal

- Results from high titres of maternal TSH-R stimulating antibodies which cross the placenta
- Usually when ♀ is euthyroid from previous treatment with radioiodine or thyroidectomy (anti-thyroid medications cross the placenta and can protect the fetus)
- Occurs in up to 10% of ♀ with a current or past history of Grave's disease
- Features (most of which can be assessed by USS) include:
  - Fetal tachycardia
  - Hydrops
  - Fetal growth restriction
  - Fetal goitre
  - Accelerated bone maturation
- Treat with maternal administration of anti-thyroid drugs

Neonatal

- This typically presents soon after delivery
- Most commonly occurs when ♀ were taking PTU or carbimazole as the neonate loses the placental transfer of the anti-thyroid medication but the TSH-R stimulating antibodies remain in the neonatal circulation for up to 3 mths
- Untreated neonatal hyperthyroidism is associated with a mortality rate of up to 15%

Postpartum thyroiditis

Background

- Thyroid dysfunction occurring in the 1st 6 mths postpartum
- Develops in 30–50% of ♀ who have TPO antibodies
- Twice as common in ♀ with T1DM
- Lymphocytic infiltration of the thyroid gland results in release of stored T_4 (Table 12.10):
  - Causes an initial period of transient hyperthyroidism
  - This phase can last up to 2 mths and may not have clinical effects
  - 2nd phase of hypothyroidism results from ↓ T_4 stores and the immune destruction of the thyroid cells

Treatment

- Treatment should be guided by symptoms rather than biochemistry:
  - β blockers for hyperthyroid phase
  - Short course of levothyroxine when hypothyroid

Prognosis

- Often remits after 1 yr
- 25% chance of hypothyroidism in later life
- Risk of recurrence in future pregnancy is 70%
- Risk of permanent hypothyroidism is 5% per year for antibody-positive ♀ so annual TFTs are advisable

Other causes

See Table 12.11.

Table 12.10 Phases of postpartum thyroiditis

	Typical onset	Duration	Features	Management
Hyper-thyroid phase	1–4 mths postpartum	Up to 2 mths	Usually mild features of hyper-thyroidism including small goitre	Distinguish from Grave's disease by repeating TFTs in 4 wks, TSH-R stimulating antibodies ± uptake scan[a] Symptomatic treatment
Hypo-thyroid phase	3–8 mths postpartum	4–6 mths	Hypothyroid symptoms	Levothyroxine

[a] This will require interruption of lactation and is often impractical with a baby.

Table 12.11 Other causes of thyroiditis

	Characteristic features	Clinical presentation
Autoimmune	• Atrophic: no goitre • Hashimoto's: goitre present; gross lymphocytic and fibrotic changes	• Hypothyroidism (most common) • Euthyroid (occasional) • Hyperthyroidism (transient and uncommon)

De-Quervain's (subacute/granulomatous)	Possibly viral in origin, multinuclear giant cells on histology	• Evidence of preceding infection
		• Systemic features of:
		  • Lethargy
		  • Arthralgia
		  • Pain

Reidel's thyroiditis (chronic fibrosing)	Extensive fibrosis leading to hard consistency of the thyroid	• Usually euthyroid
Infectious	• Acute painful thyroid associated with fever • Associated with bacterial infection such as *S. aureus*, *E. coli* or streptococcal infection • More rarely with fungal infection or TB	• Usually euthyroid
Radiation induced	An occasional complication of radioiodine use in treatment of Grave's disease	• Transient exacerbation of hyperthyroidism
Drug induced	Associated with use of • Amiodarone • Interleukin-2 • Interferon-α • Lithium	• Drug dependent—e.g. amiodarone can cause hypothyroidism or hyperthyroidism

Thyroid storm

Background
- Also known as thyrotoxic crisis
- A rare, acute, potentially life-threatening, hypermetabolic state seen in hyperthyroidism

Precipitants
- Acute infection
- Postpartum
- Exposure to contrast media
- Withdrawal of anti-thyroid medications
- Stressful event, e.g. surgery

Clinical features of thyroid storm
- Fever (often >40°C)
- Tachycardia
- Alteration in mental status, i.e. delirium
- Severe signs of hyperthyroidism
- Congestive cardiac failure
- AKI
- GI disturbance (vomiting and/or diarrhoea, jaundice)

Laboratory findings
- Leucocytosis
- AKI
- ↑ alkaline phosphatase (difficult to assess in pregnancy)
- Mild hypercalcaemia
- Thyroid hormones are usually ↑ but may not be grossly elevated

Management of thyroid storm in pregnancy
⚠ Pregnancy does not alter the management of this emergency.

- Appropriate location of the ♀ depends on gestation, need for fetal monitoring, and likelihood of potential intervention—may need intensive care admission
- Standard anti-arrhythmics can be used if tachyarrhythmia present
- β blockers, e.g. propranolol 160–480 mg daily (for symptom control)
- PTU 200–300 mg QDS via nasogastric tube
- K^+ iodide 60 mg QDS via nasogastric tube after starting PTU:
  - Inhibits thyroid hormone release
- High-dose steroids, e.g. prednisolone 40 mg daily or hydrocortisone 50 mg QDS IM (can block T_4 to T_3 conversion)

Thyroid nodules

Background

- Thyroid nodules are common, affecting 5% of ♀ in their reproductive years

⚠ A small proportion of thyroid nodules are malignant
- Differential diagnosis:
  - Solitary toxic nodule
  - Subacute (de Quervain's) thyroiditis
  - Bleed into a cystic lesion

Investigations

- TFTs and thyroid antibodies
- Thyroglobulin level: ⚠ suggests malignancy if >100 mcg/L
- USS:
  - Cystic nodules are more likely to be benign than solid nodules
  - Fine needle aspiration for cytology should be performed if >1 cm
- Biopsy (if solid lesion)

⚠ **Symptoms or signs suggestive of malignancy**
- Past history of radiation to neck or chest
- Fixed lump
- Lymphadenopathy
- Rapid growth of painless nodule
- Voice change
- Neurological involvement such as Horner's syndrome

Management of thyroid nodules in pregnancy
- In TSH-dependent tumours, levothyroxine should be given to ensure TSH is undetectable or suppressed
- Surgical resection can be performed in the 2nd and 3rd trimesters if indicated

▶ Majority of papillary or follicular cancers are slow growing, so it may be possible to defer surgical resection until after delivery

Hypercortisolaemia (Cushing's syndrome)

Excessive cortisol production can occur from a variety of causes.

Causes
- ACTH dependent:
  - ↑ ACTH secretion from the anterior pituitary (Cushing's disease)
  - Ectopic ACTH secretion
- ACTH independent:
  - ↑ cortisol production from adrenals, e.g. adrenal adenoma, carcinoma, or hyperplasia
- Pseudo-Cushing's:
  - Alcoholism
  - Severe depression
- Iatrogenic:
  - Exogenous steroids (including inhaled corticosteroids)

Diagnosis
⚠ Random or 9 am cortisol is of no diagnostic value
- ACTH level
- Serum K⁺
- 24 hr urinary free cortisol
- Midnight cortisol (cortisol <50 nmol/L when sleeping)
- Dexamethasone suppression testing:
  - Overnight (1 mg at midnight then serum cortisol at 9 am)
  - Low dose (0.5 mg every 6 hrs for 48 hrs), should ↝ cortisol <50 mmol/L but will not suppress pituitary ACTH
  - High dose (2 mg every 6 hrs for 48 hrs) will suppress in pituitary ACTH excess but not if ACTH secretion is exogenous
- Visual fields if pituitary adenoma suspected
- Imaging of pituitary and/or adrenals (MRI with contrast)

Pregnancy
- Untreated disease causes oligo- or amenorrhoea and infertility
- If previously completely treated, does not affect pregnancy
- Most are adrenal or pituitary adenomas, rarely adrenal carcinomas
- ↑ urinary free cortisol and non-suppression on a low-dose dexamethasone suppression test may be normal in pregnancy
- Non-suppression on a high-dose test is likely to indicate adrenal hypercortisolaemia
- In untreated disease:
  - ↑ risk pre-eclampsia and GDM
  - Poor wound healing
  - Preterm delivery and fetal loss
- Neonatal adrenal insufficiency (suppression by ↑ maternal cortisol)
- Treatment <20 wks associated with ↑ live birth rate
- Surgical resection can be performed in pregnancy

Signs and symptoms of hypercortisolaemia

Normal for pregnancy
- Weight gain
- Fatigue
- Glucose intolerance
- ↑ BP
- Mood disturbance

Specific to hypercortisolaemia
- Striae (red/purple rather than pale)
- Proximal myopathy
- Osteopenia/osteoporosis
- Hyperandrogenism, e.g. hirsutism, acne
- Bruising

Treatment
See Table 12.12.

Table 12.12 Treatment for hypercortisolaemia in pregnancy

Drugs	
Metyrapone	• Sometimes used • Severe ↑ BP and pre-eclampsia reported
Ketoconazole	• Used in 2nd or 3rd trimester • Associated with fetal growth restriction • No congenital malformations
Mitotane	⚠ Should be avoided
Etomidate	• Used in refractory hypercortisolaemia in non-pregnant individuals ⚠ No data to support use in pregnancy
Surgical resection	
• Trans-sphenoidal resection of pituitary adenoma	
• Laparoscopic adrenalectomy	

Primary hyperaldosteronism

Background

- A common and probably underdiagnosed cause of hypertension
- Classic combination of ↑ BP and ↓ K⁺ only occurs in 40% of cases
- Causes include:
  - Aldosterone-secreting adrenal adenomas (Conn's syndrome)
  - Bilateral adrenal hyperplasia
  - Aldosterone-secreting carcinoma (rare)

Clinical features

- ↑ BP
- ↓ K⁺ (only in 40% of non-pregnant individuals)
- ↓ renin activity in the presence of ↑ aldosterone
- Imaging: MRI of adrenals may identify bilateral hyperplasia or focal lesion
- Adrenal vein sampling can clarify if there is unilateral secretion of aldosterone

Pregnancy

- Rarely reported in pregnancy but probably under-diagnosed
- Progesterone competitively inhibits Na^+/K^+ exchange in the distal renal tubule:
  - May reduce the incidence of ↓ K⁺ during pregnancy
  - May exacerbate 1° hyperaldosteronism postpartum
- Associated with:
  - ↑ hypertensive disorders of pregnancy including gestational hypertension and pre-eclampsia
  - Placental abruption
  - Preterm delivery

Management of 1° hyperaldosteronism in pregnancy

- Antihypertensives, in particular mineralocorticoid receptor antagonists:
  - Spironolactone has potent anti-androgen effects, but use could be considered after confirmation of a ♀ fetus
  - Eplerenone does not have anti-androgen action and has been used in a few pregnancies with no adverse fetal effects reported
- Amiloride can be used as an alternative K⁺-sparing diuretic
- K⁺ supplementation as needed
- Surgical resection of adenoma

Adrenal insufficiency

Background
- Characterized by glucocorticoid and mineralocorticoid deficiency
- Common causes include:
  - Autoimmune adrenal insufficiency (Addison's disease)
  - TB
- Often associated with other autoimmune conditions

Clinical features
- Symptoms (Box 12.5)
- Signs include:
  - Postural ↓ BP
  - Hyperpigmentation of skin folds or scars (from ↑ ACTH which has structural homology with melanocyte-stimulating hormone)*
  - Vitiligo
  - Loss of body hair (loss of adrenal androgens)
- Biochemical abnormalities include:
  - ↑ K^+* and ↓ Na^+
  - Hypoglycaemia
  - Renal impairment
- FBC may show a neutrophil leucocytosis or eosinophilia
- Adrenal antibodies aids diagnosis but absence does not exclude it
* These features do not occur in pituitary insufficiency.

Pregnancy
- Well-controlled disease should not alter the course of pregnancy
- Symptoms ↑ from normal pregnancy, investigations are warranted
- Breastfeeding is not affected

Management of adrenal insufficiency in pregnancy

Diagnosis
- Cortisol ↑ towards term, so levels may be within normal range despite adrenal insufficiency
- Short Synacthen® test may be falsely reassuring due to changes in cortisol-binding globulin and adrenal response to ACTH
- If clinical concern and normal stimulation test, glucocorticoids should be started and confirmatory tests performed postpartum

Treatment
- Glucocorticoid at pre-pregnancy dose, ↑ if unwell or symptomatic
- Stress-dose steroids (higher oral dose or alternative route if unable to take orally) may be required for intercurrent illness (Table 12.13)
- Parenteral steroids are required at delivery
- After delivery, ↓ glucocorticoid gradually back to pre-pregnancy dose as the physiological diuresis can cause significant ↓ BP
- Mineralocorticoid replacement at pre-pregnancy dose, can be safely omitted at delivery (if on high doses of glucocorticoids)

Box 12.5 Signs and symptoms of adrenal insufficiency

Normal for pregnancy
- Nausea
- Vomiting
- Weakness
- ↓ Na$^+$

Specific to adrenal insufficiency
- Weight loss
- Hyperpigmentation
- Excessive ↓ Na$^+$ (greater than expected in pregnancy)
- Hypoglycaemia

Table 12.13 Requirements for stress dose steroid administration

HPA axis suppression status	Steroid exposure	Advice
Confirmed	• Documented adrenal or pituitary insufficiency on formal testing	Give stress-dose steroids
Unknown	• Equivalent of 5–20 mg prednisolone daily for >3 wks in last year	Give stress-dose steroids **Or** ACTH stimulation test and treat if inadequate response (of limited diagnostic use in pregnancy)
Likely	• Equivalent of ≥20 mg prednisolone daily for >3 wks in last year	Give stress-dose steroids
Unlikely	• Equivalent of <5 mg prednisolone daily for any length of time • Alternate-day steroids for any duration • Any dose of steroids for <3 wks	No need for stress-dose steroids

HPA, hypothalamic–pituitary–adrenal.

Stress-dose steroids
- Hydrocortisone 50–100 mg TDS–QDS depending on nature of stressful stimulus (operation/illness)
- IM route preferred

Congenital adrenal hyperplasia

Background

A group of autosomal recessive disorders caused by various enzymatic defects in adrenal steroid biosynthesis, which → accumulation of precursors proximal to the deficient enzyme:

- 21-hydroxylase deficiency (95%)
- 11β-hydroxylase deficiency (5%)
- 17α-hydroxylase deficiency (very rare)
- 3β-hydroxysteroid dehydrogenase deficiency (very rare)

Diagnosis (in the mother)

- Cortisol deficiency
- Aldosterone deficiency
- Excessive levels of precursor hormones

Variable phenotype

- Severe virilization or salt-wasting presenting in the neonatal period
- Virilization of ♀ fetus (ambiguous genitalia at birth)
- Precocious puberty in a boy
- Non-classic CAH presents in adulthood with hirsutism and menstrual irregularity

Pregnancy

- Genetic counselling should be offered to all couples after an affected pregnancy (chance of future affected pregnancy is 1 in 4)
- Continue glucocorticoid and mineralocorticoids during pregnancy and give stress-dose steroids if required
- ♀ fetus is at risk earlier than antenatal diagnostic tests can be performed, so dexamethasone should be started as soon as pregnancy confirmed:
  - Dexamethasone crosses placenta suppressing fetal ACTH so ↓ risk of masculinization and neuroendocrine effects if fetus ♀
  - Majority of fetuses will be unaffected so unnecessary exposure
  - Mother may become cushingoid as a result

Effects on pregnancy

- Subfertility
- ↑ spontaneous miscarriage rate
- ↑ risk of GDM
- ↑ risk of gestational hypertension and pre-eclampsia

Effects on the fetus

⚠ Risk is to a ♀ fetus homozygous for the affected alleles

- Depends on partner carrier status (autosomal recessive transmission) therefore preconception testing may be possible

Effects on labour

- Cephalopelvic disproportion from android pelvis (↑ risk of caesarean section)
- Impact of previous surgery for virilization (physical and psychological)

Antenatal diagnosis options
(If partner testing shows mutation, or is not performed.)

Initial fetal sex determination
- Cell-free fetal DNA
- CVS (>10 wks)
- Amniocentesis (≥16 wks)
- USS assessment of fetal sex

Diagnostic tests for affected fetus
- CVS (>10 wks):
  - Gene probe for specific mutations in the gene encoding the 21-hydroxylase enzyme
- Amniocentesis (≥16 wks):
  - 17-hydroxyprogesterone and androgen levels in amniotic fluid
  - HLA typing of amniotic cells

Catecholamine-secreting tumours

Background

See Table 12.14.
- These can either be:
  - Phaeochromocytomas (adrenomedullary tumours)
  - Paragangliomas (extra-adrenal medullary neural crest derivatives, e.g. organ of Zuckerkandl)
- 15–20% bilateral (more likely in familial syndromes)
- 10% malignant (more likely in paragangliomas)
- Hormones produced include:
  - Adrenaline (small adrenal and organ of Zuckerkandl tumours*)
  - Noradrenaline (larger adrenal tumours and paragangliomas secrete this only as they lack PNMT)
  - Dopamine (very rare)
  - Other products, e.g. PTH, ACTH, neuropeptide Y, VIP

▶ *Phenylethanolamine-N-methyl transferase (PNMT) is required for adrenaline production from noradrenaline and is dependent on cortisol, so adrenaline production occurs in corticomedullary tumours but not others.

Clinical features

Symptoms and signs may be sustained or paroxysmal:
- ↑ BP
- Cardiac:
  - Palpitations, chest pain, postural ↓ BP
- GI:
  - Abdominal pain, constipation, nausea
- Neurological:
  - Headaches, visual disturbance, seizures
- Systemic features:
  - Sweating, flushing, pyrexia

Examination can be normal, but there may be:
- Sinus tachycardia
- Hypertension
- Hypoglycaemia

Precipitants

- Exercise
- Surgery
- Pressure on abdomen
- Drugs:
  - Anaesthetics
  - Analgesics, e.g. morphine, fentanyl
  - Metoclopramide
  - Phenothiazines
  - Tricyclic antidepressants
  - Contrast media

Table 12.14 Syndromes associated with phaeochromocytoma

	Features	Mutation location	Incidence of phaeochromocytoma	Other screening considerations
Familial phaeochromocytoma syndromes (autosomal dominant)	• Strong family history of phaeochromocytoma • Absence of features of other genetic conditions	Mutations in the SDHAF2/SDHB/SDHC/SDHD genes	High	
Neurofibromatosis type 1 (autosomal dominant)	• Café-au-lait spots • Cutaneous neurofibromas • Inguinal/axillary freckling • Optic nerve gliomas • Lisch nodules (iris hamartomas) • Tumours such as neurofibromas/medullary thyroid carcinoma/carcinoid/phaeochromocytomas	NF1 gene on chromosome 17	0.5–1%	• Clinical examination • Serum calcium • Serum calcitonin
Von Hippel-Lindau syndrome	Type 1 (not associated with phaeo/paragangliomas) • Cerebellar haemangioblastoma • Retinal angiomas • Renal cell carcinoma • Renal cysts • Pancreatic cysts and tumours	VHL gene on chromosome 3	25%	• Ophthalmoscopy • MRI posterior fossa • Renal ultrasound

Table 12.14 Continued

	Features	Mutation location	Incidence of phaeochromocytoma	Other screening considerations
	Type 2 (associated with phaeo/paragangliomas) • 2A: does not feature renal carcinoma • 2B: phaeo/paraganglioma and features of type 1 • 2C: phaeo/paraganglioma without other VH-related lesions			
Multiple endocrine neoplasia (MEN) type IIA	• Hyperparathyroidism • Medullary thyroid carcinoma • Phaeochromocytoma	RET proto-oncogene	50%	• Serum calcium • Serum calcitonin
Multiple endocrine neoplasia (MEN) type IIb	• Marfanoid body habitus • Mucosal neuromas • Medullary thyroid carcinoma • Phaeochromocytoma	RET proto-oncogene	50%	• Clinical examination • Serum calcitonin

Investigations

- Urinary free metanephrines (metanephrine and and normetanephrine):
  - Breakdown products of adrenaline and noradrenaline
  - At least two 24 hr collections
  - Affected by medications including α blockers, β blockers (e.g. labetalol needs to be stopped for 4 days before testing), tricyclic antidepressants, metoclopramide, theophylline, methyldopa
- Urinary catecholamines (adrenaline and noradrenaline):
  - Episodic secretion of catecholamines from tumours compared to the continuous release of metanephrines means measurement of the latter is preferable
- Urinary vanillylmandelic acid (VMA):
  - Another catecholamine metabolite
- Plasma metanephrines:
  - Similar sensitivity and specificity compared to urinary metanephrines but not widely available
  - Elevated by caffeine, exercise, nicotine, and some drugs
- Imaging (ideally MRI)

Pregnancy

- Very rare in pregnancy
- Can be mistaken for hypertensive disorders of pregnancy

⚠ Unrecognized phaeochromocytomas have a mortality rate of up to 50% at the time of labour or induction of anaesthesia

- ↑ uterine size can exert pressure on tumours especially extra-adrenal sites:
  - Haemorrhage of tumour tissue
  - Hypertensive crisis
- Catecholamines can cause utero-placental vasoconstriction → placental insufficiency or abruption
- Maternal mortality:
  - 4% of treated cases
  - 17% of untreated ♀
- Fetal mortality:
  - 11% in diagnosed cases
  - 26% in undiagnosed cases

Management of catecholamine-secreting tumours in pregnancy

- MDT input
- Avoid medication that may precipitate a hypertensive crisis

Pharmacological therapy

- α blockade (phenoxybenzamine 10 mg BD ↑ to 20 mg QDS) **before** β blockade starts to avoid precipitating a hypertensive crisis due to unopposed α-adrenergic stimulation
- β blockade after 24–72 hrs (propranolol 40 mg TDS)

Surgery

- Surgery can be performed <23 wks, but >23 wks can usually be delayed until delivery
- Open or laparoscopic adrenalectomy
- Performed after sufficient α and β blockade
- Phenoxybenzamine (IV preferred but oral used if IV unavailable) is given for 3 days before surgery

Delivery

- Caesarean section preferred to minimize catecholamine surges, can perform adrenalectomy at the same time
- Specialist anaesthetic input is strongly recommended

Hyperparathyroidism

Background
- Common causes of 1° hyperparathyroidism:
  - Parathyroid adenoma (85%)
  - Hyperplasia (14%)
  - Carcinoma (<1%)
- Can be associated with other endocrine conditions, e.g. MEN type I and II
- 2° hyperparathyroidism from appropriate ↑ in PTH production in response to ↓Ca^{2+}, e.g. chronic renal impairment
- 3° hyperparathyroidism is autonomous production of PTH resulting from continued stimulation of the parathyroid gland, e.g. in long-standing chronic renal impairment

---

Clinical features
- Majority of patients are asymptomatic
- Patients with symptoms have ↑ Ca^{2+} and/or end-organ damage (osteoporosis, renal calculi, renal impairment, pseudo-gout, pancreatitis)

Investigations
- Serum Ca^{2+}
- Vitamin D level (↑ Ca^{2+} may be masked by vitamin D deficiency)
- Serum phosphate
- PTH (should be ↓ in the presence of hypercalcaemia, therefore normal or ↑ PTH is abnormal indicating autonomous production)
- 24 hr urinary Ca^{2+} (►► familial hypocalciuric hypercalcaemia)

Management of hyperparathyroidism in pregnancy

Diagnosis
- Identification of ↑ Ca^{2+} in pregnancy can be difficult:
  - Total Ca^{2+} can appear normal due to ↓ albumin concentration
- Isotope studies contraindicated in pregnancy
- USS can be used to identify adenomas

Treatment
- Conservative management (good fluid intake, regular monitoring)
- Surgical resection of the adenoma for those with high Ca^{2+} levels, end-organ damage, symptoms, or younger patients
- Medical treatment of 2° or 3° involves optimization of the Ca^{2+}/ vitamin D axis with phosphate binders, etc.
- Parathyroidectomy can be performed in pregnancy
- If surgery is not performed, management involves maintaining hydration and administering oral phosphates

Complications of hyperparathyroidism in pregnancy

Maternal
- ↑ BP ± pre-eclampsia (up to 25%)
- Pancreatitis
- ↑ Ca^{2+} crises

Fetal
- Mortality (up to 40% when maternal ↑ Ca^{2+} is severe, i.e. >3.5 mmol/L)
- Miscarriage
- Fetal growth restriction
- Neonatal tetany
- Neonatal death

Hypercalcaemic crisis

⚠ Rare but potentially life-threatening endocrine emergency characterized by high levels of Ca^{2+} (usually >3.5 mmol/L) and multiorgan dysfunction related to ↑ Ca^{2+}, particularly CNS and GI disturbance.

Treatment
- Hydration with regular assessment of fluid balance:
  - Add in diuretic if fluid overload occurs
- Calcitonin:
  - Does not cross placenta, has been used safely in pregnancy
  - Most useful in 1st 24–36 hrs
- Glucocorticoids:
  - Effective if ↑ Ca^{2+} due to cause other than hyperparathyroidism
- Cinacalcet:
  - Suppresses PTH secretion
  - Very small number of reported cases in pregnancy show no fetal complications
- Bisphosphonates:
  - Concerning animal data
  - Small number of published cases in pregnancy when ↑ Ca^{2+} is unresponsive to other therapies

Hypoparathyroidism

Background
- Uncommon but can → life-threatening ↓ Ca^{2+}
- Most commonly seen after thyroid or parathyroid surgery
- Autoimmune hypoparathyroidism can be associated with other abnormalities, e.g. type 2 polyglandular autoimmune syndrome

Causes
- Parathyroid gland damage:
  - Autoimmune
  - Surgical
  - Radiation
- Failure of PTH secretion (functional hypoparathyroidism):
  - ↓ Mg^{2+}
- Failure of PTH action:
  - Pseudohypoparathyroidism
- Failure of parathyroid development:
  - Di George syndrome

Pregnancy
- Severe ↓ Ca^{2+} has been associated with miscarriage and preterm delivery, probably from ↓ Ca^{2+}-related uterine irritability
- Maternal ↓ Ca^{2+} → fetal parathyroid hyperplasia and associated skeletal changes
- Maternal ↑ Ca^{2+} as a result of overtreatment can → suppression of fetal parathyroid hormone production which may → neonatal ↓ Ca^{2+}

Management of hypoparathyroidism in pregnancy
- Close monitoring of Ca^{2+} (e.g. every 2–4 wks)
- Maintenance of normal Ca^{2+} is important
- Oral Ca^{2+} supplementation
- Oral vitamin D supplementation:
  - Doses likely to need ↑ (monitor Ca^{2+} monthly and titrate)
  - Calcitriol or alfacalcidol preferred
  - ↓ early in the postpartum period
- Treatment of acute hypocalcaemia as in non-pregnant ♀:
  - Ca^{2+} gluconate bolus then infusion (NB short half-life)
  - Oral Ca^{2+}
  - Ensure normal Mg^{2+} concentration
- Inform paediatricians at delivery
- Close monitoring of serum Ca^{2+} following delivery (several cases of ↑ Ca^{2+} while breastfeeding have been reported, even in the absence of supplementation, a likely result of parathyroid hormone-related peptide production by lactating mammary epithelial cells)

Vitamin D deficiency

Background

- Very common in the UK (a recent study identified insufficient vitamin D levels in 50% of the adult population, and 16% had severe deficiency in winter and spring)
- Majority of vitamin D derived from skin exposure to sunlight
- Dietary insufficiency can occur but ↓ generally due to:
  - ↑ high SPF use
  - Indoor lifestyle
  - UK latitude and climate

Pregnancy

- Pregnancy and lactation are periods of ↑ bone turnover and Ca^{2+} loss, which can result in worsening of previously unidentified bone loss
- ↑ risk of maternal:
  - Osteomalacia
  - Myopathy
  - Bone loss
- ↑ risk to offspring of:
  - ↓ fetal skeletal mineralization
  - Neonatal tetany from ↓ Ca^{2+}
  - Neonatal rickets
- Supplementation improves maternal and neonatal vitamin D status

☞ Currently no data to show supplementation improves maternal or fetal outcomes.

Risk factors for Vitamin D deficiency

Sun exposure

- ♀ who remain covered when outdoors
- ♀ of South Asian, African, Caribbean, or Middle Eastern family origin

Dietary or metabolic

- ♀ who eat a diet low in vitamin D, e.g. a vegan diet
- Medications such as antiepileptic drugs
- Malabsorption
- Obesity
- Kidney or liver dysfunction

Management of vitamin D deficiency in pregnancy

- NICE recommends ♀ are advised about the importance of vitamin D during pregnancy and may choose to take vitamin D (10 mcg = 400 units daily)
- RCOG advocates 1000 IU/day for ♀ at high risk of ↓ vitamin D
- If ↓ vitamin D is demonstrated, treat with one of these regimens:
  - 20,000 IU colecalciferol weekly
  - 10,000 IU ergocalciferol twice weekly for 4–6 wks
  - Daily treatment of 2000–4000 IU can also be used
- There is no evidence that therapeutic doses are teratogenic
- Larger than normal doses of vitamin D may be required in:
  - Intestinal malabsorption
  - Chronic liver disease
  - Hypoparathyroidism

Types of vitamin D preparation
See Table 12.15.

Table 12.15 Types of vitamin D preparation

Name	Alternative name	Examples
Ergocalciferol	Vitamin D_2	Non-proprietary: • Tablets (97 mg Ca^{2+}, 10 mcg ergocalciferol) • 250 mcg tablets
Colecalciferol	Vitamin D_3	• Combination preparations of calcium and colecalciferol (e.g. 600 mg Ca^{2+}, 400 units[a] colecalciferol) • Colecalciferol alone (800, 1000, 3,200 or 20,000 unit[a] preparations)
Alfacalcidol	1α hydroxycholecalciferol	• 0.25, 0.5, or 1 mcg capsules • Usual dose 0.25–1 mcg OD
Calcitriol	1,25 dihydroxycholecalciferol	• 0.25 mcg capsules • Usual dose 0.5–1 mcg OD

[a] 10 micrograms = 400 units.

➲ NICE. Antenatal care for uncomplicated pregnancies (CG62): ℜ https://www.nice.org.uk/guidance/cg62

➲ RCOG. Vitamin D in pregnancy: ℜ https://www.rcog.org.uk/globalassets/documents/guidelines/scientific-impact-papers/vitamin_d_sip43_june14 pdf

Lipid abnormalities

Background

- 1° hyperlipidaemias are classified according to the Fredrickson criteria (Table 12.16)
- Defects can occur in any part of the lipid metabolism pathway
- 2° hyperlipidaemia can result from other medical conditions

---

Causes of 2° hyperlipidaemia

- DM
- Drugs including oestrogens, thiazides
- Hypothyroidism
- Renal impairment
- Nephrotic syndrome
- Alcohol intake
- Postprandial hyperlipidaemia can occur but is viewed as a normal response to eating food

---

Management of lipid abnormalities in pregnancy

Diagnosis
- Not practical in pregnancy due to:
  - Physiological ↑ in normal pregnancy
  - Normal ranges are unknown in the pregnant population

Treatment
- Hypercholesterolaemia:
  - Stop statin, niacin, and ezetimibe
  - Low-fat diet
  - Bile acid sequestrants can be considered
- Hypertriglyceridaemia:
  - Low-fat diet
  - Options include omega 3, fibrates

⚠ Statins are generally contraindicated in pregnancy, however pravastatin (more hydrophilic than other statins) has been used in some studies of obstetric antiphospholipid syndrome without complication. It is less potent than other statins and is likely to be of limited therapeutic use in ♀ with significant lipid abnormalities.

▶ If history of coronary artery disease or pancreatitis treat as described, but consider lipophoresis for hypertriglyceridaemia.

Table 12.16 Fredrickson classification for primary hyperlipidaemias

Type			Defect		Clinical features	Treatment options in non-pregnant ♀	Appearance of blood
Type I	A	Familial hyperchylomicronaemia	↓ lipoprotein lipase	↑ chylomicrons	• Skin xanthomas • Hepatosplenomegaly • Lipaemia retinalis • Acute pancreatitis	• Diet	Creamy top layer
	B	Familial apoprotein CII deficiency	Altered Apo C2				
	C		LPL inhibitor in blood				
Type II	A	Familial hypercholesterolaemia	LDL receptor deficiency	↑ LDL	• Xanthelasma • Arcus senilis • Tendon xanthomas	• Statins • Niacin • Bile acid sequestrants	Clear
	B	Familial combined hyperlipidaemia	↓ LDL receptor and ↑ Apo B	↑ LDL ↑ VLDL		• Statins • Niacin • Fibrate	Turbid
Type III		Familial dysbetalipoproteinaemia	Defect in Apo E2 synthesis	↑↑↑ IDL	• Tuboeruptive • Palmar xanthomas	• Fibrates • Statins	Turbid
Type IV		Familial hypertriglyceridaemia	↑ VLDL production and ↓ VLDL elimination	↑ VLDL	• Can cause pancreatitis	• Fibrate • Niacin • Statins	Turbid
Type V			↑ VLDL production and ↓ LPL	↑ VLDL ↑ chylomicrons		• Niacin • Fibrate	Creamy top layer and turbid bottom

Beaumont et al. *Bull World Health Organ* 1970;43(6):891–915. https://www.ncbi.nlm.nih.gov/pubmed/4930042

Metabolic acidosis

Background
- A metabolic acidosis is the most common acid–base disturbance encountered in pregnant ♀
- Identification of a metabolic acidosis often prompts a rapid diagnosis of 'sepsis' but it is important to approach methodically to ensure that other causes are not missed

Approach
See Fig. 12.1 and Table 12.17.
   To calculate the anion gap:

$$\text{Anion gap} = \left(Na^+ + K^+\right) - \left(Cl^- + HCO_3^-\right)$$

Normal value is <16 mmol/L.

Table 12.17 Metabolic acidosis

Mechanism of acidosis	↑ Anion gap	Normal anion gap
↑ Acid production	<ul><li>Lactic acidosis</li><li>Ketoacidosis:<ul><li>DM</li><li>Starvation</li><li>Alcohol associated</li></ul></li></ul>	
Exogenous acid ingestion	<ul><li>Methanol</li><li>Ethylene glycol</li><li>Aspirin</li></ul>	
↓ Bicarbonate or precursors		<ul><li>Diarrhoea or other intestinal losses (e.g. stoma drainage)</li><li>Type 2 RTA</li><li>Following treatment for ketoacidosis</li><li>Carbonic anhydrase inhibitors</li></ul>
↓ Renal acid excretion	<ul><li>Chronic kidney disease</li></ul>	<ul><li>Some cases of chronic kidney disease</li><li>Type 1 RTA</li><li>Type 4 RTA</li></ul>

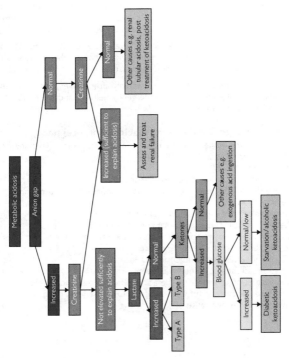

Fig. 12.1 Approach to metabolic acidosis: an assessment tool.

Starvation ketoacidosis

- ♀ in pregnancy are more prone to ketosis (↑ in 3rd trimester)
- Often follows a short period of vomiting or fasting
- Blood glucose is often in the normal range
- The acidosis can be severe
- Glucose administration is the mainstay of treatment, to ↑ endogenous production of insulin and suppress ketosis

⚠ Concern about glucose administration and potential precipitation of Wernicke's in these ♀ is probably misplaced, as they have a very short duration of vomiting compared to ♀ with hyperemesis gravidarum. However, IV Pabrinex® or oral thiamine can be given if in doubt.

⚠ Pregnant ♀ can develop a significant metabolic acidosis, in contrast to starvation ketoacidosis in non-pregnant individuals where the pH does not usually fall below 7.3 even after prolonged fasting.

⚠ The metabolic abnormalities resolve rapidly after delivery but can often be treated medically, thus avoiding emergency delivery and the morbidity associated with preterm delivery.

Management of starvation ketoacidosis in pregnancy

- Ketone testing (urine and/or capillary) in late pregnancy if vomiting
- Arterial blood gas analysis in ♀ with:
  - Ketonuria (≥2+)
  - Ketonaemia (≥1 mmol/L) and/or are unwell
- Treated with 10% dextrose as an infusion alongside fluids used for resuscitation
- Insulin, alongside dextrose if required, if the glucose levels ↑ or ketones remain ↑, but this is not always required
- Regular repeated assessment of capillary ketone measurement ± arterial blood gas to assess response
- Consider admission to HDU or ITU
- Regular assessment of fetal well-being
- Consideration of delivery if the acidosis fails to respond to these measures or evidence of fetal compromise
- Investigation of the cause of the vomiting

Metabolic alkalosis

- A pure metabolic alkalosis is rare in pregnancy
- The commonest cause is GI loss of H^+ from severe vomiting
- Fetal morbidity has been described including:
  - Fetal metabolic alkalosis
  - Respiratory distress
  - Irritability

Causes

See Box 12.6.

Box 12.6 Causes of metabolic alkalosis

Exogenous administration
- Alkali administration (e.g. milk–alkali syndrome)
- IV penicillin
- Current use of diuretics

Low urinary chloride (<20 mEq/L)
- Loss of gastric secretions, e.g. vomiting, villous adenoma
- Congenital chloridorrhoea
- Following an episode of hypercapnia
- Previous diuretic treatment

↑ *urinary chloride without ↑ BP*
- Hypokalaemia
- Hypomagnesaemia
- Bartter's syndrome
- Gitelman's syndrome

↑ *urinary chloride with ↑ BP*

↓ plasma renin activity ↓ aldosterone level	• Cushing syndrome (or steroid use) • Congenital adrenal hyperplasia • 11β-hydroxysteroid dehydrogenase deficiency • Liquorice consumption • Congenital adrenal hyperplasia • Liddle's syndrome
↑ plasma renin activity ↑ aldosterone level	• Renal artery stenosis • Diuretic use • Renin-secreting tumours
↓ plasma renin activity ↑ aldosterone level	• Primary hyperaldosteronism (adrenal adenoma, bilateral adrenal hyperplasia or rarely adrenal carcinoma)

Obesity

- The incidence of obesity is ↑ every year
- Obesity is associated with ↑ risk of maternal death
- The WHO definitions are:
  - Normal: BMI = 18.5–24.9 kg/m^2
  - Overweight: BMI = 25–29.9 kg/m^2
  - Obese: BMI = ≥30 kg/m^2

Maternal risks

- ↑ BP and pre-eclampsia associated with an ↑ booking BMI as well as excessive weight ↑ in pregnancy
- Obese ♀ are:
  - >3× more likely to develop GDM
  - 2× more likely to have thromboembolic disease
  - ↑ risk of instrumental delivery or caesarean section
  - ↑ risk of 3rd-degree perineal tears
  - ↑ risk of PPH
  - Prone to ↑ rates of postnatal complications, e.g. wound infection, lower respiratory tract infection, PPH

Fetal risks

- Miscarriage
- Stillbirth
- Macrosomia (independent of GDM)
- ↑ risk of obesity later in life
- Congenital abnormalities

Management of obesity in pregnancy

Prior to pregnancy
- Counselling regarding weight loss and lifestyle changes
- 5 mg folic acid prior to conception
- Advise on weight optimization
- Inform of risks of obesity in pregnancy
- Explain that weight loss between pregnancies ↓ the risk of stillbirth, hypertensive complications, and fetal macrosomia

During pregnancy
- 5 mg folic acid OD until 12 wks
- Vitamin D supplementation
- Referral to:
  - Consultant obstetrician
  - Anaesthetist
  - Dietician
- N.B. The threshold for referral varies between centres
- Encourage to monitor diet with a view to maintaining the same weight throughout pregnancy rather than gaining weight:
  - As the majority of readily available weight management advice is not suitable in pregnancy, advise ♀ to follow a GDM diet if they are unsure what they can eat, for the majority of obese ♀ this will → weight loss
- Weight loss drugs should not be used in pregnancy
- VTE risk assessment
- ↑ vigilance for pre-eclampsia (using the appropriate size BP cuff)
- ↑ vigilance for GDM:
  - Oral GTT at 24–28 wks
- ↑ vigilance for both macrosomia and IUGR:
  - May need serial USS to monitor growth as symphysis–fundal height measurement may not be accurate
  - May require USS at 36 wks for presentation (to prevent an undiagnosed breech) if unable to palpate fetus accurately
- Review regarding moving and handling considerations for labour and delivery
- Active management of 3rd stage particularly important in obese ♀ as ↑ risk of PPH

Postpartum
- ↑ risk of infection following caesarean section
- Specialist breastfeeding advice often useful as obesity is associated with low breastfeeding rates

↪ RCOG (2018). Care of women with obesity in pregnancy (green-top guideline no. 72):
ℰ https://www.rcog.org.uk/en/guidelines-research-services/guidelines/gtg72/

Infectious diseases

Group A *Streptococcus*

Background
- *Streptococcus pyogenes*—an aerobic Gram-positive coccus
- Most common bacterial cause of acute pharyngitis ('strep throat')
- Up to 30% of population are asymptomatic carriers (skin or throat)
- Easily spread—person to person or droplet

⚠ Can cause severe illness in pregnancy that can be insidious in onset, can cause a rapid deterioration, and can be fatal, ∴ a high index of suspicion is required

Diseases caused by GAS
- Pharyngitis
- Impetigo
- Cellulitis and other infections of soft tissue and muscle
- Scarlet fever
- Rheumatic fever
- Toxic shock syndrome
- Postpartum endometritis

Clinical features
- Often a personal or family history of sore throat or respiratory illness
- Symptoms can be non-specific but include vomiting, diarrhoea, and fever
- Complications including septic shock, DIC, and multiorgan failure can occur

---

Advice about prevention of GAS in pregnancy
- There may be transfer from the throat or nose to the perineum via the hands when using the toilet or changing sanitary towels
- Antenatal education should raise awareness of this and the importance of good personal hygiene including washing hands **before**, as well as after, using the toilet or changing sanitary towels

---

Fetal risks
⚠ If maternal peripartum infection with invasive GAS, inform neonatologist and start prophylactic antibiotics for the neonate.

Management of GAS in pregnancy

- A high clinical suspicion is required and empirical antibiotics started early if GAS infection is suspected
- Early involvement of intensive care services
- A decision about delivery timing and mode has to be individualized, and depends on:
  - Gestation
  - Assessment of fetal well-being
  - Degree of maternal resuscitation required

⬧ MBRRACE-UK 2017 report: ℛ https://www.npeu.ox.ac.uk/mbrrace-uk/reports/confidential-enquiry-into-maternal-deaths

⬧ RCOG. Green-top guidelines nos. 64a and 64b: ℛ https://www.rcog.org.uk/en/guidelines-research-services/guidelines/

Group B *Streptococcus*

Background
- Common bowel commensal
- Vaginal carriage occurs in up to 20% ♀
- Most frequent cause of early-onset, severe neonatal infection (incidence 1:2000 live births)
- Up to 70% of babies from affected mothers will be colonized at delivery but only 1% of these develop symptoms of sepsis

Clinical features
No signs or symptoms.

Diagnosis
- Carriage is confirmed by culture from a LVS or perianal swab
- Active infection is confirmed by culture of the organism on culture of blood, urine, or CSF

Fetal risks
Associated with preterm pre-labour rupture of membranes and preterm delivery.

Neonatal risks

⚠ Early-onset GBS infection (<4 days from delivery) has ~20% mortality rate and may present with:
- Pneumonia
- Septicaemia
- Meningitis

⚠ Late-onset infection (>7 days) is not associated with maternal GBS carriage:
- Carries a mortality rate of ~20%
- Of those surviving, 50% will have serious neurological sequelae, such as cortical blindness and deafness

---

Management of GBS in pregnancy

⚠ Routine antenatal screening: not currently recommended by RCOG.

Intrapartum prophylaxis advised if:
- History of previous neonatal GBS infection
- Incidental finding of GBS in urine or on vaginal swab

Intrapartum prophylaxis (in absence of positive swabs) should be considered if:
- Prematurity (<37 wks)
- Prolonged rupture of membranes (>18 hrs)
- Pyrexia in labour

Intrapartum antibiotics
- IV benzylpenicillin as soon as possible after onset of labour and at least 2 hrs before delivery
- IV clindamycin if penicillin allergic

➲ RCOG (2017). Early-onset GBS disease (green-top guideline no. 36): ℰ https://www.rcog.org.uk/en/guidelines-research-services/guidelines/gtg36/

Syphilis

Background
- Caused by *Treponema pallidum*, a spirochaete bacterium
- STI
- Currently relatively rare in the UK, but ↑
- At-risk groups include ♀ who have another sexually transmitted disease, sex workers, or those living in an area with high prevalence

Clinical features
- Infected individuals can be asymptomatic (particularly ♀ with 1° infection as they may not notice a cervical or vaginal chancre)

1° infection
- Painless ulcer ('chancre') at site of initial infection which resolves spontaneously after 3–6 wks
- Often associated with regional lymphadenopathy

2° infection
- Systemic infection, occurring weeks to months after the 1° infection
- Features include lymphadenopathy, systemic symptoms (fever, malaise, myalgia), rash, liver abnormalities, and transient proteinuria
- Spontaneous resolution is common

Late infection (tertiary syphilis)
- Can occur up to 30 yrs after initial infection, and in the absence of a clinically apparent 1° or 2° infection
- Cardiovascular (aortitis), neurological (tabes dorsalis), and granulomatous lesions ('gumma') can occur

Diagnosis
- All pregnant ♀: routine screening at the 1st antenatal visit
- High-risk ♀: repeat later in pregnancy (e.g. 28 and 32 wks)

Fetal risks
- The spirochaete can cross the placenta and is associated with preterm delivery and stillbirth
- Congenital syphilis defects, including:
  - 8th nerve deafness
  - Hutchinson's teeth
  - Saddle nose
  - Sabre shins

> ## Management of syphilis in pregnancy
> - Treatment with penicillin:
>   - <16 wks—prevents virtually all congenital infection
>   - >16 wks—still effective in most cases
> - Contact tracing with testing ± treatment should be offered
> - Assess for other STIs ± refer to genitourinary medicine clinic

Testing for syphilis

Non-treponemal specific tests
- Venereal disease research laboratory test
- Rapid plasma reagin

Treponemal-specific tests
- *Treponema pallidum* haemagglutination assay
- Fluorescent treponemal antibody absorption
- *T. pallidum* enzyme immunoassay

⚠ False-positive results are common and can occur in SLE, TB, leprosy, malaria, or IV drug users.

▶ A reactive result requires further confirmatory testing, ideally a treponemal-specific test looking at a different antigen.

Listeria monocytogenes

Background
- Rare, affecting about 1:10,000 pregnancies in the UK
- Found in soft cheese, pâté, undercooked meat, and shellfish
- Gram-positive, rod-shaped bacterium
- ↑ incidence of infection in pregnant ♀

Clinical features
- Non-specific so a high clinical suspicion is required
- Produces gastroenteritis often accompanied by flu-like symptoms
- Can cause meningitis

Diagnosis
- Confirmed by culture of the organism from bodily fluid samples
- Stool culture not routinely required for suspected systemic infection, and should only be sent if gastroenteritis is present (special culture medium required so essential to mention possible diagnosis)
- Listeria meningitis can be confirmed by CSF culture
- MRI advised where listeria meningitis is suspected

Fetal risks
- Crosses the placenta causing chorioamnionitis, and miscarriage or preterm labour

Neonatal risks
- Neonatal infection may be:
  - Generalized septicaemia
  - Pneumonia
  - Meningitis

Management of listeria in pregnancy
- High index of suspicion
- Treatment is with high-dose amoxicillin
- In penicillin allergic ♀, alternatives such as co-trimoxazole can be used
- Fetal monitoring depending on gestation

Influenza

Background

- In pregnancy is associated with ↑ mortality compared to non-pregnant ♀
- Varies with the strain of virus and uptake of vaccination
- ♀ with underlying medical conditions including asthma are at ↑ risk of severe infection

Clinical features

- Appear 2–3 days after exposure:
  - Sore throat
  - Fatigue
  - Loss of appetite
  - Cough
  - Headache
  - Weakness
  - Muscle ache
  - Insomnia
  - Shortness of breath

Influenza vaccination

- Advised for all:
  - Pregnant ♀ at any gestation to provide both maternal protection and passive immunity to neonate
  - Healthcare professionals involved in care of pregnant ♀
- Inactivated vaccines are preferred

Management of suspected influenza in pregnancy

Assess severity
- Examination including:
  - Hypoxia
  - Tachypnoea
  - Abnormalities on chest auscultation
- CXR:
  - Bilateral infiltrates
  - Evidence of consolidation suggestive of 2° bacterial infection

Mild infection
- Diagnosis is clinical
- Supportive with hydration
- Paracetamol to relieve symptoms
- Rest, stay off work

Potentially severe infection
⚠ Consider hospital admission if ♀ is breathless, has an abnormal CXR, signs of severe infection, or has an underlying medical condition predisposing her to severe infection
- Swabs of throat, nose, or nasopharynx for viral PCR; point-of-care rapid antigen tests are available in some hospitals
- Blood cultures
- Empirical antibiotics
- Antivirals (oseltamivir or zanamivir) are ideally started within 48 hrs of symptom onset but can be considered if symptoms started between 3–5 days prior to presentation

Herpes simplex virus

Background

- HSV1 is a DNA virus that most commonly causes mucosal lesions such as cold sores, but is ↑ being associated with genital herpes
- HSV2 is a DNA virus that most commonly causes genital infection
- Spread by person-to-person contact
- After the initial infection the virus remains latent and can be reactivated, often in response to a stress or immunocompromise
- Incubation ~2–7 days
- Individual may be infectious even when apparently asymptomatic

Clinical features

1° infection

- Most are asymptomatic
- Typical vesicular lesions can be very painful and last for 10–14 days
- Distribution of lesions is usually isolated to 1 area of the body
- Systemic symptoms can occur at the time of initial infection and include fever and lethargy/malaise
- 1° genital infection can cause vulvitis that can be severe enough to cause urinary retention

Recurrent infection

- Systemic symptoms are less common
- Local lymphadenopathy can occur
- Appearance of typical lesions is usually heralded by prodromal symptoms such as tingling or pain
- Episodes are of shorter duration than 1° infection

Other manifestations (more commonly seen with HSV1 than HSV2)

- Vesicles may be absent
- Encephalitis
- Fulminant hepatitis
- Sacral radiculopathy
- Transverse myelitis
- 1° ocular infection

⚠ Immunocompromised individuals are more at risk of disseminated infection and ↑ frequency of reactivation.

Diagnosis

- Usually made on the history appearance of the typical rash
- Vesicle swabs can be diagnostic
- Viral PCR assays can also be used
- Acute and convalescent antibody levels can be performed but may be difficult to interpret

Management of 1° genital herpes in pregnancy

- Refer to genitourinary medicine clinic to confirm diagnosis with PCR
- 5 days of aciclovir (400 mg TDS) may ↓ severity and duration of the 1° attack (IV if immunocompromised or severe infection)
- Paracetamol and 2% lidocaine gel for symptomatic relief
- Assess for other STIs

1st- or 2nd-trimester infection

- Refer for obstetric care
- If undelivered for 6 wks, manage expectantly and anticipate vaginal delivery if genital lesions are no longer present
- Offer further aciclovir from 36 wks (↓ herpetic lesions at term and hence the need for delivery by caesarean section)
- No evidence for management of ♀ with rupture of membranes at term, but expediting delivery to minimize the duration of potential exposure to HSV is often advised

3rd-trimester infection

- Aciclovir 400 mg TDS PO should be continued until delivery
- Caesarean should be recommended for all ♀ developing 1° genital herpes in the 3rd trimester, particularly those developing symptoms within 6 wks of expected delivery, as the risk of neonatal transmission is very high at 41%
- Aciclovir should be given intrapartum (IV 5 mg/kg TDS) and to the neonate (IV 20 mg/kg TDS) for ♀ opting for vaginal delivery

⚠ 15% of ♀ presenting with 1° infection will actually have recurrent herpes so type-specific HSV antibody testing is advisable.

▶ Presence of antibodies of the same type as the HSV isolated from genital swabs would confirm the episode to be a recurrence.

Management of recurrent genital herpes in pregnancy

- Risk of neonatal HSV is low, even if lesions present at the time of delivery (0–3% for vaginal delivery)
- Vaginal delivery should be anticipated in the absence of other obstetric indications for caesarean section
- Consider daily suppressive aciclovir (400 mg TDS) from 36 wks (32 wks if HIV positive)
- FBS or FSE may ↑ the risk of neonatal HSV infection; however, given the small background risk (0–3%) of transmission, the ↑ risk associated with invasive procedures is unlikely to be clinically significant so they may be used if required
- In the case of preterm pre-labour rupture of membranes <34 wks, expectant management is appropriate, including oral aciclovir 400 mg TDS

⮕ BASH and RCOG. Management of genital herpes in pregnancy guidelines: ✍ https://www.rcog.org.uk/globalassets/documents/guidelines/management-genital-herpes.pdf

Herpes simplex virus: complications

Maternal

- Often presents with encephalitis, hepatitis, disseminated skin lesions, or a combination of these
- More common in pregnant and/or immunocompromised ♀
- Maternal mortality is high
- Co-infection with HIV results in an ↑ replication of both viruses

---

HSV encephalitis (more commonly associated with HSV1)

- Associated with significant morbidity and mortality if untreated
- Tends to occur in later pregnancy
- Symptoms include:
  - Confusion and/or ↓ conscious level
  - Fever
  - Seizures
  - Severe headache or altered behaviour
- Empirical treatment is required (high-dose IV aciclovir) and empirical antibiotics will usually be given alongside this
- Urgent lumbar puncture should be performed with CSF sent for viral PCR

Fetus

- Infection has not been shown to cause congenital defects but has been associated with miscarriage and preterm delivery

Neonate

- 1° genital herpes infection in the 3rd trimester is associated with transmission to the neonate in around 41% of ♀
- ♀ with recurrent genital herpes should be informed that the risk of neonatal herpes is low, even if lesions are present at the time of delivery (0–3% for vaginal delivery)

Neonatal herpes infection

- Occurs in 1st 2 wks of life
- 25% limited to eyes and mouth only
- 75% widely disseminated, of which:
  - ~70% will not survive
  - Many of the survivors will have long-term problems including neurodevelopmental difficulties

Varicella zoster

Background

- DNA virus
- 1° infection known as varicella or 'chicken pox'
- Spread by respiratory droplets and contact with vesicle fluid
- Incubation 10–21 days
- Infectious from 2 days before rash until all vesicles are crusted
- Seroprevalence: ~90% of UK ♀ immune
- Incidence of 1° infection in pregnancy ~3:1000 ♀
- Reactivation after initial infection known as zoster or 'shingles'

Clinical features

- Fever
- Malaise
- Maculopapular rash which becomes vesicular then crusts over

Diagnosis

- This is a clinical diagnosis based on a history of contact with chicken pox/shingles and the development of a typical rash

---

Maternal risks

⚠ Varicella in pregnancy is often more severe and may be life-threatening as a consequence of:
- Varicella pneumonia
- Hepatitis
- Encephalitis

Fetal risks

- Fetal infection rate is thought to be ~25% in all trimesters
- If <20 wks there is a 2% risk of fetal varicella syndrome with congenital defects (Table 13.1) including:
  - Skin scarring
  - Limb hypoplasia
  - Eye lesions (congenital cataracts, microphthalmia, and chorioretinitis)
  - Neurological abnormalities (intellectual disability, microcephaly, cortical atrophy, and dysfunction of bladder and bowel sphincters)

Neonatal risks

▶ Neonatal varicella is seen in babies whose mothers contracted the infection in the last 4 wks of pregnancy.

⚠ If mother develops varicella 7 days before to 7 days after delivery, it is recommended the neonate receives VZIG.

⚠ If maternal rash appears 4 days before delivery or up to 2 days afterwards, the neonate requires consideration of IV aciclovir as well as VZIG as soon as possible (this is when severe infection is most likely in the neonate, which can be fatal).

Table 13.1 Fetal risks from 1° maternal varicella infection

Gestation	Risk to fetus	Management
<20 wks	2% develop fetal varicella syndrome (FVS)	• Detailed USS at 16–20 wks, may consider termination of pregnancy if evidence of FVS seen • Neonatal ophthalmic examination
>20 and <28 wks	Very small risk of FVS	• Detailed USS 5 wks after infection • Neonatal ophthalmic examination
>28 wks	Not associated with congenital abnormality	• Fetal and neonatal surveillance
Within 4 wks of delivery	About 20% will develop neonatal varicella infection	• VZIG as soon as possible • 14 days' monitoring for signs of infection, with aciclovir if varicella develops

⊃ RCOG (2015). Chickenpox in pregnancy (green-top guideline no. 13): ℛ https://www.rcog.org.uk/en/guidelines-research-services/guidelines/gtg13/

Management of varicella in pregnancy

1° infection, with no evidence of complications
• Oral aciclovir (800 mg 5 times per day for 7 days) starting within 24 hrs of rash onset is likely to be beneficial

Severe 1° infection or evidence of complications such as pneumonitis
• Admit to hospital
• Consider IV antiviral therapy (3 x 10mg/kg/day for 5–10 days)

All cases
• Arrange follow-up for fetal monitoring (Table 13.1)

⚠ Contact with non-immune pregnant ♀ should be avoided

Varicella contact and shingles

⚠ Significant contact with varicella is defined as being in the same room for 15 mins or more, face-to-face contact or contact in the setting of a large open ward.

Exposure to varicella *and* no history of previous infection

- Send VZV serology

If IgG detected within 10 days of exposure

- Assume immunity

If IgG not detected within 10 days of exposure

- Mother requires VZIG as soon as possible
- Oral aciclovir should be prescribed if >20 wks and the rash appeared within preceding 24 hrs
- Oral aciclovir should be considered if <20 wks and the rash appeared within preceding 24 hrs

Shingles in pregnancy

- Reactivation of varicella zoster is known as shingles
- Painful vesicular rash in a dermatomal distribution
- Low risk of transmission as affected areas are often not exposed; however, viral shedding may be greater if areas exposed (e.g. ophthalmic) or if the ♀ is immunocompromised
- Treatment with oral aciclovir (800 mg 5 times per day for 7–10 days) should be prescribed

⚠ Contact with non-immune pregnant ♀ should be avoided

VZV vaccination

- Live attenuated vaccine, so should not be used during pregnancy
- Administration after delivery should be recommended to ♀ who are identified to be non-immune

Rubella

Background
- RNA togavirus
- Respiratory droplet spread—person to person (highly infectious)
- Incubation 14–21 days
- Infectious for 7 days before and after appearance of rash
- Reinfection can occur mostly with vaccine-induced immunity

Clinical features
Symptoms are only present in 50–75% of infected individuals:
- Mild febrile illness
- Maculopapular rash
- Arthralgia
- Lymphadenopathy

Diagnosis
- Paired serology (acute phase and then repeated 10–14 days later) consistent with infection if:
  - Appearance of IgM antibodies
  - ≥4× ↑ in IgG antibody titres or ↑ IgG avidity

Congenital defects associated with rubella
- Major malformations are most likely during organogenesis, with severity ↓ with advancing gestation (Table 13.2)
- Defects include:
  - Sensorineural deafness
  - Cardiac abnormalities, e.g. VSD and PDA
  - Eye lesions (cataracts, microphthalmia, and glaucoma)
  - Microcephaly and intellectual disability
- Late-developing sequelae include:
  - DM
  - Thyroid disorders
  - Progressive panencephalitis

Prevention
- 'Herd immunity' is maintained by widespread childhood vaccination
- Uptake has ↓ following concern over safety of the MMR vaccine
- Ideally ♀ should be tested before pregnancy, but routine assessment at booking identifies those at risk and in need of postnatal vaccination (universal antenatal screening is no longer offered in the UK)

⚠ Vaccine is a live-attenuated virus and contraindicated in pregnancy
- ♀ are counselled to avoid pregnancy for 10–12 wks after vaccination

➲ Public Health England (2019). Guidance on the investigation, diagnosis and management of viral illness, or exposure to viral rash illness in pregnancy. ℘ https://www.gov.uk/government/publications/viral-rash-in-pregnancy

Table 13.2 Risk of congenital defects in 1° rubella infection

Gestation	Risk of transmission (%)	Risk of congenital abnormality	Treatment
<13	80	Almost all infected fetuses	Termination of pregnancy may be offered without invasive prenatal diagnosis
13–16	50	About 35% of those infected (mainly deafness)	Fetal blood sampling may be later offered to confirm infection
>16	25	Rarely causes defects	Reassurance

Management of pregnant ♀ with rubella

- Supportive treatment; hospital admission is rarely required
- Fetal medicine assessment should be arranged urgently (Table 13.2)
- Inform PHE as rubella is a notifiable disease in the UK

Pregnant ♀ in contact with rubella

▶ Rapidly confirm rubella in the contact.

No action required if the ♀ has had:

- 2 documented doses of rubella vaccine
- At least 1 previous rubella screening test that has detected rubella IgG.

⚠ However, she must be advised to return if she develops a rash.

If these criteria are not met, test for IgM and IgG.

Rubella IgG is detected and IgM is NOT detected

- Reassure
- Advise to return if she develops a rash

Rubella IgM is detected (irrespective of IgG result)

- Not always consistent with acute infection
- Inform PHE as rubella is a notifiable disease in the UK
- Obtain further samples for IgG, rubella RNA and IgM plus avidity
- Reference testing is recommended

Neither rubella IgG nor IgM is detected

- Send further sample 1 mth after contact or if illness develops and interpret results as previously described
- Advise MMR vaccine after delivery

Measles

Background
- RNA paramyxovirus
- Respiratory droplet spread —person to person (highly infectious)
- Incubation 9–12 days
- Infectious for 2–5 days before and after appearance of rash
- Rare in the UK following the introduction of the MMR vaccine; however, is now ↑ following a ↓ in MMR uptake

Clinical features
- Significant fever
- Generalized maculopapular erythematous rash (appears 2–4 days after onset of symptoms)
- Pathognomonic Koplik's spots inside the mouth
- Symptoms such as cough, coryza, and conjunctivitis can also occur

Diagnosis
- Viral RNA detection in saliva is one way of confirming diagnosis
- Additionally, paired serology (acute phase and then repeated 10–14 days later) consistent with infection if:
  - IgM in serum taken >4 days but <1 mth after the onset of rash

Maternal risks
- Pneumonia
- Acute encephalitis
- Corneal ulceration → scarring
- A rare complication called subacute sclerosing panencephalitis can develop later in life

⚠ Measles in pregnancy can cause maternal death

The effect of maternal measles infection on the fetus
This is associated with:
- Fetal loss
- Preterm delivery

But is **not** associated with congenital malformations.

If rash appears between 6 days pre and 6 days post delivery:
- Administration of human normal immunoglobulin (HNIG) to the neonate is recommended immediately after birth or exposure (as neonatal measles has been associated with subacute sclerosing panencephalitis)

Management of a pregnant ♀ with measles

- Treatment is generally supportive, with hospital admission rarely being required (however respiratory complications require urgent review)
- Fetal medicine assessment should be arranged urgently
- Inform PHE as this is a notifiable disease in the UK

Pregnant ♀ in contact with measles

▶ Try to rapidly confirm measles in the person the pregnant ♀ was in contact with.

Factors ↑ likelihood of the contact having measles include:
- Contact took place when the ♀ was abroad
- Person with suspected measles had travelled abroad
- Person had not been vaccinated against measles
- Person has recently been hospitalized

Reassure measles risk is remote if the ♀ has had:
- 2 documented doses of measles vaccine or
- Previous test demonstrating immunity

⚠ She must be advised to return if she develops a rash.

If these criteria are not met, then send serum for IgG:

Measles IgG detected
- Reassure and no further tests required

Measles IgG not detected
- Discuss prophylaxis with HNIG with PHE
- Advise immunization with MMR vaccine after delivery

➲ Public Health England (2019). Guidance on the investigation, diagnosis and management of viral illness, or exposure to viral rash illness in pregnancy. ℬ https://www.gov.uk/government/publications/viral-rash-in-pregnancy

➲ Public Health England (2019). Guidance on Post-Exposure Prophylaxis for measles. ℬ https://www.gov.uk/government/publications/measles-post-exposure-prophylaxis

Parvovirus B19

Background
- DNA virus
- Respiratory droplet spread—person to person
- Incubation 4–20 days
- Seroprevalence: ~50% of UK ♀ immune
- Incidence of 1° infection in pregnancy <1:100 ♀

Clinical features
- Often asymptomatic
- Typical 'slapped cheek' rash (erythema infectiosum)
- Maculopapular rash
- Fever
- Arthralgia

Diagnosis
- Paired serology (acute phase and then repeated 10–14 days later) consistent with recent infection if:
  - Appearance of IgM antibodies
  - ↑ IgG antibodies

Maternal risks
- Fit and healthy ♀: minimal
- Immunocompromised ♀: risk of sudden haemolysis potentially severe enough to require blood transfusion

The effect of maternal parvovirus B19 infection on the fetus
- Fetal infection rate is thought to be ~30%
- The virus causes suppression of erythropoiesis sometimes with thrombocytopenia and direct cardiac toxicity, eventually resulting in cardiac failure and hydrops fetalis
- No congenital defects associated with parvovirus infection

⚠ About 10% of fetuses infected at <20 wks will not survive

Management of parvovirus B19 in pregnancy
- Care in specialist fetal medicine unit to monitor for development of fetal anaemia (by serial measurement of the peak systolic velocity of the fetal middle cerebral artery on USS) as this may develop many weeks after the initial infection
- Consideration of in utero RBC transfusion in severely anaemic, hydropic fetuses to prevent fetal demise
- Consideration of platelet transfusion if significantly thrombocytopenic to ↓ the risk of fetal bleeding at the time of the in utero transfusion

Pregnant ♀ in contact with parvovirus B19

- Send serum for parvovirus B19 IgM and IgG:

Parvovirus B19 IgG is detected and IgM is not detected
- Reassure
- Advise to return if mother develops a rash

Parvovirus B19 IgM is detected (irrespective of IgG result)
- Consistent with acute infection
- Send the sample for confirmatory testing (viral DNA or IgG)
- Obtain further serum (reference testing is recommended)
- Refer for management at fetal medicine unit

Neither parvovirus B19 IgG nor IgM is detected
- Send further sample 1 mth after contact or if illness develops and act on results as previously described
- Refer for specialist advice

➲ Public Health England (2019). Guidance on the investigation, diagnosis and management of viral illness, or exposure to viral rash illness in pregnancy. ℘ https://www.gov.uk/government/publications/viral-rash-in-pregnancy

Cytomegalovirus

Background
- Herpes virus
- Transmitted in bodily fluids—low infectivity
- Can remain dormant within host for life; reactivation common.
- Seroprevalence: ~50% of UK ♀
- Incidence of infection in pregnancy ~1:100 ♀

Clinical features
Asymptomatic in 95% of cases but may present with:
- Fever
- Malaise
- Lymphadenopathy
- Bloods may show atypical lymphocytosis, and mononucleosis

Diagnosis
Maternal infection
- Paired serology (acute phase and then repeated 10–14 days later) consistent with infection if:
  - Significant ↑ in IgM antibodies (may persist for up to 8 mths)
  - ↑ IgG antibody titres
- Culture/viral PCR of maternal urine can also be diagnostic but is not widely available

Fetal infection
- Culture/viral PCR of amniotic fluid (after 20 wks)

CMV-associated congenital defects
- IUGR
- Microcephaly
- Hepatosplenomegaly and thrombocytopenia
- Jaundice
- Chorioretinitis
- Later sequelae include:
  - Psychomotor retardation—reported to account for as much as 10% of intellectual disability in children <6 yrs old
- Sensorineural hearing loss

Risk of fetal infection with 1° maternal infection
- 40% of fetuses will be infected (irrespective of gestation)
- 90% of these are normal at birth, of which 20% will develop late, usually minor sequelae
- 10% of these are symptomatic, of which:
  - 33% will not survive
  - 67% will have long-term problems

Management of CMV in pregnancy
- Supportive treatment, no specific treatments reduce transmission to fetus
- As most fetuses will be unaffected, counselling about management (including termination of pregnancy) is difficult even in the face of confirmed fetal infection
- Close monitoring of fetal growth and well-being is indicated, with appropriate paediatric follow-up

Zika

Background
- Flavivirus, 1st discovered in Uganda in 1947
- Spread by day-biting mosquitoes
- Small number of cases found to be spread by sexual transmission, risk is very low
- Usually a mild and short-lived illness (2–7 days); severe disease is uncommon

Clinical features
Symptoms include:
- Fever
- Headache
- Red sore eyes and conjunctivitis
- Joint pain and/or swelling
- Muscle pain
- Rash
- Itching

Prevention
- Currently no vaccine or drug available
- 50% DEET-based mosquito repellents are the most effective and are safe in pregnancy and breastfeeding
- Avoid unnecessary travel to areas affected by Zika if pregnant or planning pregnancy (seek advice from Public Health England)

Management
See Fig. 13.1.

Fetal abnormalities in congenital Zika infection

Cranial abnormalities	Extra-cranial abnormalities
Microcephaly	Fetal growth restriction
Cerebral and/or ocular calcification	Oligohydramnios
Ventriculomegaly	Talipes
Periventricular cysts	
Callosal abnormalities	
Microphthalmia	
Cerebellar atrophy	
Vermian agenesis	
Blake's cyst	
Mega cisterna magna	
Choroid plexus cyst	
Brain atrophy → microcephaly	
Cortical and white matter abnormalities	

➔ Public Health England. Zika virus: country specific risk: ℘ https://www.gov.uk/guidance/zika-virus-country-specific-risk

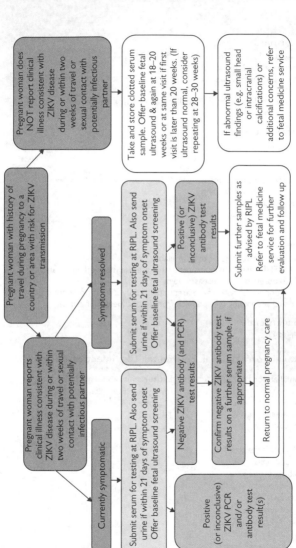

Fig. 13.1 Management of pregnant ♀ with possible infection. RIPL, Rare and Imported Pathogens Laboratory; ZIKV, Zika virus. From Zika virus risk: algorithm for assessing pregnant women (2019) ℗ https://www.gov.uk/government/publications/zika-virus-interim-algorithm-for-assessing-pregnant-women-with-a-history-of-travel, reprinted under the Open Government License V3. ℗ https://www.nationalarchives.gov.uk/doc/open-government-license (version 3/

Ebola

If the diagnosis of Ebola is being considered
- Liaise with public health (and local ID/micro services) before the patient arrives in hospital, or as soon as possible after risk identified
- Maximize the safety of all staff who are working within the high-risk area
- Follow strict infection control procedures using full personal protective equipment

Background
- Filovirus 1st recognized in 1976
- Interaction with pregnancy is poorly understood
- Incubation period is up to 21 days
- Human-to-human transmission efficiently through mucosal contact with infected body fluids
- Risk of transmission continues after death so corpses must be handled with full infection control procedures
- Can cross the placenta so likely to be transmitted to the fetus

Clinical features
Consistent with infection in an area of suspected infection
- Fever plus contact with a known case of Ebola
- Fever plus 3 of the following:

  - Headache
  - Myalgia or arthralgia
  - Dysphagia
  - Hiccups
  - Loss of appetite
  - Dyspnoea
  - Diarrhoea
  - Lethargy
  - Vomiting
  - Dyspepsia

- Any person with unexplained bleeding

Treatment
- IV access early (to avoid sharps injury if patient becomes distressed)
- Supportive care with focus on electrolyte and fluid replacement
- If possible, treat complications such as refractory shock, hypoxia, haemorrhage, septic shock, multiorgan failure, and DIC
- Manage distressing symptoms
- Consider empirical antibacterial and antimalarial treatment
- No curative treatment available, some experimental therapies and vaccinations are being developed
- Manage pregnancy after patient has tested negative for Ebola (after 4 days of being symptomatic)

Postnatally
- No evidence that ♀ who survive and subsequently become pregnant pose a risk for virus transmission
- Semen in ♂ who survive continues to contain virus for at least 3 mths following recovery

Obstetric management in ♀ with Ebola infection

⚠ Likelihood of baby surviving in an infected mother is very low ∴ fetal monitoring not advised and emergency caesarean section is not indicated for fetal reasons.

It is recommended to:
- Deliver in high-risk area
- Anticipate vaginal delivery, healthcare practitioner to be to one side to avoid direct splash of bodily fluids
- Minimize vaginal examinations and avoid artificial rupture of the membranes
- Do not perform an episiotomy
- Active 3rd stage
- Not to suture if there is a vaginal tear, use pressure instead

In utero death
- Do not induce labour until serology negative and ♀ is well
- If planned emptying of the uterus (at any stage of pregnancy), it is recommended to use mifepristone and/or misoprostol
- Placenta and stillborn child must be disposed of in accordance with high-risk material protocol

Live birth
- Unlikely
- Assume baby is Ebola +ve and highly contagious

Lactation
- Breast milk is likely to be infected, consider lactation suppressant, e.g. cabergoline
- If not feasible, provide breast pump with clear instructions for safe disposal of the infected milk, and a weaning technique with the aim of ceasing lactation
- Appropriate counselling on high chance of neonatal death
- On discharge give supplies to assist with re-entry into community:
  - Medicines including iron supplements
  - Nutritional supplements
  - Clothing
  - Hygiene pads
  - Family planning advice

➜ WHO. Ebola publications: case management, infection prevention, and control: ℘ http://www.who.int/csr/resources/publications/ebola/infection-prevention/en/

Other viral infections

Epstein–Barr virus

- Infectious mononucleosis is a common presentation of 1° EBV
- A generalized maculopapular rash may occur (particularly if ampicillin or a similar antibiotic has been taken)
- 1° infection in pregnancy carries no specific risk to the fetus

Enteroviruses

- Coxsackie virus groups A and B, echovirus, and enterovirus 68–71
- Wide range of manifestations including:
  - Meningitis
  - Rash
  - Febrile illness
  - Myocarditis
- No clear causal relationship evident for adverse fetal or neonatal outcome

▶ Hand, foot, and mouth is caused by an enteroviral infection
- 1° infection or contact with it in pregnancy is not known to have any adverse consequences for the fetus

HIV and pregnancy

Background

- In the UK, >10% of the estimated total of individuals living with HIV are unaware of their infection
- Those diagnosed late have an ↑ risk of death in the 1st year after diagnosis compared to those diagnosed early
- The risk of MTCT in the UK is <0.1% and improved after the introduction of routine antenatal screening in 1999
- High viral loads (VLs) ↑ rate of MTCT
- Pregnancy does not alter the course of the infection
- Antiretroviral Pregnancy Registry provides the best data on teratogenicity and 1st-trimester antiretroviral therapy exposure (⅏ http://www.apregistry.com)

⚠ Many partners of HIV positive ♀ are unaware of the diagnosis, so care needs to be taken when communicating in pregnancy with judicious documentation in handheld notes, and a local system to flag the information should the mother be admitted as an emergency

➲ British H IV Association (BHIVA) guidelines: ⅏ http://www.bhiva.org/guidelines.aspx

Management

See Table 13.3.

Table 13.3 Classes of antiretroviral drugs

Class of drug	Examples	Potential problems
Nucleoside analogue reverse transcriptase inhibitors	Zidovudine (ZDV, previously AZT) Lamivudine (3TC) Didanosine (ddl) Stavudine (d4T) Abacavir (ABC) Tenofovir Emtricitabine	• All generally well tolerated, but reported cases of - Anaemia - Nausea and vomiting - ↑ transaminases - Hyperglycaemia • Lactic acidosis is a possibility when d4T and ddl are combined
Non-nucleoside analogue reverse transcriptase inhibitors	Nevirapine (NVP) Delavirdine Efavirenz	• Greatest experience is with NVP, but although well-tolerated there is an association with deranged liver function in ♀ with good CD4 counts • Rash is also reported
Protease inhibitors	Ritonavir Indinavir Nelfinavir Saquinavir	• Hyperglycaemia is a risk with new-onset diabetes or exacerbation of existing diabetes • Diarrhoea with nausea, vomiting, and altered taste • Altered liver function reported
HIV-1 integrase strand transfer inhibitor		• Depression • Hyperglycaemia • Changes in body fat distribution

HIV: pre-pregnancy counselling

This depends on both the status of their partner and their individual VL (Table 13.4).

Table 13.4 Pre-pregnancy counselling for couples with HIV

	Positive ♀, negative ♂	Positive ♂, negative ♀	Positive ♀, positive ♂
Antiretroviral therapy	Recommended, but not essential if using artificial insemination	Recommended	Recommended for both
Timed ovulatory condomless sex	Recommended only if VL <50 c/mL	Recommended only if VL <50 c/mL	Recommended unless 1 or both partner detectable HIV RNA + discordant resistance
Pre-exposure prophylaxis for conception	Consider if HIV-positive partner's HIV RNA not suppressed	Consider if HIV-positive partner's HIV RNA not suppressed	Not recommended
Artificial insemination using non-spermicidal condoms	Recommended	NA	NA
Sperm washing	Not recommended	Not recommended unless detectable HIV RNA (suppressive ART 1 choice)	Not recommended
Sperm donor	Consider if ♂ subfertility	Consider if ♂ subfertility	Consider if ♂ subfertility
Egg donor	Consider if ♀ subfertility	Consider if ♀ subfertility	Consider if ♀ subfertility

Source: data from Waters L et al. (2017) BHIVA/BASHH/FRSH guidelines for the sexual & reproductive health of people living with HIV: https://www.bhiva.org/file/zryuNVwnXcxMC/SRH-guidelines-for-consultation-2017.pdf

HIV: antenatal management

Combination antiretroviral therapy (cART)

- All HIV-positive ♀ should start cART during pregnancy and continue lifelong (regardless of CD4 count)
- cART should be commenced:
  - Within the 1st trimester if VL >100,000 copies/mL (c/mL) and/or CD4 cell count <200 cells/mm³
  - As soon as they are able to do so in the 2nd trimester, by 24 wks at the latest
- Treatment is started as recommended in the BHIVA guidelines
- An integrase inhibitor-based regimen is suggested as the 3rd agent of choice in ♀ with high baseline VL (>100,000 c/mL), where cART is being started late in pregnancy or where it is failing to suppress the virus
- No dose alterations are routinely advised in pregnancy
- Zidovudine monotherapy can be used in ♀ declining cART who have a baseline VL of <10,000 c/mL and a CD4 >350 cells/mm³ and who consent to a caesarean section

Hepatitis B or C co-infection

- Requires management alongside a clinician experienced in co-infection, with hepatology input if significant cirrhosis
- Vaginal delivery can be supported if the ♀ has fully suppressed HIV VL on cART, irrespective of HBV/HCV VL

Special circumstances

- Invasive prenatal diagnostic testing should not be performed until after maternal HIV status is known, and ideally deferred until VL <50 c/mL
- If not on cART and the invasive diagnostic test procedure cannot be delayed until VL <50 c/mL, ♀ can start cART to include raltegravir and be given a single dose of nevirapine 2–4 hrs prior to the procedure
- External cephalic version can be performed in HIV-positive ♀

Late presentation

- ♀ presenting in labour/with rupture of membranes/requiring delivery without a documented HIV result must be recommended to have an HIV diagnostic point-of-care test
- A reactive point-of-care test result must prompt interventions to prevent MTCT without waiting for formal serological confirmation
- If presenting after 28 wks, ♀ should start cART without delay as per BHIVA guidelines

⚠ An untreated ♀ presenting in labour at term should be given a combination of treatments (➔ see BHIVA guidelines).

Antenatal management of HIV

▶ All cases of HIV in pregnancy (diagnosed before or during pregnancy) in the UK should be reported to the national study of HIV in pregnancy and childhood (even if the pregnancy is not continued to term)

▶ Cases can be reported online at: ℜ https://www.ucl.ac.uk/nshpc/pregnancies-hiv-positive-women

- Newly diagnosed ♀ do not require other baseline tests in addition to routine antenatal screening
- HIV resistance testing prior to treatment initiation (except in ♀ presenting late)
- Sexual health screening with treatment of infection according to British Association for Sexual Health and HIV guidelines
- Encourage to continue cART post delivery
- ♀ who either conceive on cART should have a minimum of 1 CD4 count at baseline and 1 at delivery
- In ♀ who commence cART in pregnancy:
  - CD4 cell count should be performed at initiation
  - VL should be performed 2–4 wks later, at least once every trimester, at 36 wks, and at delivery
  - LFTs should be performed at initiation of cART and at each antenatal visit
- If VL not suppressed (to <50 c/mL) at 36 wks with cART:
  - Review adherence and concomitant medication
  - Perform resistance testing if appropriate
  - Consider therapeutic drug monitoring
  - Optimize to best regimen
  - Consider intensification
- Fetal USS should be carried out as per national guidance
- The combined screening test for trisomy 21 is recommended as this has the best sensitivity and specificity and will minimize the number of ♀ who may need invasive testing
- Non-invasive prenatal testing should be considered for ♀ with a high-risk result as this may ↓ the need for invasive procedures

➲ British HIV Association guidelines: ℜ http://www.bhiva.org/guidelines.aspx

➲ British Association for Sexual Health and HIV guidelines: ℜ https://www.bashh.org/guidelines

HIV: intrapartum

Mode of delivery

- This should depend on:
  - VL at 36 wks
  - Presence/absence of obstetric complications
  - Chronology of an individual's treatment and response to treatment

⚠ Vaginal delivery does not require any modifications to standard intrapartum care

VL <50 c/mL

- No obstetric complications → support vaginal delivery (including vaginal birth after a caesarean section)
- Caesarean section for obstetric indication only

VL 50–399 c/mL

- Consider elective caesarean section (depending on factors including VL and trajectory, treatment duration, adherence, and obstetric issues)

VL ≥400 c/mL

- Elective caesarean section advised at 38–39 wks

Rupture of membranes

⚠ In all cases of term pre-labour rupture of membranes, delivery should be expedited.

VL <50 c/mL

- Immediate induction of labour is recommended
- Low threshold for treatment of intrapartum pyrexia

VL 50–999 c/mL

- Consider caesarean section (depending on factors including actual VL and trajectory, treatment duration, adherence, obstetric issues)

VL >1000 c/mL

- Immediate caesarean section recommended

⚠ If rupture of membranes between 34–37 wks, GBS prophylaxis advised.

Preterm pre-labour rupture of membranes at <34 wks
- IM steroids administered as per national guidelines
- Optimize virological control
- Delivery timing and mode based on MDT discussion

Intrapartum IV zidovudine if:
- VL >1000 c/mL + labour/rupture of membranes/admission for elective caesarean section
- VL unknown + not on treatment + labour/rupture of membranes

▶ Not required if VL <1000 c/mL + on cART.

HIV: postnatal concerns

Neonatal management
- Post-exposure prophylaxis should be started within 4 hrs of birth
- Neonate should be risk stratified by the paediatric team so as to decide length and type of post-exposure prophylaxis treatment.
- Co-trimoxazole prophylaxis for *Pneumocystis jirovecii* pneumonia is recommended from 1 mth of age if HIV PCR is positive at any stage or if the infant is confirmed to be diagnosed with HIV

⚠ This should only be stopped if HIV infection is subsequently excluded

Postnatal management and follow-up
- All ♀ are recommended to continue cART postpartum
- ♀ should be followed up at 4–6 wks

Breastfeeding
- Use of formula milk eliminates the risk of HIV exposure after birth
- If not breastfeeding, the use of cabergoline to suppress lactation should be considered
- ♀ on cART with VL <50 c/mL and good adherence, who choose to breastfeed can be supported in this, but there is a low risk of MTCT

➲ British HIV Association guidelines: ℐ http://www.bhiva.org/guidelines.aspx

Malaria

Background

- Protozoan infection (75% *Plasmodium falciparum,* others include *P. vivax,*
  P. ovale, and *P. malariae*)
- Not endemic in the UK but commonly imported
- Spread by the sporozoite-bearing female *Anopheles* mosquito

Clinical features

There are often no specific symptoms or signs, with the infection presenting
with a 'flu-like' illness, but may include:

- Fever (cyclical 'spiking')
- Rigors/chills/sweats
- Muscle pain and general malaise
- Confusion, drowsiness, and lethargy
- Features of severe malaria are shown in Box 13.1

Diagnosis

- Rapid antigen testing is now in widespread use
- Thick and thin blood films can also be diagnostic:
  - >3 negative smears, 12–24 hrs apart to exclude the diagnosis

Maternal risks

- Pregnancy ↑ the risk of developing severe disease
- ⚠ Infection in pregnancy can be fatal

Fetal risks

- Stillbirth, miscarriage, or preterm delivery
- Congenital malaria
- Low birth weight (2° to prematurity or IUGR)

Box 13.1 Features of severe malaria

Clinical features
- Impaired consciousness/prostration
- Respiratory distress and/or pulmonary oedema
- Seizures
- Circulatory collapse
- Abnormal bleeding, DIC
- Jaundice
- Haemoglobinuria (in absence of G6PD deficiency)

Laboratory tests
- Severe anaemia (Hb <80 g/L)
- Thrombocytopenia
- Hypoglycaemia (<2.2 mmol/L)
- Acidosis (pH <7.3)
- Hyperlactataemia
- Hyperparasitaemia (>2% parasitized RBCs)

Management of malaria in pregnancy

⚠ Malaria in pregnancy should be treated as an emergency:

- ♀ should be admitted to hospital
- Assessment of severity (Box 13.1)
- LP if suspicion of cerebral malaria
- Quinine and clindamycin is the treatment of choice for non-severe
  P. falciparum infection in the 1st trimester
- IV artesunate should be used for non-severe *P. falciparum* infection in
  the 2nd and 3rd trimesters, and all severe cases
- Antipyretics as needed
- Close monitoring for severe malaria
- Delivery plans entirely depend on the severity of the maternal illness,
  assessment of fetal well-being, and gestation, but usually malaria is
  not an indication for delivery

⚠ Placental sequestration of parasites can occur, so the placenta should
be sent for histological examination after delivery.

⚠ Risk of neonatal infection so paediatrics team should be informed at
delivery.

⚠ Notifiable condition in the UK and needs reporting to PHE.

Malaria prophylaxis in pregnancy

- Appropriate antimalarials should be taken (proguanil and chloroquine
  are most commonly used)
- Avoidance of exposure to mosquito bites:
  - Mosquito nets
  - Long sleeves and trousers (tucked into socks)
  - Insect repellents—50% DEET-based mosquito repellents are the
    most effective and are safe in pregnancy and breastfeeding

➔ RCOG. Green-top guidelines nos. 54A and 54B: ⌕ https://www.rcog.org.uk/en/guidelines

Toxoplasmosis

Background
- Protozoan parasite *Toxoplasma gondii*
- Spread by contact with cat faeces and eating undercooked meat
- Incubation <2 days
- ~20% of UK ♀ are immune
- Incidence of 1° infection in pregnancy ~1:500 ♀

Clinical features
Asymptomatic in ~80% of cases but may present with:
- Fever
- Lymphadenopathy

Diagnosis
Maternal infection

Paired serology (acute phase and then repeated 10–14 days later) consistent with recent infection if:
- Isolated very high titres of IgM antibodies (may persist up to 1 yr)
- Concurrent high IgM and IgG antibodies
- 4-fold ↑ in IgG antibodies

Fetal infection
- Diagnosed by the presence of IgM antibodies in amniotic fluid or fetal blood
- Amniocentesis is accurate only after 20 wks
- Although ultrasound signs such as cerebral ventriculomegaly can occur, most affected fetuses have a normal scan

---

Fetal risks
- Spontaneous miscarriage is common with infection in the 1st trimester (Table 13.5)
- Defects associated with 1° infection include:
  - Chorioretinitis
  - Microcephaly and hydrocephalus
  - Intracranial calcification
  - Intellectual disability

Table 13.5 Risk of congenital defects by gestation

Gestation (wks)	Risk of transmission (5)	Risk of congenital abnormality in infected fetuses (%)
<12	~17	75
12–28	~25	25
>28	65	<10

Management of toxoplasmosis in pregnancy
- Fit and healthy ♀ have minimal risk from the condition itself
- Immunocompromised ♀ have a risk of severe disseminated illness with chorioretinitis and encephalitis
- Spiramycin for maternal infection may ↓ the risk of fetal infection
- If vertical transmission occurs, combination anti-toxoplasmosis therapy is used
- Neonatal follow-up should include an ophthalmic review and cranial radiological studies
- It is usually recommended that future pregnancies are delayed until maternal IgM antibodies have been cleared

Vaccination in pregnancy

Vaccination

- Live-attenuated vaccines (e.g. rubella, polio, MMR, VZV) are contraindicated in pregnancy
- Passive immunization with specific human immunoglobulin is safe and may provide important protection (e.g. VZIG)
- ♀ who are HBsAg negative but considered at high risk should be offered vaccination in pregnancy
- Vaccinations for travel should be considered on an individual basis, and the small risk from the vaccine compared with the risk from contracting the disease
- A list of vaccinations in pregnancy is shown in Table 13.6

Table 13.6 Vaccinations in pregnancy

Infection	Issues
Cholera	Can be used in pregnancy but no specific studies of this
Hepatitis A	Can be used in pregnancy if required
Hepatitis B	Can be offered to ♀ who are HBsAg negative but considered to be at high risk
Pneumococcus	Inactivated virus, so can be used in pregnancy
Meningococcus	Safety unknown, consider if high risk
Rabies	Not contra-indicated in pregnancy and breastfeeding
Tetanus	Safe in pregnancy
Yellow fever	Safety unknown, consider if high risk

Oncology

Principles of management of cancer in pregnancy

Background
- Many malignancies occur in pregnancy, but breast, cervical, and haematological are the most common
- Malignancy is associated with maternal mortality, as shown in the MBRRACE-UK 2018 report
- Many symptoms can be non-specific and inappropriately attributed to pregnancy by the patient or healthcare professional

Imaging
- Is crucial to make a diagnosis and, if malignancy is identified, to make an accurate assessment of the stage
- Pregnancy often leads to a reluctance to perform imaging if ionizing radiation is required, but if this imaging will make a difference to the management in pregnancy then it should be performed
- Senior clinicians must be involved at an early stage

Surgery
- Often appropriate to be performed during pregnancy, but depends on gestation and whether it will affect the prognosis or management
- The nature and duration of required surgery are important factors (e.g. complex neck dissection for head and neck malignancy with a long anaesthetic is likely to be better performed after delivery)
- Fetal monitoring before and after is gestation dependent:
  - Intraoperative fetal monitoring is not commonly undertaken

Chemotherapy
- Many chemotherapeutic agents have been successfully used in pregnancy without being associated with adverse fetal outcomes
- If advice on a particular agent or regimen is required, then the UK Teratology Information Service can be helpful (http://www.uktis.org)

Radiotherapy
- Ideally should be delayed until after delivery
- In rare circumstances can be performed in pregnancy, but depends on targeted location, the intended dose, and the gestational age
- Lead shielding of the fetus is used during radiotherapy

Delivery
- Malignancy is not an absolute indication for caesarean section or preterm delivery
- For ♀ on chemotherapy, delivery planning should include sufficient time after a cycle to allow recovery of neutrophils
- It may be possible to aim for a term delivery, which ↓ the morbidity for both neonate and mother
- Many malignancies can spread to the placenta, ∴ it should be sent for histological analysis to look for micrometastases

Breast cancer

Background
- Commonest malignancy in ♀ (lifetime risk 1 in 8 in the UK)
- 15% of cases are diagnosed before the age of 45 years

Clinical features
- Most common presentation is an isolated breast lump
- Systemic features such as malaise, weight loss or sweats may occur, but this is usually in the setting of metastatic disease

---

If a breast lump is detected in pregnancy
- Refer to breast specialist team and manage as part of a MDT
- USS can be performed, ± biopsy for histology
- Cytology is often inconclusive due to associated proliferative changes
- Mammography can be performed
- If high clinical suspicion of metastatic disease, then CXR and abdominal USS can be performed

  ☙ CT is not absolutely contraindicated but pelvic CT should be avoided where possible
- If there is concern about bone involvement:
  - Plain X-rays or MRI are advisable
  - Isotope bone scan is not recommended in pregnant ♀
- The decision to continue the pregnancy should be discussed with the ♀ and her partner, considering factors including:
  - Prognosis
  - Treatment options during and after pregnancy
  - Impact on future conception

History of previous breast cancer
- Long-term survival is not adversely affected by pregnancy
- ♀ should be advised to wait at least 2 years after treatment, which is when the risk of cancer recurrence is highest
- Echocardiography may be advisable for ♀ at risk of cardiomyopathy from chemotherapy with anthracyclines
- ♀ should be reassured that there is no ↑ risk of malformation in children conceived after treatment for breast cancer

➔ RCOG (2011). Pregnancy and breast cancer (green-top guideline no. 12): ℜ https://www.rcog.org.uk/globalassets/documents/guidelines/gtg_12.pdf

Management of breast cancer in pregnancy
- Should be managed by an experienced MDT

Treatments

Surgery
- Surgery can be performed in all trimesters
- Reconstructive surgery should be delayed until after pregnancy:
  - Prevents asymmetry resulting from pregnancy-related changes
  - Avoids prolonged anaesthesia
- Sentinel node assessment using radioisotopes does not cause significant uterine radiation and can be performed if required

Radiotherapy
- Radiotherapy delayed until after delivery unless to prevent either life-threatening or organ-threatening complications, e.g. spinal cord compression
- It can be performed with fetal shielding

Chemotherapy
⚠ Systemic therapy is contraindicated in the 1st trimester
- Can be performed from the 2nd trimester onwards
- Not associated with late miscarriage, growth restriction, or organ dysfunction in the fetus
- Anthracycline regimens can be used
- Taxanes lack safety data in pregnancy and are therefore reserved for high-risk (node positive) or metastatic disease

Hormone/targeted therapy
⚠ Trastuzumab and tamoxifen are contraindicated in pregnancy and breastfeeding.

Other medications
- Antiemetics, e.g. dexamethasone and ondansetron, can be used
- G-CSF can be used in chemotherapy-related neutropenia
- VTE prophylaxis should be prescribed to all ♀ with malignancy in pregnancy unless contraindications present

Delivery timing
- At least 2 wks after the last cycle of chemotherapy is advisable, to avoid issues with neutropenia at delivery
- Administration of steroids for fetal lung maturation as normal if preterm delivery is anticipated
- G-CSF may be useful prior to delivery

Lactation
- No evidence that breastfeeding ↑ chance of recurrence
- Lactation be more difficult depending on the surgical intervention that may have been performed
- In ♀ with a recent diagnosis of breast cancer, chemotherapy plans will determine whether breastfeeding is advisable

Cervical cancer

Background
- Most commonly diagnosed gynaecological malignancy in pregnancy
- Squamous cell makes up 80% of cervical cancers in pregnancy

🔑 Diagnosis can be more challenging because of the physiological cervical changes seen in pregnancy

Clinical features
Overlap with common symptoms seen in pregnancy including:
- Postcoital bleeding (present in 50% of cases)
- Abnormal vaginal discharge (watery or pinkish)
- Pelvic/sciatic/abdominal pain
- Anaemia

If cervical cancer is suspected in pregnancy
- Cervical cytology is not recommended in pregnancy
- Colposcopy should be performed by an experienced practitioner familiar with the changes of pregnancy
- Biopsies can be taken in pregnancy but only to exclude invasion as the risk of haemorrhage is significant
- Staging with MRI is required when malignancy is confirmed

History of previous cervical cancer

Conization for precursor lesions or microinvasive disease
- There is an ↑ risk of preterm birth following excisional treatment of >1 cm of tissue
- The larger the amount of tissue removed, the greater the ↑ risk

Pregnancy after trachelectomy
- Trachelectomy is considered for 1A2/1B1 cancers only
- Management should be by an experienced MDT
- Permanent isthmic suture is placed at the time of trachelectomy
- ↑ risk of mid-trimester miscarriage and preterm delivery, often as a consequence of preterm pre-labour rupture of membranes
- Delivery should be by caesarean section

Management of cervical cancer in pregnancy

- Should be managed by an experienced MDT
- Treatment will depend on:
  - Gestational age at diagnosis
  - Stage
  - Size of the lesion
  - Wishes for future fertility

Invasive (stages IA2, IB, and IIA)

- No evidence that pregnancy accelerates the disease
- Disease-specific survival is independent of the trimester during which the diagnosis is made
- Careful counselling is required including the option of termination of pregnancy (<24 wks) to facilitate immediate treatment

🌀 Postponement of surgical treatment to enable the fetus to reach a viable age has not been demonstrated to ↑ the risk of recurrence

- Platinum-based chemotherapy and taxanes can be used after the 1st trimester
- Radical surgery can be performed immediately after caesarean delivery

Invasive (stages IIB, III, and IV)

- Rare in pregnancy
- Immediate treatment is usually recommended

Route of delivery

- Caesarean delivery should be performed for all invasive tumours

Melanoma

Background

- Most common malignancy in ♀ of childbearing age
- Pregnancy-associated skin changes can make the diagnosis more challenging as enlargement of naevi on breasts or abdomen can occur from skin growth

⚠ Darkening of existing naevi is not a normal finding

Clinical features

- Changes to a pigmented lesion including:
  - Itching
  - Darkening
  - Bleeding
  - Crusting

If melanoma is suspected in pregnancy

- New lesions should be assessed according to standard guidelines
- Enlargement of a naevus or darkening should prompt a clinical review
- Biopsies can be performed at any stage of pregnancy
- Tumours are staged by assessing their thickness, lymph node involvement, and distant spread
- Various imaging modalities can be used for staging:
  - MRI is preferred
  - CT and nuclear medicine scans can be used if they are likely to yield essential information that other scans will not (that will influence treatment plans)

History of previous melanoma

- ♀ should be advised to wait at least 2 yrs after treatment, which is when the risk of cancer recurrence is highest (especially important in thicker lesions)
- Ensure they are having appropriate follow-up (regular total body skin examination)
- Newer melanoma treatments such as checkpoint inhibitors (anti-PD1 or anti-CTLA4 such as nivolumab and ipilimumab) or BRAF inhibitors (e.g. vemurafenib) may be teratogenic so if conception occurs these should be discontinued
- If planning a pregnancy while on one of these agents, between 2 wks and 5 mths off treatment is advised prior to conception

Management of melanoma in pregnancy
- No evidence that the development of melanoma in pregnancy is associated with a worse long-term prognosis
- Surgery can be performed in pregnancy
- Sentinel node assessment using radioisotopes does not cause significant uterine radiation and can be performed in pregnancy if required
- Transplacental passage of melanoma can occur, resulting in a risk of metastatic melanoma in the fetus:
  - Placenta should be sent for histology
  - Paediatricians should be notified for neonatal assessment

Hodgkin lymphoma

Background

- One of the most common malignancies in pregnancy
- Estimated to affect 1 in 1000–6000 pregnant ♀
- Arises in B cells in germinal centres or post-germinal centres
- Reed–Sternberg cells on an inflammatory background are diagnostic
- Associated with immunosuppression and autoimmune conditions
- Pregnancy does not alter the course of Hodgkin lymphoma

Clinical features

- Asymptomatic lymphadenopathy
- Mediastinal mass
- Systemic features ('B symptoms') include fevers, night sweats, and weight loss
- Pain can occur in affected sites and be worsened by alcohol intake
- FBC may be normal, but may show cytopenias reflective of bone marrow involvement

---

If lymphoma is suspected in pregnancy

- Diagnosis should be confirmed with a lymph node core biopsy or excision biopsy (not aspirate)
- Imaging to stage the condition is required:
  - MRI preferred in pregnancy
  - PET/CT can be used if likely to yield essential information that will influence treatment plans

---

History of previous lymphoma

- ♀ should be advised to wait at least 2 years after treatment, when risk of cancer recurrence is highest (relapses in pregnancy are rare)
- History including treatments (in particular, chemotherapy doses) and most recent conclusion from haematology/oncology review
- Echocardiogram (if not recently performed) after anthracyclines
- VTE prophylaxis to be reviewed if recent treatment and any concerns about remission/relapse

---

Bleomycin and respiratory complications

⚠ Can be associated with lung damage which can be accelerated by the use of high-flow oxygen.

- Take any respiratory symptoms in ♀ on regimes including this drug seriously
- Have low threshold for further investigation such as CXR
- If oxygen is required:
  - Start at a low flow and gradually titrate to the minimum needed to achieve the target saturation
- Avoid Entonox® ('gas and air': 50% oxygen, 50% nitrous oxide)

Management of Hodgkin lymphoma in pregnancy
• Treatment depends on gestation, stage, and preferred regimen

1st trimester
• Options include termination of pregnancy, or use of a single agent, i.e. vinblastine, or use of ABVD (doxorubicin, bleomycin, vinblastine, and dacarbazine)

2nd and 3rd trimesters
• In early disease and near term, delivery can be expedited
• If treatment is required, ABVD does not ↑ adverse outcomes
• Radiotherapy with adequate shielding does not ↑ adverse outcomes, but should only be done before delivery *in extremis*

Other therapies
• Antifungals:
  • Amphotericin is considered the safest antifungal in pregnancy and is recommended if treatment is required
• Prophylaxis for *Pneumocystis jirovecii*:
  • Co-trimoxazole (trimethoprim and sulfamethoxazole) can be used in pregnancy (after the 1st trimester)
• Antivirals:
  • Not routinely recommended alongside ABVD chemotherapy
• Blood products:
  • Should be CMV negative and irradiated
• DVT prophylaxis:
  • Should be prescribed to all pregnant ♀ with active malignancy

Delivery plans
• Should be individualized and depend on timing of chemotherapy:
  • Aiming for delivery at term is reasonable unless clear indications for preterm elective delivery are present
  • Delay of >2 wks following chemotherapy is best to allow time for the neutrophil count to recover prior to delivery
  • Caesarean section is required for obstetric indications only

Non-Hodgkin lymphoma
• Less common in pregnancy as it is more likely to occur in older individuals, however AIDS-related NHL is an ↑ problem particularly in low-income countries
• Treatment principles are similar to that of Hodgkin lymphoma

Acute leukaemia

For chronic myeloid leukaemia, see 'Chronic myeloid leukaemia', p. 352.

Background

- Less common than lymphoma (affects ~1 in 75,000 pregnancies)
- About 2/3 of cases are acute myelocytic leukaemia and the remainder acute lymphocytic leukaemia
- Development of leukaemia in pregnancy is associated with significant mortality and treatment delays can contribute to a worsening of maternal and fetal prognosis

Clinical features

- Non-specific symptoms can overlap with features of normal pregnancy such as fatigue and breathlessness
- Bleeding can occur as a result of thrombocytopenia or coagulopathy
- Laboratory testing can show anaemia, thrombocytopenia, or abnormal coagulation parameters; the white cell count may be very raised due to the presence of blasts
- A blood film may identify blast cells

Management of acute lymphocytic leukaemia in pregnancy

⚠ It is both possible and appropriate to treat acute lymphocytic leukaemia in pregnancy:

- In the 1st trimester, discussion about termination of pregnancy should be undertaken given the importance of adequate treatment and the high chance of maternal and fetal morbidity if not
- Very steroid responsive:
  - High-dose steroids for 1–2 wks may prolong the pregnancy to a more favourable gestation for delivery
- There are a variety of chemotherapeutic agents used as part of induction, consolidation, and maintenance regimens
- Intrathecal therapy is often used (intrathecal methotrexate is used in non-pregnant individuals, but alternatives to this are usually used in pregnancy)

Acute promyelocytic leukaemia

- Type of AML associated with DIC and bleeding complications
- Treatment with all-trans retinoic acid (ATRA) should be started as soon as possible

⚠ ATRA not advised in the 1st trimester due to teratogenicity so termination of pregnancy vs continuation must be discussed

⚠ If continuing with the pregnancy, an anthracycline should be used and ATRA initiated in the 2nd trimester

Management of AML in pregnancy

◆ Tyrosine kinase inhibitors for those who are BCR-ABL ('Philadelphia chromosome') positive, are advised against in pregnancy.

1st trimester
- Termination of pregnancy should be discussed to facilitate the early commencement of optimal treatment

2nd and 3rd trimesters
- Decision for treatment and delivery needs to be individualized
- Delivery of a pancytopenic mother is undesirable ∴ where possible induction treatment should be commenced with an elective delivery after the mother has recovered
- A standard induction regimen can be used (daunorubicin and cytarabine '3 + 10' schedule)

Other therapies
- High-dose steroids:
  - No dose adjustment required
  - Monitoring for hyperglycaemia should be commenced
- Antifungals:
  - Amphotericin is considered the safest antifungal in pregnancy and is recommended if treatment is required
- Prophylaxis for *Pneumocystis jirovecii*:
  - Co-trimoxazole (trimethoprim and sulfamethoxazole) can be used in pregnancy (after the 1st trimester)
- Antivirals:
  - Aciclovir can be used in pregnancy if indicated
- Blood products:
  - Should be CMV negative and irradiated
- DVT prophylaxis:
  - Should be prescribed to all pregnant ♀ with active malignancy

Delivery considerations
- Timing depends on gestation and chemotherapy plans
- A delay of >2 wks following chemotherapy is best to allow time for the neutrophil count to recover prior to delivery
- Caesarean section is required for obstetric indications only
- Anaesthetic input is important as regional analgesia and anaesthesia may be contraindicated in the presence of significant neutropenia, thrombocytopenia, or coagulopathy
- Active management of the 3rd stage is advised due to the ↑ risk of bleeding
- Paediatric team should be informed and present at delivery

➲ British Society for Haematology (2015). Management of AML in pregnancy: ℛ https://b-s-h.org.uk/guidelines/guidelines/management-of-aml-in-pregnancy/

Preserving fertility

Treatment-related risk of infertility

- Targeting of rapidly dividing cells means that there is always a risk of damage to oocytes
- Risk varies greatly between type of malignancy and the nature and dose of the chemotherapeutic agents that are used (Tables 14.1 and 14.2)
- Sometimes treatment can be delayed to allow time for fertility-preserving interventions, e.g.:
  - Ovarian or oocyte preservation
  - IVF resulting in embryos that can be stored

❖ This is not appropriate if delay in treatment initiation could significantly impact the prognosis

Table 14.1 Risk of infertility with treatment

Low <20%	Medium/high risk	Very high risk >80%
• Acute lymphocytic leukaemia	• AML	• Total body irradiation
• Wilm's tumour	• Osteosarcoma	• Pelvic abdominal radiotherapy
• Brain tumour radiotherapy <24 Gy	• Ewing's sarcoma	• Metastatic Ewing's sarcoma
• Soft tissue sarcoma stage 1	• Soft tissue sarcoma stage II/III	• Soft tissue sarcoma (very high stage)
• Hodgkin lymphoma (low stage)	• Hodgkin lymphoma (high stage)	• Hodgkin lymphoma (pelvic radiotherapy/relapse)
	• NHL	• Chemotherapy pre bone marrow transplantation
	• Breast cancer	
	• Brian tumour with high-dose chemotherapy	
	• Neuroblastoma	

Table 14.2 Risk of oocyte depletion

Low risk	Intermediate risk	High risk
• Methotrexate	• Doxorubicin	• Cyclophosphamide
• Bleomycin	• Cisplatin	• Busulfan
• Fluorouracil	• Carboplatin	• Melphalan
• Actinomycin		• Chlorambucil
• Mercaptopurine		• Dacarbazine
• Vincristine		• Procarbazine
		• Ifosfamide

Late effects of cancer treatment

Cardiotoxicity
- Most common concern after exposure to chemotherapeutic agents
- Related to a number of drugs, particularly anthracyclines, where the development of cardiac complications appears to be dose dependent
- Trastuzumab can also be related to acute cardiomyopathy (where chest pain or ↑ troponin levels may be noted) or a late cardiomyopathy, similar to inherited dilated cardiomyopathy
- If there is a history of cancer treated with these agents, then further details should be sought (e.g. total dose) and an echocardiogram performed

Neurological
- Cancer treatments can be associated with peripheral and central nervous system consequences such as peripheral neuropathy and cognitive issues respectively
- Unlikely to cause a problem in pregnancy or have their trajectory altered by pregnancy

Fertility
- The impact of previous cancer treatment on fertility is discussed elsewhere (➔ see 'Preserving fertility', p. 505)

Malignancy risk in the offspring
- In general, the risk of malignancy in the offspring is not ↑ unless the maternal cancer was part of an inherited syndrome
- If an inherited syndrome is identified, genetics referral is appropriate (depending on the exact details of the syndrome)

Neutropenic sepsis

Background

- Neutropenic sepsis can occur after use of some chemotherapeutic agents

⚠ Maternal sepsis is associated with significant maternal mortality

Significant chorioamnionitis can occur with minimal maternal signs initially:
- This carries a high risk of fetal morbidity and mortality and can rapidly progress to threaten maternal life
- Emptying the uterus irrespective of gestation can be a life-saving measure in this situation

Definition

NICE define neutropenic sepsis as:
- A temperature ≥38°C
  Or:
- Symptoms/signs consistent with sepsis
  In:
- A person receiving chemotherapy with a neutrophil count <0.5 × 10⁹/L

Management of neutropenic sepsis in pregnancy

- Inform oncology team
- Inform ITU team depending on severity of illness
- Bloods including:
  - FBC
  - U&E
  - LFTs
  - CRP
  - Lactate
  - Blood cultures
- Cultures of other sites (e.g. wound, urine) if indicated by history or examination
- Fluid assessment and administration of IV fluid resuscitation
- Empirical antibiotics, e.g.:
  - Piperacillin and tazobactam
  - ± An aminoglycoside
  - ✿ Consult local guidelines and consider clinical situation
- Gestation-appropriate fetal monitoring
- Delivery decision has to be individualized, depending on:
  - Severity of maternal illness
  - Gestational age of the fetus and fetal monitoring status

Dermatology

Common skin changes in pregnancy

Hyperpigmentation

- Linea nigra (dark, vertical line down the middle of abdominal skin)
- ↑ pigmentation of melanocytic naevi ('moles')
- Striae gravidarum (stretch marks)
- Darkening of nipple, areola, and genital skin

Pruritus gravidarum

- Generalized itching which can be severe
- No rash (the only skin lesions are excoriations 2° to scratching)
- Occurs towards end of pregnancy
- Important to exclude obstetric cholestasis

Telogen effluvium

- Excessive shedding of hair 1–5 mths after delivery
- Affects somewhere between 40% and 50% of ♀
- Usually temporary

Nail changes

- Longitudinal ridging
- Fragility

Vascular changes

- Palmar erythema
- Telangiectasia
- Venulectasia
- Angiomas
- Spider naevi

Greasier skin

- ↑ sebaceous gland activity (2° to maternal androgens)

Appearance of skin tags

- Most commonly on the neck and in the axillae and groin area

Melasma

- Hyperpigmentation of sun-exposed skin

Acne

- Often flares in 3rd trimester (↑ circulating androgens)
- Can be distressing and disfiguring for the mother
- Management includes topical treatments (including benzoyl peroxide and azelaic acid), topical antibiotics, or oral erythromycin
- The fetus can have acne neonatorum (if maternal androgens cross the placenta)

⚠ Retinoids are teratogenic and should be avoided in pregnancy

➔ Images of all conditions are available online: ⅋ https://www.dermnetnz.org/topics/skin-problems-in-pregnancy/

Causes of pruritus in pregnancy
- Atopic eruption of pregnancy
- PEP
- PG
- Urticaria
- Scabies
- Cholestasis
- Iron deficiency

Steroids
See Table 15.1 for topical steroids.

Table 15.1 Topical steroids

Potency	Examples
Mild	• Hydrocortisone 1%
Moderate	• Betamethasone valerate 0.025%
	• Clobetasone butyrate 0.05%
Potent	• Betamethasone valerate 0.1%
	• Hydrocortisone butyrate 0.1%
	• Mometasone furoate 0.1%
Ultrapotent 🔴	• Clobetasol propionate 0.05%

🔴 A 2015 Cochrane review concluded that the prolonged exposure to potent or ultrapotent topical steroids in pregnancy *may* be associated with an ↑ risk of low birthweight babies so their use should be minimized where possible (🔗 https://www.cochrane.org/CD007346/SKIN_safety-topical-steroids-pregnancy)

Atopic eruption of pregnancy

Background

- Also known as:
  - Eczema in pregnancy
  - Prurigo of pregnancy
  - Pruritic folliculitis of pregnancy
  - Papular dermatoses of pregnancy
- Most common pregnancy-related rash and can develop early on
- Seen more frequently in ♀ with atopy or a history of eczema

Clinical features

E-type atopic eruption of pregnancy

- 2/3 of cases
- Widespread eczematous changes on the face, neck, chest, and flexural surfaces

P-type atopic eruption of pregnancy

- Papular lesions on the trunk and limbs
- Prurigo nodules on shins and arms

Recurrence of both types in future pregnancy is common.

Fetal risks

- No fetal morbidity but the infant is at ↑ risk of atopic skin disease

> **Management of atopic eruption of pregnancy**
>
> - Emollients
> - Topical steroids
> - Antihistamines
> - Phototherapy (UVB) or oral steroids may be needed in severe cases

➔ Images and an information leaflet are available online: ℘ https://www.dermcoll.edu.au/atoz/atopic-eruption-pregnancy/

Polymorphic eruption of pregnancy

Background
- Also known as pruritic urticarial papules and plaques of pregnancy
- Occurs in ~1 in 200 pregnancies
- >75% occur in 1st pregnancy with low risk of recurrence

Clinical features
- Pruritic eruption across lower abdomen
- Urticarial papules begin in abdominal striae then coalesce into plaques, then spread more distantly to buttocks and thighs
- Usually starts in the 3rd trimester and resolves at delivery or up to a month afterwards
- Spares the umbilicus

▶ Can be distinguished from PG as PEP spares the umbilicus but PG does not.

Fetal risks
- No associated fetal morbidity

Management of PEP
- Antihistamines
- Emollients
- Topical steroids (mild to moderate potency)
- Systemic steroids rarely required

⮕ Images are available online: ℬ https://www.dermnetnz.org/topics/polymorphic-eruption-of-pregnancy/

⮕ A patient leaflet is available online: ℬ http://www.bad.org.uk/shared/get-file.ashx?id=227&itemtype=document

Pemphigoid gestationis

Background
- Rare cause of pruritus in pregnancy
- IgG antibodies bind to bullous pemphigoid antigen 2 in the hemidesmosomes of the basement membrane zone causing damage and blister formation
- Can occur in 1st or subsequent pregnancy
- Recurrence in future pregnancies can be earlier and ↑ severity
- Postpartum flare seen in up to 75%, can take up to a year to resolve
- Can recur with menstruation and oral contraceptives

Clinical features
- Pruritic erythematous urticarial papules and plaques with ring-like patterns develop, followed by vesicles and bullae
- Usually starts around the umbilicus and then spreads to thighs, breasts, palms, and soles
- Typically occurs in the 2nd or 3rd trimester but has been reported earlier and postpartum

▶ Can be distinguished from PEP as PEP usually spares the umbilicus but PG does not.

Fetal effects
- Severe disease associated with preterm delivery and low birthweight
- Antibodies can cross the placenta causing a mild rash in the neonate

Diagnosis
- Skin biopsy:
  - Direct immunofluorescence demonstrates the antibodies at the basement membrane zone in all affected ♀ (not seen with PEP)
  - Indirect serum immunofluorescence may identify the antibodies

Management of PG in pregnancy
- Urgent input from Dermatology, as the treatment options include:

Mild disease
- Emollients
- Topical steroids (➋ see Table 15.1, p. 511)

Severe disease (with bullae)
- Systemic steroids (up to 1 mg/kg/day prednisolone)

Refractory disease
- IVIg
- Pulsed methylprednisolone

➋ Images are available online: ℘ https://www.dermnetnz.org/topics/pemphigoid-gestationis/

➋ A patient leaflet is available online: ℘ https://www.bad.org.uk/shared/get-file.ashx?id=224 &itemtype=document

Erythema nodosum

Background
- More common in ♀ than ♂
- Occurs most frequently in the childbearing years
- Can be triggered by pregnancy and the oral contraceptive pill
- Hypersensitivity reaction triggered by several conditions including:
  - Streptococcal infection (most common cause)
  - Sarcoidosis
  - IBD
  - Malignancy
  - TB
  - Many cases are idiopathic

Clinical features
- Tender, red or violet subcutaneous nodules
- Usually in the pretibial region but less frequently occur on other parts of the legs or buttocks
- Can last up to 8 wks
- Systemic features can also occur prior to the onset of the skin lesions, including:
  - Fever
  - Malaise
  - Arthralgia
- Skin biopsy shows panniculitis without features of vasculitis

Management of erythema nodosum in pregnancy
- Careful history (medications, travel, illnesses) and examination for underlying cause (including throat)
- Consider CXR if sarcoid or TB a possibility
- Consideration of testing for streptococcal infection or TB depending on the clinical history
- Mainstay of management is supportive care as the lesions tend to resolve spontaneously
- Severe cases may require oral steroids

➲ Images are available online: ℛ https://www.dermnetnz.org/topics/erythema-nodosum/

Erythema multiforme

Background

- A rare condition which occurs in ♀ less frequently than ♂
- Commonest ages are the 3rd to 4th decade, i.e. overlapping with childbearing years
- Usually a self-limiting condition with resolution seen over weeks
- Can be triggered by pregnancy
- Many other causative factors have been suggested which include:
  - Viral infections (HSV is the most common)
  - *Mycoplasma pneumoniae* infection
  - Drugs (<10% of cases) such as antibiotics, NSAIDs, and AEDs
  - Malignancy
  - Sarcoidosis

Symptoms

- Eruption of papules, macules, and vesicles in a symmetrical distribution, including the classic 'target' lesion
- Papules sometimes develop at trauma sites ('Koebner phenomenon')
- Rash often lasts 2–4 wks
- Mucosa of the mouth, eye, and genitalia can also be involved which can be very painful

Management of erythema multiforme in pregnancy

- Identification of the underlying cause is key
- If severe and involving oral mucosa, treatment options include:
  - Topical local anaesthetic agents
  - Analgesic/anti-inflammatory mouthwashes

➔ Images are available online: ℘ https://www.dermnetnz.org/topics/erythema-multiforme/

Pemphigus vulgaris

Background
- Can worsen in pregnancy or present *de novo*
- Autoimmune condition featuring antibodies to the epidermal proteins desmoglein 3 or 1

Clinical features
- Flaccid blisters or erosions on the trunk and limbs
- Often also involves the oral and genital mucosae

Fetal effects
- Neonatal pemphigus:
  - Results from antibody transfer across the placenta
  - More likely if the mother has oral involvement (the desmoglein 3 profile in the oral mucosa is the same as that in the fetal skin)
- No correlation between severity in mother and the neonate

Management of pemphigus vulgaris in pregnancy
- The diagnosis is based on clinical features but skin biopsy can be performed if there is diagnostic uncertainty
- Discussion with Dermatology as treatment options include:
  - Oral steroids
  - Plasmapheresis/plasma exchange
  - Dapsone
  - Azathioprine

➲ Images are available online: ℛ https://www.dermnetnz.org/topics/pemphigus-vulgaris/

Psoriasis

Background

- This is a common skin condition associated with systemic manifestations (➔ see 'Psoriatic arthropathy', p. 276)

Different manifestations

Chronic plaque psoriasis

- Commonest type of psoriasis
- Typical symmetrical psoriatic plaques on extensor surfaces or on scalp
- In many ♀ this improves in pregnancy

Guttate psoriasis

- This features small psoriatic plaques and papules
- Can occur after acute streptococcal infection
- Most commonly occurs in children and young adults

Pustular psoriasis of pregnancy

- Previously known as impetigo herpetiformis
- Rare, life-threatening variant of generalized pustular psoriasis
- Sudden onset of erythema, scaling, and superficial pustules which can be very extensive
- Can be associated with systemic manifestations including:
  - Fever
  - Diarrhoea
  - Hypocalcaemia
  - Tetany
  - Malaise
- Typically occurs in 3rd trimester or early postpartum period
- Symmetrical erythematous plaques are seen with rings of sterile pustules at the edges
- Begins on flexures and spreads, and usually involves the trunk and limbs, sparing the hands, feet, and face

Management of psoriasis in pregnancy

- Bloods for:
  - FBC (leucocytosis may be seen)
  - U&Es (hypocalcaemia particularly) if unwell with pustular psoriasis of pregnancy
- Treatment options then depend on:
  - Type of psoriasis
  - Distribution and extent of lesions
  - Gestation (or breastfeeding status if postpartum)

Treatment options for psoriasis in pregnancy

Topical agents
- Emollients
- Topical steroids:
  - Low to moderate potency preferred initially
  - Reserve more potent steroids for those who do not respond
- Topical calcineurin inhibitors:
  - Not that effective but can be used in pregnancy if required

⚠ Tazarotene is a topical retinoid and should not be used in pregnancy.

Phototherapy
- Narrowband UVB phototherapy (wavelength 311 nm) can be used safely
- Usually instituted in addition to topical agents
- Can ↑ the chance of melasma developing

Systemic treatments
- Ciclosporin
- Sulfasalazine:
  - Can be used in pregnancy
  - 5 mg folic acid OD should be prescribed during therapy
  - Is of limited use in the treatment of psoriasis
- Oral steroids:
  - Only used in pustular psoriasis of pregnancy, as risk of flare when treatment stopped

Biologics
(➲ See Table 8.11, p. 3.)
- Being ↑ used in non-pregnant ♀ with psoriasis
- Adalimumab, etanercept, and infliximab can be used
- Ustekinumab (targeting IL-12 and IL-23):
  - Is an effective treatment for psoriasis
  - Use in pregnancy is limited to case reports but there were no complications
- Secukinumab (targeting IL-17A):
  - Newer biological therapy for use in severe psoriasis
  - No complications reported in small series of pregnant ♀

⚠ Methotrexate should be avoided in pregnancy or when planning to conceive

⚠ Acitretin is an oral retinoid and it is recommended that pregnancy is avoided for 3 years following the last dose

Perinatal mental health

Overview

- 10–20% of ♀ develop a mental health problem during pregnancy or the year after birth
- Risk of a severe mental health problem is greater in the immediate postpartum than at any other point in a ♀'s life
- Vulnerable ♀ have a higher rate of mental health problems compared to the general population
- Suicide is the leading cause of direct maternal death in the year after birth
- Perinatal mental health problems ↑ risk of psychological and developmental problems in the offspring
- Of the ♀ who die 2° to perinatal mental health problems, improvements to care would make a difference to outcome in a substantial number

Role of maternity service

- Screen for mental health problems
- Liaise with GP, e.g. inform of pregnancy, explicitly enquire about mental health, and alert if mental health problems escalate
- Enquire about current mental health throughout pregnancy and early postpartum
- Refer ♀ at risk of severe mental health problems to specialist care
- Refer ♀ with mental health problems to appropriate specialist care
- ↓ impact of physical health problems on mental health
- Collaborate with all elements of the perinatal mental health service

Screening for mental health problems in pregnancy

⚠ All pregnant ♀ should be screened for mental health problems taking note of:

- Past or present severe* mental health problem
- Past or present treatment by a specialist mental health service, including inpatient care
- Severe perinatal mental health problem in a 1st-degree relative

⚠ ♀ may not disclose mental health problems due to anticipated discrimination, self-perceived resilience, fear of negative perception of them as a mother, fear of custody loss, or the very nature of the mental health problem.

*A severe mental health problem is defined by NICE as severe and incapacitating depression, psychosis, schizophrenia, bipolar affective disorder, schizoaffective disorder or postpartum psychosis.

➔ NICE (2014). Antenatal and postnatal mental health (CG192): ℞ https://www.nice.org.uk/guidance/cg192/

Mental health

Definition

A state of well-being in which every individual realises his or her own potential, can cope with the normal stresses of life, can work productively and fruitfully, and is able to make a contribution to her or his community. (WHO, 2014)

- Good mental health is not just the absence of mental health problems

Determinants of mental health

- Mental health is influenced by biological, psychological, and social factors (Fig. 16.1)
- These factors:
  - Threaten or protect mental health
  - Impact and accumulate, over the whole life course
  - Interact dynamically and with significant complexity

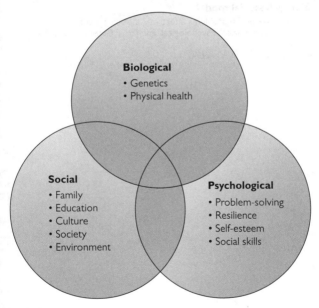

Fig. 16.1 Determinants of mental health.

Cause and effect

- Social deprivation ↑ risk of mental health problems

Risk factors for mental health problems include:

- Poverty
- Unmanageable financial debt
- Homelessness
- Poor quality, insecure, and overcrowded housing
- Unemployment and unstable employment
- Exposure to violent or unsafe environments
- Being a victim of crime
- Being a survivor of physical and/or sexual violence

▶ Mental health problems impact on social factors, e.g. employment, relationships:

- Bi-directional dynamic between mental health problems and social factors
- Can create a 'spiral of adversity'
- The same bi-directional dynamic is also seen with mental health and biological and psychological factors

⚠ Complex relationship between cause and effect

Biopsychosocial model

- To manage health problems effectively, including mental health problems, biological, psychological, and social factors must all be addressed
- A MDT approach is needed

General principles

- All ♀ with a mental health problem should have an individualized care plan which:
  - Is written in collaboration and shared with the ♀ and the MDT
  - Should state who is responsible for coordinating care, and who is responsible for each aspect of care

Preconception considerations

- Review current and previous mental health problems (diagnosis, severity, recency of acute episodes, previous response to medication)
- Refer to perinatal mental health service

Biological

- Review current contraception
- Ensure also receiving normal antenatal care, including folic acid and vitamin D (doses depending on risk factors and local guidelines)
- Review current interaction between mental health and physical factors, psychological factors, and social factors

Psychiatric medications and pregnancy

- Discuss risk versus benefit of current medication:
  - Risk of relapse if medication stopped
  - Risk to the ♀, infant, and family of not treating the mental health problem
  - Risk of fetal and/or infant exposure
  - Risk to the ♀ from medication, e.g. overdose
  - Risk versus benefit of changing medication
  - Risk versus benefit of non-pharmacological interventions
- If commencing or changing medication:
  - Consider the ♀'s previous response to medication
  - Use lowest risk profile for the ♀, fetus, and infant
  - Use lowest effective dose
  - Use as few drugs as possible
  - Avoid depot medication (unless history of non-adherence to oral medication)

➔ NICE (2014). Antenatal and postnatal mental health (CG192): ⌕ https://www.nice.org.uk/guidance/cg192/

General considerations in pregnancy and postpartum

- Manage all ♀ with a history of a severe mental health problem as high risk
- Monitor regularly for symptoms of relapse or deterioration

Biological

- Continue to review risk versus benefit of medication throughout pregnancy and postpartum

⚠ Avoid sudden discontinuation of medication on diagnosis of pregnancy, as may not remove risk of teratogenicity and may → sudden relapse or ↑ risk

- Organize detailed USS ± fetal echocardiogram if medication has a significant risk of teratogenicity
- Serial USS if ↑ risk of IUGR or SGA
- Monitor infant for adverse medication effects

Psychological

- Assess attitude of ♀ towards pregnancy
- Assess mother–infant attachment and relationship

Social

- Ensure continuity of care in pregnancy and postpartum
- Enhanced postnatal care:
  - Monitor for relapse
  - Additional and/or extended appointments with midwife
  - Comprehensive handover to health visitor and GP

⚠ Ensure ongoing support to ♀ if loss of custody

⊅ NICE (2014). Antenatal and postnatal mental health (CG192): ℬ https://www.nice.org.uk/guidance/cg192/

Depression

Prevalence

- Common: 100–150 in 1000 pregnant ♀ have a mild–moderate depressive problem; severe in 30 of 1000 pregnant ♀
- A depressive episode is traditionally classified as postnatal depression if onset is within 4–6 wks of birth

▶ The extent to which postnatal depression is a separate clinical entity to depression at any other time is subject to debate.

Clinical features of depression

- Low mood
- ↓ energy and/or ↓ activity
- Anhedonia and/or loss of interest in usual activities
- ↓ in concentration
- ↑ fatigability
- Disturbed sleep, e.g. early waking
- ↓ appetite
- ↓ self-esteem and/or self-confidence
- Feelings of guilt and/or worthlessness

These features:

- Pervade all aspects of life
- Show little day-to-day variation, i.e. present most of the day, nearly every day
- Do not respond to changes in circumstances
- May be accompanied by 'somatic' symptoms, e.g. psychomotor retardation, agitation, weight loss, loss of libido

▶ Severity is dependent on the number of symptoms and their impact on the activities of daily life.

Differential diagnosis

▶ Not all ♀ referred with 'depression' have the clinical condition:

Baby blues

- Emotional changes following birth (not pathological)
- Affects ≥50% of ♀ postpartum
- Mild depressive symptoms, which last <10 days
- Self-resolving; does not require medical treatment

Sadness

- Emotional state, i.e. an inherent aspect of the human experience
- Not a pathological condition, does not require medical treatment
- Not usually pervasive, may resolve with a change in circumstances
- No clinically significant impairment or distress

Grief

- ♀ may experience profound loss in pregnancy, e.g. bereavement including stillbirth, financial loss, loss of physical health

Management of depression in pregnancy

Biological

(➲ See 'Psychotropic medications' Table 16.5, p. 555.)

⚠ If antidepressants stopped during pregnancy ↑ risk of relapse

⚠ After starting, ↑ risk of suicidal ideation in those <25 yrs, but active treatment of depression ↓ overall risk of suicide

- 1st line—SSRIs
- If severe depression consider ECT

⚠ Do not use monoamine oxidase inhibitors: ↑ risk of congenital malformations, ↑ risk of hypertensive crisis

Psychological

- Facilitated self-help if mild or moderate depression
- High-intensity psychological intervention if moderate or severe depression, e.g. cognitive behavioural therapy
- Risk assessment for self-harm and suicide (➲ see p. 551)

Social

- Advice on sleep hygiene
- Support to ↓ social isolation, e.g. antenatal classes, baby groups
- ↓ impact of detrimental socioeconomic factors, e.g.:
  - Insecure housing → contact local housing officer
  - Domestic violence → domestic violence advocacy
- Enhanced postnatal care:
  - Monitor for relapse
  - Additional and/or extended appointments with midwife
  - Comprehensive handover to health visitor and GP

Impact of depression on pregnancy

Depression has far-reaching effects on the family unit as a whole.

Maternal
- ↑ risk of maternal death:
  - ↑ risk of suicide
  - Most common diagnosis prior to maternal suicide
- ↑ risk of maternal morbidity:
  - Self-neglect, including poor diet
  - ↑ risk of substance use
  - ↑ risk of self-harm
- ↑ risk of substandard antenatal care:
  - ↑ difficulty attending appointments 2° ↓ energy and/or ↓ activity

Fetal
- ↑ risk of fetal morbidity:
  - ↑ risk of spontaneous miscarriage
  - ↑ risk of low birthweight
  - ↑ risk of preterm birth

Offspring
- ↑ risk of neonatal/infant morbidity
- Impact on mother–infant attachment and relationship with ↑ risk in the offspring of:
  - Depression
  - Emotional problems
  - Symptoms of ADHD and conduct disorders
  - Impaired cognitive function
  - Schizophrenia
  - Maltreatment 2° to other adults
  - Underweight and stunting (low and middle-income countries) and overweight (high-income countries)

Family
- ↑ risk of paternal depression in postpartum period
- Impact on father–infant attachment and relationship

Electroconvulsive therapy
- Potential treatment for severe depression, e.g. if medication has been tried but not proven effective, life-threatening dehydration or malnutrition, or acute suicidal ideation
- Provides rapid resolution of symptoms
- Neuromodulatory treatment with induction of bilateral generalised seizure required for beneficial effect
- Requires anaesthesia and muscle relaxant
- Evidence on complication rate is limited

⚠ ↑ risk of VTE

Schizophrenia

Prevalence
- 0.7% adult population have schizoaffective disorder or schizophrenia

---

Clinical features of schizophrenia
- Characterized by a pattern of signs and symptoms
- Severe impact on occupational and/or social functioning
- Most individuals require support with daily living

Distortions of thinking
- Formal thought disorder, e.g. switching from one topic to another such that communication is substantially impaired
- Thought insertion, withdrawal, broadcasting, or echo
- Delusions of control, influence, or passivity

Distortions of perception
- Hallucinatory voices commenting on, or discussing, the individual, in the 3rd person

Inappropriate or blunted affect
- ↓ emotional expression
- Laughing in the absence of an appropriate stimulus

Impact of pregnancy on schizophrenia
- Pregnancy is probably not protective against psychosis
- ↑ risk of relapse in year following birth

Risks of schizophrenia in pregnancy
- Unplanned pregnancy
- Maternal death (suicide, sudden cardiac death)
- ↑ risk maternal morbidity (co-morbidities, i.e. obesity, T2DM, cardiovascular and respiratory disease, poor self-care, including poor nutrition, substance use)
- ↓ engagement in health maintenance, e.g. GDM screening
- Antipsychotic-related weight gain, T2DM, hypertension, ECG abnormalities, e.g. QTc prolongation
- GDM 2° to atypical (2nd-generation) antipsychotics
- Substandard antenatal care (difficulty attending appointments, poor communication with healthcare professionals)
- Fetal death and morbidity (low birthweight, preterm birth)
- Infant death and morbidity
- Impact on mother–infant attachment and relationship

→ MBRRACE-UK 2017 report: ℘ https://www.npeu.ox.ac.uk/mbrrace-uk/reports/confidential-enquiry-into-maternal-deaths

Management of schizophrenia in pregnancy

Biological
- Advice on diet and nutrition
- Review risk versus benefit of antipsychotic (➲ see 'Psychotropic medications', Table 16.5, p. 555)
- Baseline ECG
- Monitor weight gain
- Screen for GDM—oral GTT
- If catatonia, and severe physical risk to ♀ or fetus, consider ECT

⚠ Do not prescribe valproate to ♀ of childbearing age

Psychological
- Cognitive behavioural therapy
- Family intervention

Social
- Consider home visits
- May require assessment of activities of daily living
- Encourage and support to ↓ social isolation, e.g. antenatal classes, baby groups
- Consider safeguarding assessment if significantly impaired functioning and/or significant risk to infant, e.g. worrying content of psychotic symptoms
- Enhanced postnatal care:
  - Monitor for relapse
  - Additional and/or extended appointments with midwife
  - Comprehensive handover to health visitor and GP

Bipolar affective disorder

Prevalence
- 2% of the adult population

Clinical features of bipolar effective disorder

≥2 episodes of significant disturbance of mood and activity levels:
- Mania (or hypomania)
- Depression
- Significant impact on employment and socioeconomic status

Features of mania
- Elevated mood
- ↑ energy
- Overactivity
- Pressure of speech
- ↓ need for sleep
- Unable to sustain attention
- Inflated self-esteem, with grandiose ideas
- Loss of normal social inhibitions, → inappropriate/out-of-character behaviour

Features of depression
→ See p. 527.

Impact of pregnancy on bipolar affective disorder
- Pregnancy does not protect from recurrence
- ⚠ Growing evidence that birth is a trigger for relapse

Impact of bipolar affective disorder on pregnancy
- ↑ risk of maternal death (higher lifetime risk of suicide)
- ↑ risk maternal morbidity (obesity, substance use, postpartum psychosis)
- Antipsychotic-related weight gain, T2DM, hypertension, ECG abnormalities, e.g. QTc prolongation
- Gestational diabetes (GDM) 2° to atypical (2nd-generation) antipsychotics
- Obstetric complications e.g. induction of labour, caesarean section, instrumental delivery
- Unplanned pregnancy
- Neonatal morbidity (preterm birth, ↑ risk of neonatal hypoglycaemia)

→ MBRRACE-UK 2017 report: ℛ https://www.npeu.ox.ac.uk/mbrrace-uk/reports/confidential-enquiry-into-maternal-deaths

Management of bipolar affective disorder in pregnancy

Biological

⚠ Do not prescribe valproate to ♀ of childbearing age
- Prior to conception: if taking an anticonvulsant or lithium, consider switching to a mood-stabilizing antipsychotic
- Review risk versus benefit of mood stabilizer

⚠ If prophylactic mood stabilizers are stopped, ↑ risk of relapse, ↓ time to relapse, ↑ length of relapse

- Consider specific issues with medications:
  - Advise on diet and nutrition (monitor weight gain)
  - Antipsychotics: screen for GDM (GTT)
  - Lithium: careful fluid balance monitoring in labour
  - Antidepressants: risk of inducing mania

⚠ Consider ECT if mania and severe physical risk to ♀ or fetus

Psychological

- Self-monitoring using mood diaries
- Structured individual, group, and family interventions:
  - Depression: cognitive behavioural therapy, interpersonal therapy, couples therapy
- Monitor and actively prepare for potential postpartum psychosis:
  - Raise awareness that stressors, irregular activity patterns, and sleep disturbance can trigger relapse
  - Create list of early warning signs
  - Create treatment plan to initiate if early warning signs detected, including care plan for infant
  - Monitor for prodromal symptoms/signs immediately after birth

⚠ Red flags for relapse and/or postpartum psychosis include:
  - Recent significant change in mental state
  - Emergence of new symptoms
  - New thoughts or acts of violent self-harm
  - New and persistent expressions of incompetency as a mother
  - Estrangement from the infant

⊃ MBRRACE-UK 2017 report: ℘ https://www.npeu.ox.ac.uk/mbrrace-uk/reports/confidential-enquiry-into-maternal-deaths

Social

- Explore options to ↓ potential life stressors
- Sleep hygiene
- Support to ↓ social isolation, e.g. antenatal classes, baby groups
- Enhanced postnatal care:
  - Monitor for relapse
  - Additional and/or extended appointments with midwife
  - Comprehensive handover to health visitor and GP

Postpartum (puerperal) psychosis

- Postpartum period associated with ↑ risk for a manic or psychotic episode compared with other times of life
- The term 'postpartum psychosis' is not strictly a diagnosis; it does not appear in international classification systems
- Evidence indicates an association with bipolar affective disorder
- Recovery can take up to 6–12 mths

Incidence

- 0.1–0.25% in the general population

Clinical features of puerperal psychosis

- Onset often within 2 wks of birth, and most within a few days
- Sudden onset and rapid deterioration
- Severe symptoms of mania and/or depression (➔ see pp. 527, 532):
  - Mood can swing rapidly from one extreme to the other
  - Delusions, especially paranoid delusions, e.g. of persecution, being dead, grandeur, contact with God, child exchange, death of child
- Hallucinations, e.g. auditory 2nd person—'That's not your baby'
- Confusion or perplexity is common
- Evidence for a prodromal phase before onset of overt psychosis:
  - Frequently hypomanic in nature, e.g. excited, giggly, chatty
  - Difficult to recognize, unless specifically monitored for, as can be easily attributable to the ♀ 'coping well'

Risk factors for puerperal psychosis

- Previous episode of:
  - Postpartum psychosis: risk 25–50%
  - Bipolar affective disorder: risk 25–50%
  - Bipolar affective disorder and family history of postpartum psychosis: risk >50%
- 1st-degree family history of postpartum psychosis or bipolar affective disorder
- ▶ 50% of ♀ have no history to suggest high risk
- Primiparity is the only known obstetric risk factor

Differential diagnosis

- Delirium, e.g. 2° to sepsis:
  - If diagnostic uncertainty, ensure MDT involvement with consultant obstetrician and consultant psychiatrist

➔ MBRRACE-UK 2017 report: ⅋ https://www.npeu.ox.ac.uk/mbrrace-uk/reports/confidential-enquiry-into-maternal-deaths

Management of puerperal psychosis
⚠ Psychiatric emergency

Early identification
- At booking, identify high-risk ♀

If history of bipolar affective disorder (→ see p. 532):
- Monitor and actively prepare for potential postpartum psychosis:
  - Raise awareness that stressors, irregular activity patterns, and sleep disturbance can trigger relapse
  - Create list of early warning signs
  - Create treatment plan to initiate if early warning signs detected, including care plan for infant
  - Monitor for prodromal symptoms/signs after delivery

⚠ Red flags for relapse and/or postpartum psychosis include:
- Recent significant change in mental state
- Emergence of new symptoms
- New thoughts or acts of violent self-harm
- New and persistent expressions of incompetency as a mother
- Estrangement from the infant

→ MBRRACE-UK 2017 report: ⌘ https://www.npeu.ox.ac.uk/mbrrace-uk/reports/confidential-enquiry-into-maternal-deaths

Biological
- Antipsychotics
- Antidepressants
- Mood stabilizers

Psychological
- Ongoing assessment of mother–infant attachment and relationship
- Discuss any concerns the ♀ may have and provide information, support, and treatment, e.g. referral to parent–infant mental health service

Social
- Admission to mother and baby unit
- Support to the partner/family
- Enhanced postnatal care:
  - Monitor for relapse
  - Additional and/or extended appointments with midwife
  - Comprehensive handover to health visitor and GP

Future pregnancy
- >60% of ♀ will have a further episode not related to pregnancy

⚠ Avoiding future pregnancy will not necessarily avoid future mental health problems

Generalized anxiety disorder

Prevalence
- 5.9% of the adult population

Clinical features
- Generalized and persistent anxiety
- Not restricted to any set of circumstances—'free floating'
- The 2-item Generalized Anxiety Disorder scale (GAD-2) can be used to screen for anxiety disorders
- Differences between GAD and normal worries are outlined in Table 16.1

Impact of GAD on pregnancy
- ↑ risk of maternal morbidity:
  - Physical symptoms of GAD may be inappropriately attributed to a physical health problem → over-investigation, overtreatment, and potential exacerbation of the existing anxiety
  - Symptoms of a physical health problem may be inappropriately attributed to GAD → under-investigation and lack of treatment
- Impact on mother–infant attachment and relationship → ↑ risk of neonatal/infant morbidity including:
  - ↑ risk of emotional problems, ADHD, and conduct disorders
  - Impaired cognitive function
  - Schizophrenia
- ↓ ability of ♀ to encourage confidence in her children

Table 16.1 Differences between GAD and non-pathological anxiety

GAD	Non-pathological anxiety or 'normal worries'
Anxiety is excessive/out of proportion to the likelihood or impact of the event	Anxiety is proportionate to the likelihood or impact of the event
Anxiety interferes with other tasks or activities	Anxiety can be 'put aside'
Anxiety is perceived as overwhelming	Anxiety is perceived as manageable
Anxiety is accompanied by physical symptoms, e.g. dizziness, epigastric discomfort, muscular tension, palpitations, sweating, trembling	Anxiety is not usually accompanied by physical symptoms

Management of GAD in pregnancy

Biological
- ↓ caffeine intake
- Consider SSRIs
- Risk of harmful substance use and dependence syndrome
- ⚠ Only offer benzodiazepines for short-term treatment of severe anxiety

Psychological
- Low-intensity psychological intervention (facilitated self-help, psychoeducational groups)
- High-intensity psychological intervention (cognitive behavioural therapy, applied relaxation)

Social
- Advice on sleep hygiene
- Encourage and support to ↓ social isolation, e.g. antenatal classes, baby groups
- Enhanced postnatal care:
  - Monitor for relapse
  - Additional and/or extended appointments with midwife
  - Comprehensive handover to health visitor and GP

Blood, injury, and injection phobia

This is an example of a phobic anxiety disorder, which features:
- Symptoms of anxiety are evoked in *situations* that are well-defined and not currently dangerous
- Anxiety, and anticipatory anxiety, are out of proportion to the actual danger posed by the *situation*
- *Situation* is avoided or endured with dread
- Focus is often on a specific symptom, e.g. palpitations, but associated with 2° fear of dying or losing control

Prevalence
- 7.2% of pregnant ♀
- High prevalence among 1st-degree relatives

Clinical features of BII phobia
- 80% experience vasovagal syncope or pre-syncope
- ▶ Most other specific phobias generate a 'fight or flight' response

---

Impact on pregnancy
- 2 maternal deaths partly attributable to BII phobia in UK since 2000:
  - Declining regional anaesthesia → gastric aspiration at time of caesarean section under general anaesthetic
  - Declining thromboprophylaxis → pulmonary embolism
- ↑ risk of maternal death and/or morbidity:
  - From anaesthesia
  - 2° to declining blood tests, e.g. failure to diagnose anaemia, alloimmunization
  - 2° to declining injections, e.g. haemorrhage 2° to no injectable uterotonics; hyperglycaemia as a result of declining insulin
  - Physical symptoms may be inappropriately attributed to a physical problem → over-investigation and overtreatment
  - Symptoms of a physical health problem may be inappropriately attributed to the phobia → under-investigation and lack of treatment
  - Avoidance of clinical environment may → delay in booking antenatal care
  - ↑ risk of neonatal death and/or morbidity as a result of declining regional anaesthesia, avoidance of clinical environment, e.g. declining hospital birth against maternity care advice

Management of BII phobia in pregnancy

Biological
- Anaesthetic review
- Consideration of the use of local anaesthetic cream and fine-bore needles
- Presence of senior clinician

Psychological
- Low-intensity psychological intervention (facilitated self-help)
- High-intensity psychological intervention (exposure-only cognitive behavioural therapy)

Social
- Consider use of less overtly clinical environments for appointments, e.g. community centres, home visits
- Support to attend appointments in clinical environments
- Consider home birth or birth in midwifery-led unit
- Choice of birth partner, if birth partner also has BII phobia discuss the impact of this as well as potential solutions, e.g. self-referral of birth partner for therapy, presence of 2nd birth partner

⚠ If the ♀ achieves partial or complete resolution of her phobia during pregnancy, ensure any previous omissions in her maternity care are addressed, e.g. re-offer screening for blood-borne viruses.

⚠ If the phobia is severe and remains resistant to treatment, consider the creation of an **advanced directive**.

Tocophobia

Prevalence
- Anxiety relating to birth is common
- Broad spectrum from non-pathological anxiety to tocophobia
- May affect up to 14% of pregnant ♀ to some degree
- 1° and 2° tocophobia are defined in Table 16.2

> **Clinical features of tocophobia**
> - Fear may be focused on specific aspects of birth, e.g.:
>   - Abandonment by healthcare professionals during birth
>   - Fear of mistreatment and/or obstetrical violence
>   - Loss of autonomy and control
>   - Medical interventions
> - Avoidance may be of any aspect of birth, e.g. talking about birth
> - Assessment tools may aid diagnosis, e.g. Wijma Delivery Expectancy/Experience Questionnaire (W-DEQ)

Impact on pregnancy
- ↑ risk of maternal morbidity:
  - Avoidance of preparation for birth
  - Refusal of appropriate medical interventions
- ↑ risk of social isolation:
  - Avoidance of antenatal classes
- ↑ risk of pregnancy loss:
  - Termination of pregnancy, even if desires a family
- ↑ risk of neonatal/infant morbidity
- Impact on mother–infant attachment and relationship

Management of tocophobia in pregnancy

Biological
- If elective caesarean section requested:
  - Detailed risk versus benefit discussion with ♀
  - Ensure ongoing discussion as pregnancy progresses

Psychological
- Low-intensity psychological intervention (facilitated self-help):
  - If associated with PTSD offer high-intensity psychological intervention (e.g. trauma-focused cognitive behavioural therapy, eye movement desensitization and reprocessing)

Social
- Consider home birth
- Emphasis on continuity of care
- Enhanced counselling if considering termination of pregnancy
- If a history of physical and/or sexual violence is disclosed:
  - Acknowledge bravery of disclosure
  - Encourage to contact support organizations, e.g. Rape Crisis
  - A safeguarding assessment may be necessary
- Encourage and support to join local support networks, e.g. antenatal classes, baby groups
- Enhanced postnatal care:
  - Monitor for relapse
  - Additional and/or extended appointments with midwife
  - Comprehensive handover to health visitor and GP

Table 16.2 Primary and secondary tocophobia

1° tocophobia	2° tocophobia

• Develops before pregnancy:
  • Often since childhood or adolescence
• Sometimes associated with:
  • Childhood sexual abuse
  • Observing or hearing about negative experiences of birth
	• Following a pregnancy event experienced as negative or traumatic
	• Sometimes related to PTSD

Obsessive–compulsive disorder

Prevalence

- 1.3% of the adult population

Clinical features of OCD

- Obsessional thoughts which are nearly always distressing:
  - Ideas, images, or impulses—often relating to contamination, symmetry, and/or aggression
  - Enter the individual's mind repeatedly, 'intrusions'
  - Recognized as own mind but unable to resist them
- Ruminations—indecisive, endless, consideration of alternatives, resulting in an inability to make day-to-day decisions
- Compulsive acts—stereotyped behaviours or mental acts, e.g. mentally repeating a certain phrase, which do not result in completion of a useful task:
  - Intended to prevent an objectively unlikely event
  - If resisted → ↑ anxiety

'Intrusive' thoughts versus 'obsessional' thoughts
- Intrusive thoughts, doubts, and images are normal
- Content can be indistinguishable from obsessional thoughts, e.g. 'I am going to stab my baby', is a common, intrusive thought
- Intrusive thoughts can be critically appraised, dismissed, and do not motivate compulsive acts

---

Impact on pregnancy

⚠ Risk does not arise from the obsessional thought(s):
- No recorded cases of a ♀ with OCD carrying out their obsession
- Risk arises from the unintended consequences of acting on compulsions

---

⚠ Risk of misdiagnosis

- Obsessional thoughts misdiagnosed as delusions →:
  - Misdiagnosis of postpartum psychosis
  - Inappropriate harmful management, e.g. separating ♀ and baby
  - Distress, ↑ avoidance, and ↑ compulsive behaviours in ♀
- Sexual fantasy of sex offender misdiagnosed as obsessional thoughts → possible sexual abuse of child

⚠ Risk assessment **must** involve a perinatal mental health specialist

---

Risks to pregnancy
See Table 16.3.

Management of OCD in pregnancy

Biological
- Consider SSRIs

Psychological
- Cognitive behavioural therapy
- Careful balance between ensuring best practice maternity care and accommodating compulsive acts, e.g.:
  - If non-attendance at appointments 2° to compulsive acts, consider offering home visits

Social
- Sensitive enquiry regarding obsessional thoughts:
  - ♀ may be reluctant to discuss these, e.g. may fear custody loss
- Sensitive and appropriate safeguarding assessment if concerns about impaired functioning and/or risk to infant
- Encourage and support to ↓ social isolation, e.g. antenatal classes, baby groups
- Enhanced postnatal care (monitor for relapse, additional and/or extended appointments with midwife, comprehensive handover to health visitor and GP)
- Appropriate support for partner/family, e.g. partner may be enmeshed in compulsive acts → significant exhaustion

Table 16.3 Examples of risks from compulsive behaviours

Obsessional or ruminative thought	Compulsive act	Impact from unintended consequence
'My baby is going to be stillborn'	• Repeatedly checking fetal movements	• Sleep deprivation • Maternal morbidity, e.g. depression • Repeated hospital attendance • ↑ risk of poor relationship with healthcare professionals
'My baby is going to die from contamination'	• Avoidance of others	• Social isolation
	• Cleaning rituals	• Delayed response to infant feeding cues as repeatedly sterilizing bottle/ washing breast • Irritation of newborn skin from repeated use of cleaning products
'I am going to suffocate my baby'	• Minimal handling of infant	• Impact on mother–infant attachment and relationship • Maternal death 2° suicide: • ♀ takes her own life to protect her child

Anorexia nervosa

Background
- 0.6% of adult population
- Pregnancy affects body shape and eating behaviour, which can be challenging for ♀ with a current/history of an eating disorder
- Residual symptoms are common
- Amenorrhea is common in very underweight ♀ but infertility should not be assumed

---

Clinical features of anorexia nervosa
- Dread of fatness and flabbiness of body contour persists as an intrusive, overvalued idea
- Deliberate weight loss, with a self-imposed low weight threshold
- Weight loss is achieved by:
  - Restricted diet and/or excessive exercise
  - Induced vomiting and purging
  - Manipulation of medication, e.g. insulin, levothyroxine
  - Use of appetite suppressants, diuretics, and/or enemas

Impact on pregnancy

Maternal risks
- ⚠ Highest mortality rate of all mental health problems
- ↑ risk of maternal death (e.g. suicide, sudden cardiac death)
- Maternal morbidity including:
  - Physical health complications
  - Hyperemesis gravidarum
  - Substance use
  - Depression and anxiety

Infant risks
- ↑ risk of SGA, low birthweight:
  - Nutritional issues including feeding difficulties, poor growth
  - Impact on mother–infant attachment and relationship

Physical health complications of anorexia nervosa
- Arrhythmias, including bradycardia
- Aspiration pneumonia
- Cerebral atrophy
- Gastroparesis
- Hypoglycaemia
- Mitral valve motion abnormalities
- Pancytopenia
- Pericardial effusion
- Refeeding syndrome
- Thyroid function abnormalities

Management of anorexia nervosa in pregnancy

Preconception
- Psychoeducation about body image
- Nutritional counselling
- If active eating disorder, or receiving active treatment, advise to delay pregnancy until in remission or recovered

Biological
- Advice on nutrition, diet, and exercise
- If purging, provide information on the safety of drugs in pregnancy, consider SSRI
- Baseline medical investigations, e.g. ECG, FBC, liver function, renal function, electrolytes, glucose, thyroid function
- Baseline vital signs, e.g. pulse, temperature
- Anaesthetic review

▶ Standard dose–effect calculations may not be appropriate for very low BMI ♀ in late pregnancy
- Serial USS to monitor for fetal growth restriction
- Monitor weight and BMI, consider admission if failure to gain adequate weight
- Monitor fluid balance intrapartum as ↑ risk of dehydration
- Monitor infant weight and growth

Psychological
- Individual eating disorder-focused cognitive behavioural therapy
- 'Maudsley Anorexia Nervosa Treatment for Adults' model
- Specialist supportive clinical management
- Eating disorder-focused focal psychodynamic therapy
- Assess mother–infant attachment and relationship:
  - Discuss any concerns the ♀ may have and provide information, support, and treatment, e.g. referral to parent–infant mental health service

Social
- Enhanced postnatal care:
  - Monitor for relapse
  - Additional and/or extended appointments with midwife
  - Comprehensive handover to health visitor and GP
- Referral to specialist midwife for breastfeeding support

Bulimia nervosa

Prevalence
- 1% of the adult population

Clinical features
- Excessive preoccupation with the control of body weight
- Repeated bouts of overeating
- Purging behaviours (self-induced vomiting, use of stimulant laxatives, diuretics, and/or enemas)
- Often previous history of anorexia nervosa

Impact on pregnancy

Maternal risks
- ↑ risk maternal death (suicide, or 2° to electrolyte and acid–base abnormalities, e.g. arrhythmias)
- Physical health complications:
  - Cathartic colon syndrome
  - Diarrhoea
  - Gastric acid reflux
  - Haemorrhoids
  - Oedema
  - Rectal prolapse
- Substance use
- Depression/anxiety

Fetal risks
- Neonatal morbidity including ↑ risk of large for gestational age

Management

Biological
- Advice on diet and nutrition
- Baseline medical investigations, e.g. ECG, electrolytes
- Review risk versus benefits of fluoxetine
- If purging, provide information on the safety of drugs in pregnancy
- Monitor weight and BMI
- Serial USS to monitor fetal growth
- Monitor infant weight and growth

Psychological
- Bulimia nervosa-focused guided self-help
- Eating disorder-focused cognitive behavioural therapy
- Assess mother–infant attachment and relationship:
  - Discuss any concerns the ♀ may have and provide information, support, and treatment, e.g. referral to parent–infant mental health service

Social
- Enhanced postnatal care:
  - Monitor for relapse
  - Additional and/or extended appointments with midwife
  - Comprehensive handover to health visitor and GP
- Referral to specialist midwife for breastfeeding support

Personality disorder

- The personality of an individual encompasses how they perceive, think, feel, and relate to others
- Social convention dictates the normal range of these behaviours
- An individual with a personality disorder has deeply ingrained and enduring behaviour patterns that fall outside the normal range
- These behaviour patterns:
  - Usually evident since childhood or adolescence
  - Result in inflexible responses to a range of personal and social situations
  - Cause the individual significant distress and social disruption

Prevalence

- 4.4% of the adult population

Emotionally unstable personality disorder (EUPD)

Background
- Affect 0.4% of ♀
- Associated with traumatic events in childhood including neglect and physical and/or sexual abuse

---

Clinical features of EUPD

- Chronic feelings of emptiness
- Incapacity to control behavioural explosions
- Intense and unstable interpersonal relationships
- Liability to outbursts of emotion
- Tendency to self-destructive behaviours, e.g. suicide gestures
- Tendency to act impulsively without considering the consequences
- Tendency to quarrelsome behaviour
- Unpredictable and capricious mood

Impact on pregnancy

- ↑ risk of maternal death (mainly suicide: 60–70% of individuals with EUPD make suicide attempts)
- ↑ risk of maternal morbidity, e.g. substance use, self-harm, depression
- ↑ risk of substandard antenatal care (2° to ↑ risk of dysfunctional relationships with healthcare professional):
  - ↑ risk of socioeconomic deprivation, e.g. unemployment
  - ↑ risk of neonatal/infant morbidity (emotional and behavioural problems, difficulty responding sensitively to infant's needs)

Management of personality disorders in pregnancy

Biological
- Risk assessment following any episode of self-harm (➔ see p. 551)

Psychological
- Specialist long-term psychological therapies focusing on relationship to oneself and/or to others, e.g. cognitive analytical therapy
- Assess mother–infant attachment and relationship

Social
- Emphasis on continuity of care
- Clear and consistent boundaries, e.g. relationships with healthcare professionals, appointment times
- If a history of physical and/or sexual violence is disclosed:
  - Acknowledge bravery of disclosure
  - Encourage to contact relevant support organizations, e.g. Rape Crisis
- Encourage and support to ↓ social isolation, e.g. antenatal classes, baby groups
- Consider socioeconomic factors, e.g. insecure housing, domestic violence
- Consider safeguarding assessment if significantly impaired functioning and/or significant risk to infant
- Enhanced postnatal care:
  - Monitor for relapse
  - Additional and/or extended appointments with midwife
  - Comprehensive handover to health visitor and GP

Self-harm

- Defined by NICE as self-injury or poisoning, irrespective of motive
- Broader definitions include self-neglect, exposure to unnecessary physical risk, and excessive exercising

Prevalence

- 8.9% of ♀ have self-harmed without suicidal intent:
  - Steep ↑ in reporting since the year 2000
- 8.0% of ♀ have made a suicide attempt, i.e. self-harm with suicidal intent

Function(s) of self-harm

- Express extreme distress
- Cope with extreme distress
- Relieve unbearable tension
- Punish oneself
- Communicate with others, e.g. express anger, punish others, 'cry for help'

Relationship to suicide

- Self-harm is a strong risk factor for suicide
- Level of suicidal intent ranges from little or no suicidal intent to definite suicidal attempt
- 1 in 25 people presenting to hospital for self-harm will die by suicide within 5 years

---

Management of self-harm in pregnancy

⚠ Inform all relevant healthcare professionals, including GP

⚠ Advise ♀ and her partner and/or family to seek further help if deterioration of situation

Biological
- Assess likely risk and refer as appropriate, e.g. to emergency department

Psychological
- Assess function of self-harm, risk, and suicidal intent
- Psychological therapy, e.g. cognitive behavioural therapy, psychodynamic therapy, problem-solving

Social
- Be supportive and non-judgemental
- If referred to emergency department, consider transport and need for supervision

Suicide

⚠ Leading cause of maternal death in the year after pregnancy
- 0.52 per 100,000 pregnant ♀
- Majority of deaths were by violent means, suggesting the majority of ♀ were clear in their intention
- Most common prior diagnosis was recurrent depressive disorder
- Risk factors are outlined in Table 16.4

Extended suicide

- Death of the baby with the mother
- Very rare

Red flags

- Recent significant change in mental state or new symptoms
- New thoughts or acts of violent self-harm
- New and persistent expressions of incompetency as a mother or estrangement from the infant

Suicide risk assessment

- Are they feeling hopeless, or that life is not worth living?
- Have they made plans to end their life?
- Have they told anyone?
- Have they carried out any acts in anticipation of death, e.g. cancelled a subscription
- Do they have the means for a suicidal act?
- What support do they have?

▶ No evidence asking about suicidal thoughts ↑ a ♀'s risk

⚠ Do not assume responsibility for a child is a protective factor

Source: data from *Clinical Guide: Assessment of suicide risk in people with depression*. Centre for Suicide Research, Department of Psychiatry, University of Oxford.

⮕ MBRRACE-UK 2017 report: ⌕ https://www.npeu.ox.ac.uk/mbrrace-uk/reports/confidential-enquiry-into-maternal-deaths

Table 16.4 Risk factors for suicide

Specific for depression	Other factors
• Family history of mental health problems • Previous suicide attempts, including self-harm • Severe depression • Anxiety • Feelings of hopelessness • Personality disorder • Harmful substance use	• Family history of suicide or self-harm • Physical health problem, especially if recently diagnosed, chronic, or painful • Exposure to suicidal behaviour, including via media • Recent discharge from psychiatric inpatient care • Access to potentially lethal means of self-harm/suicide

Source: data from *Clinical Guide: Assessment of suicide risk in people with depression*. Centre for Suicide Research, Department of Psychiatry, University of Oxford.

Treatment without consent

Mental Capacity Act 2005

Treatment for **any health problem** can be given **without** consent if a ♀ >16 yrs lacks capacity and the treatment is in her best interest.

⚠ ♀ >16 yrs are assumed to have capacity unless there is evidence to the contrary ∴ lack of capacity must be demonstrated.

Mental Health Act (MHA) 1983

Treatment for a **mental health problem** can be given **without** consent if a ♀ is detained under Section 2 or 3 of the MHA 1983.

⚠ A ♀ can be detained (often referred to as 'being sectioned') if:
• She needs assessment and/or treatment for a mental health problem (even if her capacity is not impaired)
AND
• The health problem is sufficiently severe to need assessment or treatment in a mental health hospital, i.e. there is risk to either her health or safety, or that of another person (and if so detention may be in the best interests of the other person/public rather than the ♀)
AND
• She is **unable** or **unwilling** to agree to admission

Common section types

• Section 2 can last up to 28 days and is for assessment and treatment
• Section 3 can last up to 6 mths, but can be renewed, and is for treatment
• A Section can only be discharged (ended) by the ♀'s psychiatrist, a legally-defined relative (but this can be overridden) or a specially appointed panel

Limitations

⚠ A **physical health problem** cannot be treated under the MHA unless:
• It is causing the mental health problem, e.g. treatment of hypothyroidism causing depression
• It is directly caused by the mental health problem, e.g. life-threatening dehydration in anorexia nervosa

Mental health versus mental capacity

• Treating someone without their consent is a weighty decision
• Legally imperative that the correct piece of legislation is used
• A ♀ can be subject to both the MHA and the Mental Capacity Act, at the same time, for distinct aspects of their care

⚠ If there is doubt about the correct piece of legislation or the situation is highly complex, seek psychiatry advice, and consider formal legal advice and/or a court referral.

Mother and baby unit

- Specialist psychiatric inpatient unit
- Provides assessment and care for mothers with severe and/or complex perinatal mental health problems
- Infant can be admitted with the ♀

Admission should be considered:

- If a pregnant ♀ has:
  - Symptoms or signs of psychosis
  - New or persistent beliefs of inadequacy as a mother
  - Pervasive guilt or hopelessness
  - A rapidly changing mental state
  - Significant estrangement from the infant
  - Suicidal ideation
- If there is a risk of harm to others, including the infant
- At a time of anticipated high risk, e.g. postpartum if a ♀ has a previous history of bipolar affective disorder and postpartum psychosis

Additional considerations

- Physical healthcare needs of the ♀ and/or infant (can these be provided in this location?)
- Likely 1° caregiver of the infant (is a joint admission in the best interests of the infant if the ♀ is unlikely to be the 1° caregiver?)

➔ MBBRACE-UK 2015 report: ⟋ https://www.npeu.ox.ac.uk/mbrrace-uk/reports/confidential-enquiry-into-maternal-deaths

Psychotropic medications

See Table 16.5.

Table 16.5 Psychotropic medications in pregnancy and breastfeeding

Drug		Ability to conceive	Pregnancy outcome	Breastfeeding
Selective serotonin reuptake inhibitors (SSRI)		No data	• Not major teratogens • Possible ↑ risk of cardiac malformations (especially with paroxetine), persistent pulmonary hypertension of the newborn • ↑ risk of neonatal withdrawal syndrome • Some evidence for ↑ risk of autism spectrum disorders	• Usually reasonable to continue with drug used in pregnancy • If starting treatment—consider sertraline as low rate of reported adverse effects
Anxiolytics	Benzodiazepines	No data	• Some evidence for ↑ risk of malformations (including oral clefts) and delayed psychomotor development • ↑ risk of preterm birth, low birthweight, SGA, caesarean section. 'floppy baby syndrome'	• Avoid if possible, if necessary use a drug with a short half-life • Consider lorazepam
	Z-drugs	No data	• Zolpidem may ↑ risk of preterm birth, low birthweight, caesarean section	• Avoid if possible, if necessary use a drug with a short half-life

Drug		Ability to conceive	Pregnancy outcome	Breastfeeding
Antipsychotics	1st generation (typical)	If ↑ prolactin then ↓ fertility	• Minimal risk of teratogenicity • ↑ risk of preterm birth, low birthweight, neonatal withdrawal syndrome, neonatal dyskinesia • ↑ risk of neonatal jaundice with phenothiazines • Possible ↑ risk of caesarean section, stillbirth	• Usually reasonable to continue with drug used in pregnancy
	2nd generation (atypical)	If ↑ prolactin then ↓ fertility	• Unlikely to be major teratogens • Potential ↑ risk of malformations with risperidone • Possible ↑ risk of ↑ birthweight • ↑ risk of neonatal withdrawal syndrome • ↑ risk of intensive care admission and low birthweight with olanzapine • ↑ risk of hyperglycaemia and ketosis with olanzapine/clozapine • Possible ↑ risk of caesarean section, stillbirth	• Usually reasonable to continue with drug used in pregnancy ⚠ Clozapine—contraindicated as risk of agranulocytosis and seizures—advise against breastfeeding and continue with clozapine
Lithium		No data	• Risk of major malformation • ↑ risk of neonatal readmission within 28 days of birth • Neonatal goitre, hypotonia, lethargy, and cardiac arrhythmia have been reported	• Not absolutely contraindicated, seek specialist advice to individualize decision

Substance use

Prevalence

- ~1% of pregnant ♀ have problematic drug use
- ~1% of pregnant ♀ have problematic alcohol use

Clinical features

Harmful use

- A pattern of psychoactive substance use causing damage to physical and/or mental health

Dependence syndrome

- Behavioural, cognitive, and psychological phenomena that develop after repeated substance use, typically including:
  - Strong desire to take the substance
  - Difficulties in controlling use of the substance
  - Persistence in using the substance despite harmful consequences
  - Higher priority given to substance use than other activities
  - ↑ tolerance
  - Physical withdrawal state

Screening

- Use a validated tool to screen for substance use, harmful use and dependence syndrome, e.g. Alcohol, Smoking, and Substance Involvement Screening Test

---

Assessment of substance use

- Types of substance used (including prescribed, over the counter)
- Quantity
- Frequency of use
- Pattern of use
- Routes of administration (including any injecting)
- Sources of substances obtained
- Attitude of ♀ to substance
- Previous abstinence(s)
- Previous treatments(s)

Impact of substance abuse on pregnancy

Maternal risks

- ↑ risk of maternal death (overdose, suicide, violence, accidental)
- Chronic physical health problem 2° substance use, e.g. HIV
- Anaemia 2° to poor maternal nutrition
- Infections and sequelae (injection site-related skin infections and/or abscesses, including botulism, tetanus and anthrax, bacterial endocarditis, dental caries and periodontal disease, TB)
- Blood-borne virus infection (including HIV, hepatitis C, hepatitis B) 2° to injecting practices and/or prostitution
- VTE, e.g. smokers, IV drug users
- Difficult venous access and the impact on treating maternal health problems that depend on venous access, e.g. PPH
- ↑ risk of substandard antenatal care (delayed presentation, chaotic engagement with services, failure to disclose substance use due to fear of prejudice, stigma, loss of custody)

Social issues

- ↑ risk of socioeconomic deprivation 2° to unpredictable lifestyle:
  - Partner and/or social network also involved in substance use
  - Rejection by family/social networks
  - Loss of employment
  - Criminal activity including prostitution, arrest and imprisonment
  - Homelessness
  - Interpersonal violence

Offspring risks

- ↑ risk of neonatal/infant death or morbidity:
  - Vertical transfer of blood-borne viruses
  - Neonatal withdrawal syndrome
- ↑ risk of poor mother–infant attachment and relationship:
  - 80% rate of relapse following abstinence in pregnancy
  - ↓ emotional availability
  - Chaotic family life
  - Maternal prioritization of substance use over needs of infant
- Accidental or deliberate injury to the infant can result from:
  - Maternal somnolence or intoxication
  - Effect of maternal drug-seeking behaviour, e.g. leaving infant alone
  - Physical abuse and/or neglect
  - Exposure to criminal behaviour and/or drug paraphernalia
  - Ingestion of substances/maintenance therapy, including deliberate supply by ♀

Principles of management of substance abuse in pregnancy

- Pregnancy provides a window of opportunity and may act as a catalyst for change, e.g. ♀ may accept treatment if ↓ likelihood of custody loss
- Overarching aim is to retain the ♀ in a treatment programme, achieve stability in all areas of life and ↓ chaos, abstain from illicit drugs, and ↓ associated harmful behaviours
- Refer to substance misuse service even if continuing to use illicit drugs, ♀ have better antenatal care and better general health

Biological

- Maternal:
  - Maintenance treatment or detoxification
  - Monitoring for substance use, e.g. carbon monoxide monitoring
  - Organize detailed USS ± fetal echocardiogram if substance use is associated with teratogenicity
  - Serial USS if ↑ risk of IUGR
  - Advice on diet and nutrition
  - Review current or previous physical health complications of substance use
  - Review venous access
  - Refer for dental assessment and treatment
  - VTE risk assessment
  - Screen for blood-borne viruses, including hepatitis C
- Offspring:
  - Hepatitis B vaccination if mother is an IV drug user
  - Monitor infant for adverse substance effects
  - Risk assessment for breastfeeding (nature of substance, risk of exposure to substance in breast milk, HIV status)

Psychological

- Offer psychological intervention to all ♀ using substances, e.g. cognitive behavioural therapy, contingency management
- Assess mother–infant attachment and relationship

Social

- Emphasis on continuity of care
- Assertive and proactive engagement in treatment including co-location of services and/or provide home visits
- Encourage and support to ↓ social isolation, e.g. antenatal classes, baby groups
- ↓ impact of detrimental socioeconomic factors, e.g. insecure housing, domestic violence
- Signpost to relevant support groups, e.g. Alcoholics Anonymous
- Directing partner to substance treatment programme
- Safeguarding assessment if continued harmful substance use, or significant risk of harm to infant

Tobacco smoking

- Most commonly used substance in pregnancy
- 17% of ♀ with a severe mental health problem smoke in pregnancy
- >50% of pregnant ♀ with nicotine dependence have a mental health problem

Risks to the fetus

- Leading preventable cause of fetal morbidity and mortality
- ↑ risk of:
  - Miscarriage
  - Stillbirth
  - IUGR
  - Low birthweight
  - Preterm birth
  - Placental abruption
  - Congenital malformation

Risks to the child

- ↑ risk of:
  - Neonatal death
  - Sudden infant death syndrome
  - Illnesses in later life including diabetes, obesity, asthma, and cancer
  - ↑ risk of behavioural or neurodevelopmental disorders

Smoking cessation in pregnancy

- Higher proportion of ♀ stop smoking during pregnancy than at any other times in their lives
- Advise all ♀ to stop smoking, not just cut down
- Evidence-based smoking cessation programmes include structured self-help, cognitive behavioural therapy, and motivational interviewing
- Smoking cessation programmes ↓ smoking rates and ↓ the incidence of low birthweight babies and preterm birth
- Refer all ♀ to smoking cessation if they smoke, stopped smoking in the last 2 wks, or have an exhaled carbon monoxide reading ≥7 ppm
- Nicotine replacement therapy should only be considered if cessation without replacement therapy has failed
- There is currently a lack of evidence for the safety of 'e-cigarettes', also known as 'vaping'

⚠ Bupropion and varenicline should not be used in pregnancy or breastfeeding.

Alcohol

Background
- Alcohol consumption in pregnancy is common and occurs in all sociodemographic groups
- There is no clear safe amount of alcohol that can be consumed during pregnancy, so public health campaigns advocate abstinence throughout pregnancy

Maternal risks
- Individuals do not need to be dependent on alcohol to develop long-term sequelae, which include cirrhosis, pancreatitis, neuropathy, and ↑ risk of cancer
- Alcohol dependence can → alcohol withdrawal if intake is stopped abruptly (which can be life-threatening, see Box 16.1)

Fetal risks
- Miscarriage
- Preterm birth
- Low birthweight
- Fetal alcohol spectrum disorders

⚠ These risks ↑ with ↑ alcohol intake.

Box 16.1 Acute alcohol withdrawal
⚠ Alcohol withdrawal is a medical emergency.

Clinical features
- Shivering
- Sweating
- Agitation
- Seizures
- Tremor
- Visual hallucinations

Management
- Long-acting benzodiazepine, e.g. ↓ course of chlordiazepoxide
- Thiamine supplementation
- Consider in-patient care
- No evidence on use of medications to prevent relapse in pregnancy

Opioids

Background

- **Opiates** are naturally occurring compounds derived from the opium poppy plant, e.g. morphine, codeine, heroin
- **Opioids** are all compounds that act on the opioid receptors, including opiates, but also synthetic compounds such as fentanyl, oxycodone, and methadone
- Rates of opioid dependence are ↑ globally

Maternal risks

- Infertility can occur, as the result of amenorrhoea 2° to opioid use
- Analgesia resistance

Fetal risks

- IUGR
- Placental abruption
- Preterm birth
- Stillbirth

Risks to infant

- Sudden infant death syndrome
- Neonatal respiratory depression
- Neonatal withdrawal syndrome

Management of opioid dependence in pregnancy

1st-line (maintenance) therapy

- Long-acting opioid agonist, e.g. methadone or buprenorphine to maintain stable levels
- Associated with low rates of relapse and ↓ cravings
- Can be continued in breastfeeding
- Risk of neonatal withdrawal syndrome

2nd-line (detoxification) therapy

- If maintenance therapy refused, consider pharmacological treatment of withdrawal syndrome by using a gradual ↓ in long-acting opioids to manage withdrawal syndrome
- Do not use antagonists, e.g. naloxone
- Usually only recommended in 2nd or 3rd trimester
- May be beneficial to start as inpatient
- If successful, no risk of neonatal withdrawal
- High risk of relapse
- Higher risk of adverse maternal (overdose) and fetal outcomes
- Anaesthetic review as ♀ with opioid dependence syndrome may require higher than average doses of opioids for analgesia:
  - Use of full opioid agonists, e.g. methadone, or partial agonists, e.g. buprenorphine will determine choice of analgesia

Other substances of abuse

Benzodiazepines
⚠ Abrupt cessation → severe withdrawal syndrome, i.e. seizures and psychosis
- Gradual dose ↓ using long-acting benzodiazepines
- Consider in-patient care
- Advise not to breastfeed if using high dose

Cannabis
- ↑ risk of adverse fetal outcomes including:
  - Low birthweight babies
  - Preterm birth
  - Congenital malformations
  - Neurodevelopmental problems
  - Childhood malignancy

⚠ Evidence about cannabis is confounded by tobacco use
- No safe drug for substitute prescribing

Cocaine
- Fetal risks:
  - ↑ risk of miscarriage
  - Placental abruption
  - IUGR
  - Stillbirth
  - Sudden infant death syndrome
  - Neonatal death
  - Neonatal withdrawal syndrome
- Conflicting evidence regarding teratogenicity but believed to cause:
  - Microcephaly
  - Cardiac defects
  - Limb, gut, and genitourinary defects
- No safe drug for substitute prescribing
- Advise not to breastfeed

Ophthalmology

General considerations

Physiological changes in pregnancy
- Unilateral ptosis has been reported that resolves after delivery
- Dry eyes
- Intolerance to contact lenses:
  - Drier eyes
  - ↑ corneal sensitivity
- ↓ IOP (by up to 10%)
- Change in refractive index of cornea

⚠ It is advisable not to get new glasses until ≥2 mths postpartum

General messages
- Counselling ♀ about the use of medications in pregnancy for potentially sight-threatening conditions is crucial; it is not enough to simply say they might lose their vision
- Consideration of the problem and consequences of inadequate treatment is required: central vision vs peripheral fields vs contrast sensitivity vs colour (and the impact this may have, e.g. on driving)
- The systemic absorption of most topical ocular medications is very small, so the balance will usually be in favour of continuing treatment ➋ see Tables 17.2, 17.3 and 17.4, for details
- Systemic absorption may be reduced further by punctal occlusion with a finger for a few minutes after eye drop administration

Causes of visual loss in pregnancy
- Pre-eclampsia:
  - Retinal detachment
  - Macular oedema
  - Cortical blindness (from cerebral oedema)
- DM:
  - Vitreous haemorrhage
- Optic neuropathy (ischaemic or inflammatory)
- Retinal arterial or venous occlusion
- Central serous chorioretinopathy
- Retinal detachment

Floaters
- Little black specks that float around in the visual field, often more prominent against a bright background
- Very common, and the majority, while irritating, are harmless
- Retinal detachment is the commonest cause of a sudden ↑

⚠ Urgent optometry/medical review should be advised if:
  - Sudden ↑ in number or change in appearance
  - Associated with flashing lights
  - More noticeable floaters or occur in second eye
  - Other visual symptoms occur, e.g. scotomata

Table 17.1 Causes of a painful red eye

Site	Possible cause
Conjunctiva	• Conjunctivitis
Subconjunctival	• Subconjunctival haemorrhage
Corneal	• Corneal ulcer
	• Corneal abrasion
	• Foreign body
	• Chemical burn
Sclera	• Scleritis
Intraocular	• Acute angle-closure glaucoma

Table 17.2 Topical antibiotics for ocular use

Drug	Use in pregnancy
Tobramycin	• Has been used extensively in pregnancy
Ofloxacin	• Oral quinolones tend to be avoided in pregnancy due to concerns about effects on cartilage formation; small studies have failed to confirm this
	• Lack of data about topical use so cannot be routinely recommended, but could be used if no reasonable appropriate alternative
Chloramphenicol	• Limited data about topical use, but oral use has been associated with 'grey baby syndrome' in neonates
	• Avoid use in pregnancy when possible
Fusidic acid	• No data about use in pregnancy
	• Manufacturer states it can be used in pregnancy if necessary
Gentamicin	• IV gentamicin can be used in pregnancy
	• Lack of data about topical use, but systemic absorption likely to be small ∴ can be used if no reasonable alternative
Erythromycin	Oral erythromycin safe to use in pregnancy so no problems anticipated with topical use

Conjunctivitis

Background
- Very common complaint both outside and during pregnancy
- While common in children, it can be serious in neonates and cause visual loss if untreated (⊃ see 'Ophthalmia neonatorum', p. 569)

Clinical features
- Allergic (seasonal or chronic):
  - Bilateral itchy eyes
  - ↑ lacrimation
  - Eyes usually pink rather than red
  - Can be associated chemosis
  - Other allergic symptoms present (stuffiness, sneezing)
- Infectious:
  - ↑ lacrimation
  - Discharge (bacterial often purulent, viral more watery)

Management of conjunctivitis in pregnancy

Allergic
- ↓ exposure to known triggers
- Sodium cromoglicate drops can be used in pregnancy
- Antihistamines such as chlorphenamine can also be used

Bacterial
- Not all cases require antibiotic drops
- Conservative management (good eye hygiene)
- Consider referral to ophthalmology if:
  - Associated pain
  - Contact lens wearer
  - Infection not localized to conjunctiva
  - History of recent ophthalmic procedure

Viral
- No role for antiviral treatment
- Conservative management

Ophthalmia neonatorum

- Conjunctivitis which occurs in neonates in the 1st 4 weeks of life
- Affects 1.6–12% of all neonates
- It results from contact with the mother's body fluids in the birth canal

Causes

Chemical
- A mild, self-limiting purulent discharge seen within the 1st 24 hrs of life

Bacterial
- Sexually transmitted infections:
  - *Chlamydia trachomatis* (now the most common cause of ON)
  - *Neisseria gonorrhoeae*
- Non-sexually transmitted infections:
  - *Haemophilus* species
  - *Streptococcus pneumoniae*
  - *Staphylococcus aureus*
  - *Staphylococcus epidermidis*
  - *Streptococcus viridans*
  - *Escherichia coli*
  - *Pseudomonas aeruginosa*

Viral
- Adenovirus
- HSV

Clinical features

- Purulent or mucopurulent discharge
- Crusting on the eyelashes
- Eyelid oedema
- Redness (usually bilateral)

Management of ophthalmia neonatorum

- Prompt assessment and investigation of the cause as this can → permanent visual loss if untreated
- Some bacterial causes can require several days of systemic antibiotics

⤷ The College of Optometrists. Ophthalmia neonatorum: ✎ https://www.college-optometrists. org/guidance/clinical-management-guidelines/ophthalmia-neonatorum.html

Glaucoma

Background

- Defined as an optic neuropathy, typically associated with high IOP
- Can result in permanent visual impairment if untreated
- Mostly occurs over the age of 40, but can occur in younger adults
- **Angle-closure glaucoma** is when the angle of the anterior chamber (through which the aqueous humour drains) is narrowed, ↓ drainage and hence ↑ IOP
- **Open-angle glaucoma** is when the angle is normal but the IOP is elevated, which is thought to be due to ↑ production or ↓ outflow of aqueous humour
- Other causes of glaucoma include an idiosyncratic response to steroids, 2° to inflammation and neovascular glaucoma (vasoproliferative disease within the angle of the eye) in proliferative diabetic retinopathy or ischaemic central retinal vein occlusion
- Treatments are outlined in Table 17.3.

Table 17.3 Treatments for glaucoma

Types	Pregnancy considerations
α agonists Brimonidine (topical)	• Preferred treatment in pregnancy (including 1st trimester), reported association with neonatal apnoea so discontinue in late pregnancy and while breastfeeding
β blockers Timolol (topical)	• Oral β blockers are used in pregnancy • Neonatal bradycardia can occur but is rare • Can be continued if required
Prostaglandin analogues Latanoprost (topical) Bimatoprost (topical)	Latanoprost • PGF2α analogue, similar to those used systemically to cause uterine contractions and induce delivery • Small series in pregnancy do not show an ↑ in adverse outcomes but not usually 1st line in pregnancy Bimatoprost • PGF2α analogue but does not act on F2α receptors • Lack of data about topical use but benefits likely to outweigh theoretical risks
Anticholinergics Pilocarpine (topical)	• Adverse fetal outcomes reported in animal models, but no human studies to support this • Can be used if potential benefit outweighs theoretical risks to fetus
Carbonic anhydrase inhibitors Brinzolamide Dorzolamide (topical) Acetazolamide (oral)	• Oral preparations associated with teratogenicity in animal models, however used in pregnancy without an ↑ in adverse fetal outcomes • Oral acetazolamide used in pregnancy for IIH (need to monitor hydration, electrolytes and acid–base status) • Limited data available about topical preparations but these can be used if no alternative

Clinical features
- Acute angle-closure glaucoma (Box 17.1)
- Open-angle glaucoma is often asymptomatic, but the visual loss is progressive and irreversible

Management of chronic glaucoma in pregnancy
- IOP often ↓ by a small degree in pregnancy
- Joint management with an ophthalmologist
- Review medications
- Make an individualized plan based on severity of disease, treatment history, and treatment options
- At delivery:
  - Careful fluid balance
  - Avoidance of low BP is important to maintain ocular perfusion pressure in advanced glaucoma
- Not an indication for caesarean section

Box 17.1 Acute angle-closure glaucoma
⚠ This is a medical emergency and requires immediate referral to an ophthalmologist.

Symptoms
- Intense pain
- Red eye (➲ see Table 17.1 for other causes of a painful red eye)
- Visual loss
- Haloes around lights
- Headache
- Nausea and vomiting

Signs
- Circumcorneal injection (vessel dilatation around the rim of the cornea)
- Fixed, slightly dilated pupil

Management
- Analgesia
- Immediate referral to an ophthalmologist who will institute management involving pressure-lowering eye drops ± IV acetazolamide

Uveitis

Background

- Inflammatory condition of the uvea (the iris, ciliary body, and choroid)
- Related to:
  - Infections (e.g. HSV, CMV, or TB)
  - Inflammatory conditions (e.g. spondyloarthritis, psoriatic arthritis, sarcoidosis)

Clinical features

- Anterior uveitis (iritis):
  - Redness
  - Pain (often described as a 'deep ache' in the eye)
  - Constricted pupil
  - Light sensitivity
  - Watering eye
- Intermediate/posterior uveitis:
  - Redness and pain may be absent
  - Floaters and visual loss can occur

Management of uveitis in pregnancy

- Investigation for underlying associated inflammatory or infectious causes
- Anti-inflammatory treatment with topical, systemic, or biological treatments (⊕ see Tables 17.2 and 17.4)
- Intravitreal steroids can be used as normal in pregnancy; the doses are very small with negligible systemic absorption so the ♀ can be reassured

Miscellaneous conditions

Hypertensive disorders of pregnancy

(➲ See Chapter 1, p. 1.)

These can be associated with the same visual complications as hypertension in the non-pregnant individual; however, in pregnant ♀ these complications may develop rapidly as a result of pre-eclampsia.

- Visual symptoms include:
  - Flashing lights (photopsia)
  - Scotomata
  - ↓ in vision or blurred vision

⚠ Management includes urgent treatment of the underlying condition with early ophthalmology input if symptoms remain despite BP control.

Diabetic retinopathy

⚠ Retinopathy can progress very rapidly in pregnancy and be sight-threatening.

⚠ Close monitoring and prompt treatment are essential.

Types of retinal abnormality

- Non-proliferative (cotton wool spots, microaneurysms; also known as background retinopathy)
- Proliferative (new blood vessels on retina or disc)
- Macular oedema

Management of diabetic retinopathy in pregnancy

- Retinal screening every trimester and regularly for 1 yr postpartum
- Laser treatment can be performed, as can vitreoretinal surgery
- Intravitreal anti-VEGF has been used in small numbers of pregnant ♀ with no problems reported (see table 17.4)

Central serous chorioretinopathy

- A rare condition causing fluid to leak and pool under the retina that can occur in the 3rd trimester of pregnancy (predominantly occurs in ♂ otherwise)
- Causes a ↓ in visual acuity
- Can cause scotomata
- ↑ risk if steroids have been administered (topical, inhaled, or systemic)
- Usually resolves later in pregnancy or after delivery
- Can recur in subsequent pregnancies

Other pharmacological therapies

See Table 17.4.

Table 17.4 Miscellaneous agents used for the investigation and treatment of ophthalmic conditions

Class	Drug	Route	Pregnancy-specific considerations
Contrast agents for retinal angiography	Fluorescein	IV	• Limited data, but not known to be teratogenic (retinal angiography usually avoided in 1st trimester as a precaution)
	Indocyanine green	IV	• Used in studies of liver flow rate in pregnancy with no adverse fetal effects reported • Can be used in pregnancy
Antivirals	Aciclovir	Topical or PO	• Oral aciclovir is used in pregnancy for the treatment of conditions such as varicella and HSV • Lack of data about topical use but no problems anticipated
Mydriatics	Phenylephrine Tropicamide Cyclopentolate	Topical	• All considered appropriate to use in pregnancy, but repeated exposure discouraged
Anti-VEGF	Ranibizumab Bevacizumab	Intravitreal	• Systemic absorption shown by studies showing ↓ plasma VEGF following intravitreal administration (bevacizumab persisting for up to 1/12, ranibizumab for 1 day) • Small numbers of pregnant ♀ receiving anti-VEGF have been reported • Suggestion of contribution to development of pre-eclampsia in susceptible individuals, but not clear that the anti-VEGF use was causative • Can be used if the benefits to the mother outweigh the theoretical risks to the fetus
Local anaesthesia	Lidocaine	Topical	• No evidence of fetal complications from use in pregnancy
NSAID	Diclofenac	Topical or PO	• Can be used in pregnancy until 24–28 wks • Risk of premature ductus arteriosus closure if used in 3rd trimester

Index

Notes As the subject of this book is concerned with pregnancy, all entries refer to this unless otherwise stated. vs. indicates a comparison or differential diagnosis Tables, figures and boxes are indicated by t, f and b following the page number